Playing for Life

AF854782

Playing for Life

Performance in Africa in the Age of AIDS

Louise M. Bourgault

Professor, Communication and Performance Studies
Northern Michigan University

Carolina Academic Press
Durham, North Carolina

Copyright © 2003
Louise M. Bourgault
All Rights Reserved

Bourgault, Louise Manon.
Playing for life : performance in Africa in the age of AIDS / Louise M. Bourgault
p. cm.
Includes bibliographical references and index.
ISBN 0-89089-125-7
1. Performing arts--Africa. 2. AIDS (Disease)--Africa. 3. AIDS (Disease) and the arts.
I. Title.
PN2969.B68 2003
791'.096--dc21
2003040969

Cover Photo Credits:

Front Cover: Kora Player in the Gambia. Photo courtesy of the author.

Back Cover: (top) Scene from "Free Birds," a joint South-African and Dutch AIDS play. Photo courtesy of the author.

(bottom) Ethiopian Children. Photo courtesy of David Schein, Awassa Children's Project.

Carolina Academic Press
700 Kent Street
Durham, North Carolina 27701
Telephone (919) 489-7486
Fax (919) 493-5668
E-mail: cap@cap-press.com
www.cap-press.com

Printed in the United States of America.

This volume is dedicated to
the memory of the 19 million Africans
who have died of AIDS.

Contents

List of Illustrations and Maps

List of Multi-Media Clips Appearing on Compact Disk

System Requirements for Operating Compact Disk

Microsoft® Windows® 95 or higher
QuickTime 3.0 or higher
233MHz
16MB of RAM
256-color video display adapter
(millions recommended)
CD-ROM Drive

Macintosh G-3 or higher
Operating System OS8
QuickTime 3.0 or higher
400MHz
64MB of RAM
256-color video display adapter
(millions recommended)

Chapter 5 Oral Narratives

Video 1. **Griot Songs with Kora**
Djeli Mory *dit* "Fa" at the Grand Hotel, Bamako, Mali

Audio 1. **"Yiriba," AIDS Awareness for Truck Drivers**
Griots Dauda Dembélé and Hawa Dembélé, Mali

Chapter 6 Chants and Songs

Audio 1. **Ideophones of Machete from "Mother Swamp"**
Village Theatre of Gwemble, Liberia

Video 1. **Songs of Introduction and Welcome**
Catholic Diocesan Choir, Kumasi, Ghana

Video 2. **1. Shembe; 2. St. John's; 3. Durban Christian Centre; 4. International Central Gospel Church; 5. Diocesan Seminary Chapel**
1., 2., 3. Durban, South Africa; 4. Accra, Ghana; 5. Kumasi, Ghana

Video 3. **AIDS Ryhthm & Blues and Rap**
Joel Zuma and Sibongiseni Mbambo and Linda Hlongwe at AIDS Summit and Edu-Fair, South Africa

Video 4. **AIDS Ballad**
Joel Zuma and Sibongiseni Mbambo, AIDS Edu-Fair, South Africa

Video 5. **SIDA, AIDS Song**
Griotte Teme Dembélé, Bamako, Mali

Video 6. **AIDS Rap**
Abubakar Kouyaté, Wanda Records, Mali

Chapter 7 Dance

Video 1. **Sangoma Divination Dance**
Shakaland, South Africa

Video 2. **Zulu Stick Fight**
Shakaland, South Africa

Foreword

by Dr. Gilbert Doho

For the last 20 years, Theatre for Social Change, alternately known as People's Theatre or Theatre for Development, has had a tremendous impact on theatre practitioners in the developing world and on the organization and funding of political and social development projects. The goal of this movement, as outlined by Ross Kidd and Martin Byram, is to bring theatre to the people to raise their consciousness and to facilitate human and economic development (Eyoh 1994). People's Theatre has contributed a great deal in the empowerment of the disadvantaged rural and urban masses in the last 20 years. It has denounced corrupt national and international money mongers who have monopolized the knowledge, power, and wealth of the African continent. People's Theatre has led the marginalized masses in Africa to the reappropriation of their political and social rights. Indeed, Theatre for Social Change has been at the forefront of the people's struggle against man-made and natural catastrophes such as war, corruption, famine, hunger, environmental destruction, and deadly diseases such as AIDS.

Today, People's Theatre is changing hands. What began as theatrical experimentation by expatriates and alienated African intellectuals, is today being taken over by the masses. The prostitutes of Bamako, the street boys of Harare, the pygmies in the Central African rainforest, and the inhabitants of the remotest villages in Africa are all using performance to empower themselves and to castigate Africa's unaccountable kleptocratic classes.

Performances of People's Theatre raise daring and paradoxical questions. Why has Africa, so rich in natural resources, become a continent of misery? Why have so many Africans had their lives disrupted by war and genocide? Why do African leaders choose military solutions over peaceful ones? And what must Africans do to build countries where poverty, pandemic diseases, and early death are things of the past?

There is a substantial literature on Theatre for Social Change. But much of this material tends to be narrow in scope, consisting mainly of reports of People's Theatre workshops and experiments. The preponderance of this literature falls loosely into the category of the case study and is thus limited in time and space. The South African experiences by Zakes Mda (1993), the Kammiriithu odyssey by Ross Kidd (1983), the Cameroonian "Hammocks to bridges dream" by Hansel Ndumbe Eyoh (1986), or the Hausa women's struggle in Nigeria (Eyoh 1986) are essentially different versions of the same experience.

Louise M. Bourgault's *Playing for Life: Performance in Africa in the Age of AIDS* goes beyond the existing literature on Theatre for Social Change to encompass other genres of performance: oral narratives, songs and chants, dance, and of course, drama. Her book draws upon pre-existing African performance practices, arguing that these are the true foundations for social change. Her work urges African performers and scholars to delve into their own performance roots to create genuinely transformative genres. She goes so far as to posit that ritual is the foundation of a practice that can induce changes in African society. She develops an argument that relates performance to ritual in the African context. In her approach, the people take the place of ritual specialists, create roles, and act for themselves. *Playing for Life: Performance in Africa in the Age of AIDS* is a post-modern work that is holistic in its approach and continental in its relevance.

It is not surprising that Louise Bourgault is publishing a valuable work on formal and informal tools of communication. She is neither a newcomer to the field of communication nor a neophyte in Theatre for Social Change. (See Bourgault 1991). She posited long ago that the media are revolutionary weapons that can reshape power relationships and may even contribute to the redistribution of wealth on the African continent. She was among the first scholars to inspire sons and daughters of Africa to see the potential of the mass media in the emancipation of the continent (Bourgault 1995). She teaches that the media can advance the liberation of the African continent from imperialist and neo-colonial chains. But she maintains that genuine democracy in Africa cannot be sustained without the development of free and responsible print and electronic media. An informed Africa citizenry, Bourgault argues, must be the backbone of economic, political, and social development in Africa.

Playing for Life: Performance in Africa in the Age of AIDS is an ambitious and informative work, one that synthesizes concepts of Theatre for Social Change from performance and drama studies with concepts of edutainment from media studies and social marketing. Bourgault draws from the theoretical works of Schechner and Turner and then analyzes performances from other literature and from her extensive experience in Africa. She develops a theory of social change based in performance. The practice, she argues, functions like ritual.

As an African, I view performance for social change as ritual in what Westerners would call a post-modern sense. By this I mean that the fundamental purpose of ritual is to effect change in the lives of the people for whom it is performed. Theatre for Social Change functions in a similar manner and has a similar purpose. It proposes to enact a change in the lives of the people. This change must ultimately result in a redistribution of power, from top down to bottom up.

When I visit my native village of Fu'nda in the Grassfields of Cameroon every year to offer a fowl to my ancestors (i.e., to perform a ritual), I fully expect the ancestors to meet my needs. When the Bali Nyonga of Cameroon perform the annual Leila every December, they clearly expect the ritual to result in good fortune for the year to come. The blood of the animal that is sacrificed during these performances fertilizes the earth so that good things will befall the ritual enactors. To perform ritual is to anticipate for oneself and the community a fruitful harvest from the ancestors, the benefactors of our society. Theatre for Social Change, argues Bourgault, walks along the same path!

For the last 10 years, I have been witness to the miracles that theater can perform. In the politically charged atmosphere of Cameroon of the early 1990s, I observed the ability of theatre to convince the Bafounda people to destroy coffee plantations and replant the agribusiness estates with subsistence crops. In the same village, I saw a group of women succeed in opposing the sale of their secret and sacred forest to loggers and to local industrial developers. And I have even seen theatre, in Muyuka in South West Province of Cameroon, tear down ethnocentric governance. Theatre for Social Change helped a mother to denounce her own son, an unscrupulous, corrupt, and tainted politician. Within the fiction of a People's Theatre performance this mother/judge condemned the corrupt mayor of an imaginary town. When the woman later emerged from the performance arena, she stood up before the community and denounced its mismanagement by its corrupt mayor, her son. The performance and the mother's public denunciation occasioned this compromised individual to step down from office. Just a few months after the play was performed, justice took over from fiction! This incident is a prime post-modern example of both art imitating life and life imitating art. It is also a testimony to the tremendous power of Theatre for Social Change.

The author of *Playing for Life: Performance in the Age of AIDS*, Louise Bourgault is a friend of Africa. By this I do not mean she is an Africanist of the armchair variety. Nor do I mean she is a mere occasional traveler who, having visited one or a handful of countries, dares to talk about a continent with thousands of languages and cultures, a continent almost three times the size of the United States of America. Bourgault has traveled all over Africa. She has lived and worked in many African countries. She has trained journalists, helped to establish radio stations, lectured university students, evaluated development projects, and even monitored elections. She has lived the realities of the continent from Dakar to Mombassa, from Cairo to Cape Town. She has shared the *Tsuya* and *Kose* of the Nigerians, the *Achu* of the Cameroonians, the *Atkeke-poisson* of the Ivorians, and the mealies of the Southern Africans. She has interviewed people from all walks of African life from ministers and government officials, to traditional chiefs and title-holders, to ordinary people, even the marginalized. She tackles the issue of AIDS with the depth of an anthropologist and the curiosity of a journalist. She has chosen to enlighten her readers on the paradox of Africa through the lens of the AIDS pandemic. What are the past and present causes of the spread of HIV/AIDS in Africa? How can theatre help to halt the development of this deadly disease? The agony of the present day, one that translates into millions dead and millions more orphaned, spreads in all directions and cries out to all fields—virology, epidemiology, medicine, economics, politics, culture, communication, and even history and geography, for an explanation.

Playing for Life: Performance in Africa in the Age of AIDS presents Africa in a diachronic and well as a synchronic perspective. This is a broad-based work with an interdisciplinary focus that delivers historical, geographical, and cultural information about the African continent. Bourgault's intention is to explore the present so as to build a future that is firmly rooted deep in African cultures of the past. The fight against AIDS must take account of the cultural context of the epidemic. Bourgault therefore draws from pre-colonial, colonial, and post-colonial Africa to explain its present day problems. She also posits that mankind is largely responsible for the spread of the HIV/AIDS epidemic.

Bourgault assesses the role enacted by every actor in the gruesome life-drama taking place in Africa. Although colonial and neocolonial regimes carry the heaviest responsibility for creating African "mal-development," the majority of the ruled are not blameless. Traditional customs and mores see women's primary role as that of reproduction. This turns females, the more numerous gender group in most societies, into both targets and victims of HIV/AIDS. For to foster upon society the belief that girls are born to be nothing more than reproductive machines is as heinous as to bleed the national coffers dry when holding political office. Such vile positions and actions lead to the spread of poverty that both creates and justifies the sex market in most African countries. And where else can profuse sexuality lead if not to AIDS?

Bourgault is not an Afro-pessimist. *Playing for Life: Performance in Africa in the Age of AIDS* is designed to help equip Africans (and friends of Africa) for the struggle against the AIDS pandemic. Bourgault's book offers a new approach for waging a modern war against the epidemic through the use of performance for social change. The approach focuses on prevention because at least for the time being, prevention is the most efficient means to fight against the disease. The volume reviews various forms of edutainment and acknowledges their effectiveness in carrying of messages warning to potential targets of HIV/AIDS. And *Playing for Life: Performance in Africa in the Age of AIDS* is also designed to show students in the Western world what Africans are doing with performance so as to mobilize Western students to use performance effectively in their own struggle against HIV/AIDS.

Playing for Life salutes AIDS activists and is a call for action to those who doze while Africa is dying. This call summons Africans and Americans, and all people of goodwill to combat this deadly epidemic. For we are living in the "Age of AIDS." Indeed it would be self-deception to think that HIV/AIDS is only an African disease. US citizens have no cause to be complacent about HIV. The disease is on the rise in the USA as well as in Africa. This is why Bourgault also takes it upon herself to bring AIDS performance artists from Africa, such as Eager Artists of Durban, South Africa, to exhibit their preventive techniques in the United States. She hopes to disseminate performance-based approaches to combating the HIV epidemic. She hopes to bring about the world-wide movement of AIDS activists, both to demonstrate their talents and their techniques, and to issue warnings to diverse publics about the grave dangers of HIV/AIDS. We live in dangerous times. No part of this planet is safe. The spread of infectious disease is another aspect of globalization. HIV needs no visa to cross national boundaries!

These were our thoughts as Bourgault, a group of students, and I set out to create a piece of AIDS Theatre for Social Change in Marquette, Michigan in March 2001. The play, which came to be called *Phambili* (in Zulu, "Let Us Unite") drew from the energies and talents of Northern Michigan University undergraduates. The powerful message these young people created went straight to the hearts of audience members, both young and old. The post-performance discussion raised an important question many of us would prefer not to face, "Have you been tested?"

Until all the citizens of the world can be shown to be free of HIV/AIDS, the struggle against the pandemic implicates every one of us. This is in fact the final message of *Playing for Life*: *Performance in the Age of AIDS*. The author summons each and every one of us, the living, the dying, the deceased, the spirits of the gods, and of the ancestors, to join in the ultimate ritual combat of this planetary pandemic.

Gilbert Doho, *Doctorat d'état*
February 2002

Acknowledgments

The list of contributors to this volume is long indeed. In South Africa, my research was facilitated by Dr. Keyan Tomaselli and Dr. Lynn Darlymple who invited me to study the work of the DramAide Project. My research in South Africa was assisted by Musa Ndlovu, Nonhlanhla Xaba, and Joel Zuma. Other members of the DramAide team, notably Mhkonhzeni Gumede, Mdu Mbaso, Paul Botha, and the late Jerome Dludla also indulged my questions and provided much insight into the world of South African youth. I also owe a debt of gratitude to my colleagues and hosts, Costas and Jenny Criticos for providing a home and work environment that made living in Durban, South Africa, such an intellectually stimulating and rewarding experience. Other South African contacts and performers have also added to my appreciation of South African performance, especially Jerry Pooe and Eager Artists. Lindane Cele, Joel Zuma, and Sibongiseni Mbambo contributed their work to the book.

In Mali, my work was facilitated by my good friend Dennis Bilodeau of USAID. Research assistants Mountaga Ly, Jacques Keita, and Halima Konaté have also been extraordinarily helpful. Teme Dembele, Abubakar Kouyaté, Daouda and Hawa Dembelé, Yaya Coulibaly, and Mamadou Diarra contributed their creative efforts to the work. Madame Traoré at SIDA 2 & 3 furnished photographs; Madame Medina Boucoum at Plan International, Mali, shared a great deal of her insight with me. Gaoussou Mariko and Moussa Bambara, both of the U.S. Embassy were also of assistance. Philippe Bertier and Mali K7 were helpful in obtaining reprinting permissions. Some of my photographs from Liberia were taken with the help of research assistant John Momo.

A number of talented students have worked with me on parts of this project. Anthony Whitlock produced the CD that accompanies this text. Lon Markham of Talking Gorilla Productions edited the video "AIDS and the Arts in Africa," a production that provides a visual summary of this book. Wesley Oman produced many of the volume's illustrations. *Playing for Life: Performance in Africa in the Age of AIDS* has also been enriched by contributions from Duduzile Phildile Mashinini and Lawrence Kimama. April Spray, Jane Cisluycis, Diane Raven, and Brandon Wislocki provided important editorial assistance in the pre-production phase of the project. Erin Nigl's help was invaluable in producing the glossary. I also acknowledge the comments of students at Northern Michigan University who took my course on Communication and Performance in Africa. They have provided me with much useful feedback on earlier versions of *Playing for Life*.

I am extremely grateful to readers who provided critical readings of the manuscript. These include Neil Cumberlidge, Keyan Tomaselli, Gilbert Doho, David Prychitko, and Arnold Shepperson. I appreciate the support I have received from Northern Michigan University, especially the 1999–2000 sabbatical leave that permitted the initial fieldwork needed for this project. I am grateful for moral support I have received from Terry Seethoff, Sara Doubledee, and Jim Rapport. Sue Salo has given cheerful aid and countenance. Finally, I wish to acknowledge my spouse, Neil Cumberlidge, who always stands by me, backstops on the computer technology, and helps me out in a myriad of ways. Without his gracious assistance this project would undoubtedly be a far more modest one.

Other individuals and groups have been gracious enough to share their photographs with me. They include David Schein (awassachildrensproject@hotmail.com); Ann McGuigan, Childreach/Plan International (sookikis@plan.iess.com); Neil Cumberlidge; Doug Paterson; John and Louise Reber (Mfdi@mweb.co.zw); Bob Hanson; Gilbert Doho; Edie Turner; Richard Schechner; Norma Wolff; Population Services International (PSI) (info@psi.org); the Killie Campbell Collection (South Africa); Soul City (dani@soulcity.org.za); Jubilee 2000 (coord@j2000usa.org); Editions Jamana; and California Newsreel (contact@newsreel.org). I am also grateful to Steve and Sally Smith (ssmith@mfdi.org), Mary Schmidt, and to Oliver Mtukudsi. Photographs not otherwise attributed are my own.

Note: A 20 minute video tape summary of *Playing for Life: Performance in Africa in the Age of AIDS* is available from two sources.

Carolina Academic Press
700 Kent Street
Durham, North Carolina 27701

Media For Development International
184 Crescent Lane
Glenwood Springs, Colorado 81601
Ssmith@mfdi.org

Introduction

The AIDS pandemic was one of the most heart-wrenching crises of the 20th century. By the beginning of 2000, AIDS had killed an estimated 17 million people worldwide. And it had orphaned more than 11 million children. Two years into the new millennium the catastrophic AIDS figures only seem to get grimmer. AIDS has killed another three million people and has left another three million orphans. The AIDS catastrophe is expected to generate one-hundred million cases of HIV/AIDS on this planet by 2005 as the epidemic, presently centered on the African continent, takes hold of populations in Eastern Europe, India, China and elsewhere. Perhaps these regions will be luckier than Africa. Perhaps a vaccine will be discovered to prevent the development of HIV, or perhaps science will come up with a cure for this most dreaded of afflictions. Maybe we will one day look back with curiosity and some bewilderment at all our agonies and all our efforts at HIV/AIDS prevention. I know when that day comes it will be important to know how Africans tried to cope with the epidemic at the end of the 20th century. For Africa is fighting a war of attrition against the epidemic of HIV/AIDS. The HIV/AIDS conflagration is being waged on the prevention battlefront. It is largely a war of symbols, of information, education, and communication, barely the only weapons available to the African people. And because performance figures so prominently as a mode of communication in Africa, performance is a major combatant in the African HIV/AIDS campaigns.

When I first traveled to South Africa in 1997, I was impressed with the grassroots response to the tackling the AIDS epidemic. I was struck by the conviction of ordinary people that their actions could make a difference in the AIDS struggle. And I was delighted by the originality of approaches people were using to fight the AIDS epidemic. I was particularly edified by the outpouring of performative artistic talent attacking the AIDS problem. South Africans were adapting folkways—recitation, song, dance, dramatic styles, and so on, that had moved them in the past, to the information needs of AIDS prevention. A year later I had the opportunity to work in Mali training community radio broadcasters. Once again, I found artists, this time, Malian musicians and storytellers, adapting time-tested folk genres to the problems of HIV prevention. At that point, I made up my mind to return to the African continent to further study the performance techniques Africans were using for AIDS awareness. I wanted to learn more about how Africans were harnessing the performing arts to fight the terrible scourge of HIV/AIDS. And I wanted to share with readers the impressive community efforts Africans were making to save their people.

Five years later the results of my explorations have produced *Playing For Life: Performance in Africa in the Age of AIDS*. The *Playing for Life* project includes a basic text, an accompanying CD, and a video documentary. While the digital video provides moving illustrations of specific points in the book, the documentary, "AIDS and the ARTS in AFRICA," is a meta-commentary or visual summary of the book. (It also exists as a unit in its own right).

The aim of *Playing for Life* is threefold. First, I hope to provide an introduction to the study of Africa through performance suitable for undergraduate students. Second, I have attempted to supply a sampling of Africa's rich performative resources. And third, I have tried to show how Africans are working to harness the energy of performance to help solve this most terrible of contemporary problems, the AIDS pandemic.

Because the continent is so vast, I though it best to focus chiefly on the AIDS epidemic in two countries. Out of more than 45 countries I might have chosen, I selected the countries of South Africa and Mali. The choice reflected my desire to provide at least two different case views of African performance and African performative response to the AIDS crisis. The countries, so divergent from one another by most social indicators—economy, religion, geography and climate, colonial history, pre-colonial history, and nature and severity of the AIDS epidemic seemed to offer sufficient contrasts appropriate for this work. They could amply justify my desire to seize fortuitous opportunities for research that emerged in my academic career in the late 1990s.

The book is organized in the following way. Part I contains four overview chapters. Chapter 1 is an introduction to the African continent. Chapter 2 provides a review of the AIDS crisis in Africa. Chapter 3 provides thumbnail sketches of two African countries, South Africa and Mali. Chapter 4 provides a survey of performance theory and is designed to help readers consider theory as they read through the performance chapters.

Part II of *Playing for Life* contains four genre chapters and a final chapter. Chapter 5 provides a continental survey of oral narratives. Chapter 6 provides a survey of African songs and chants. Chapter 7 examines the African world of dance. Chapter 8 covers the world of African drama. Chapter 9, the concluding chapter, returns to the level of theory and attempts to create a theory of ritual, performance, and social change suitable for explaining how performance can work to shift attitudes in behaviors surrounding HIV/AIDS. In so doing, it returns to two issues that promise to be of continuing concern for much of this century: the question of gender, and the subject of globalization.

Because art in Africa is by its very nature group-oriented, African artists have produced communal responses to the terrible sickness within their communities. This response is interesting and noteworthy in its own right. African performance art, while adhering to basic conventions of genre, has always been responsive to historical process. I wanted to show how AIDS performances arise out of existing genres. This accounts for the structure of the performance chapters in Part II that start with genre surveys and end with AIDS performances.

Just as African artists are working within genre conventions, so too are they bound up within the larger socio-historical processes of their continent, their individual country of origin, and its place within the global economic order. This order has consequences in terms of the spread of the AIDS epidemic, and the resources available to counter it. And the modalities of response to the AIDS crisis exist within a geo-political and a globalizing contest. It is equally important to understand these. Besides providing a general introduction for undergraduate students, Part I of the volume serves to provide a social, political, historical and epidemiological background into which the performances fit.

In addition to maps, charts, and photographs sprinkled throughout the volume, the genre chapters have been illustrated with audio and video clips featured on the accompanying compact disk (CD). These illustrations are intended to help readers to get a feel for some of the performances about which they are reading. And because the content of some of these performances has not been exhaustively discussed in the text, the clips featured in the CD should pique the curiosity of interested readers, and stir them to seek additional information on the subjects presented.

Throughout the creation of these three interrelated projects, the text, the CD, and the video, I have also felt a good deal of open-endedness about these works. In these days of Internet resources and constantly updated databases, one never experiences the satisfying feeling academics once had of having thoroughly researched the field. Even in the time that passes between completing the writing and the appearance of the book, the field becomes ever more fluid, and with it the search for truth more elusive. This is probably even truer of the AIDS field than most because study of the AIDS pandemic, so vast in scope, so paradoxical in nature, cuts across so many disciplines. Indeed minute by minute developments in several areas of inquiry make a work of this kind outdated almost as soon as an analysis is on paper. Some of these fields include epidemiology, behavioral science, medical anthropology, virology, human geography, pharmacology, public policy, foreign policy, popular culture, theatre, mass and interpersonal communication and so on. There seems hardly an academic discipline (with the possible exception of astronomy), untouched by this pandemic.

Playing for Life: Performance in Africa in the Age of AIDS has been enriched with the inclusion of a Foreword provided by the gifted Cameroonian playwright, social activist, and friend, Dr. Gilbert Doho.

While the greatest care has been taken to ensure that all of the facts and figures presented in this work are accurate and up to date, I take full responsibility for any errors that do appear.

Louise M. Bourgault, Ph.D.
Marquette, Michigan August 16, 2002

Part I

The African Continent and the AIDS Epidemic in Context

Chapter 1

The African Continent

Africa is a continent of contrasts, a continent where ancient tradition lives beside modern day edifices; where stone age paintings are located not far from modern urban buildings. Each of Africa's 54 countries and island nations constitutes a unique configuration of history, geography, ethnography, and politics.[1] And all of these factors have impacted the performing arts traditions of Africa in a myriad of ways. This chapter will provide an overview of the African continent, one that aims to share with readers the enormous diversity of the African continent. The chapter will further review some of the major issues facing the continent today. Africa has been called the cradle of humanity and so it is fitting to make that continent the subject of study of some of the oldest and lasting forms of communication on earth.

Geography

Probably the most startling fact about Africa is its size. The African land mass could contain continental America three times and more. Africa is the world's second largest landmass, with a total area spread over 19 million square kilometers (11.8 million square miles). The distance from Tangiers, in Morocco, on the northernmost tip of the African land mass to Cape Town in the extreme south of South Africa is 8,387 kilometers (5,200 miles). This is the same distance separating Anchorage, Alaska and Panama City, Panama. The distance between the widest most points in Africa, between Dakar, Senegal and Cape Guardafui (Cape of Perfumes) in Somalia is 7,420 kilometers (4,600 miles). This is about the distance between New York and Honolulu.

The equator crosses Africa just south of Libreville, Gabon in Central Africa, passes through the Congo, the Democratic Republic of the Congo, Uganda, and

1. The countries of North Africa are Morocco, Algeria, Tunisia, Libya, and Egypt. The countries of West Africa are Benin, Burkina Faso, Cote d'Ivoire, The Gambia, Ghana, Guinea, Guinea-Bissau, Liberia, Mali, Mauritania, Niger, Nigeria, Senegal, Sierra Leone, and Togo. The region also claims the island nation of Cape Verde. The countries of Central Africa are Cameroon, Central African Republic, Chad, Republic of the Congo (Brazzaville), Democratic Republic of the Congo (Kinshasa), Equatorial Guinea, and Gabon. The region also claims the island nation of São Tomé and Príncipe. The countries of East Africa are Sudan, Eritrea, Ethiopia, Djibouti, Somalia, Uganda, Kenya, Rwanda, Burundi, Kenya, and Tanzania. The region also claims the island nations of Comoros, Seychelles, Mauritius, and Madagascar. The countries of Southern Africa are Angola, Botswana, Lesotho, Mozambique, Malawi, Namibia, South Africa, Swaziland, Zambia, and Zimbabwe.

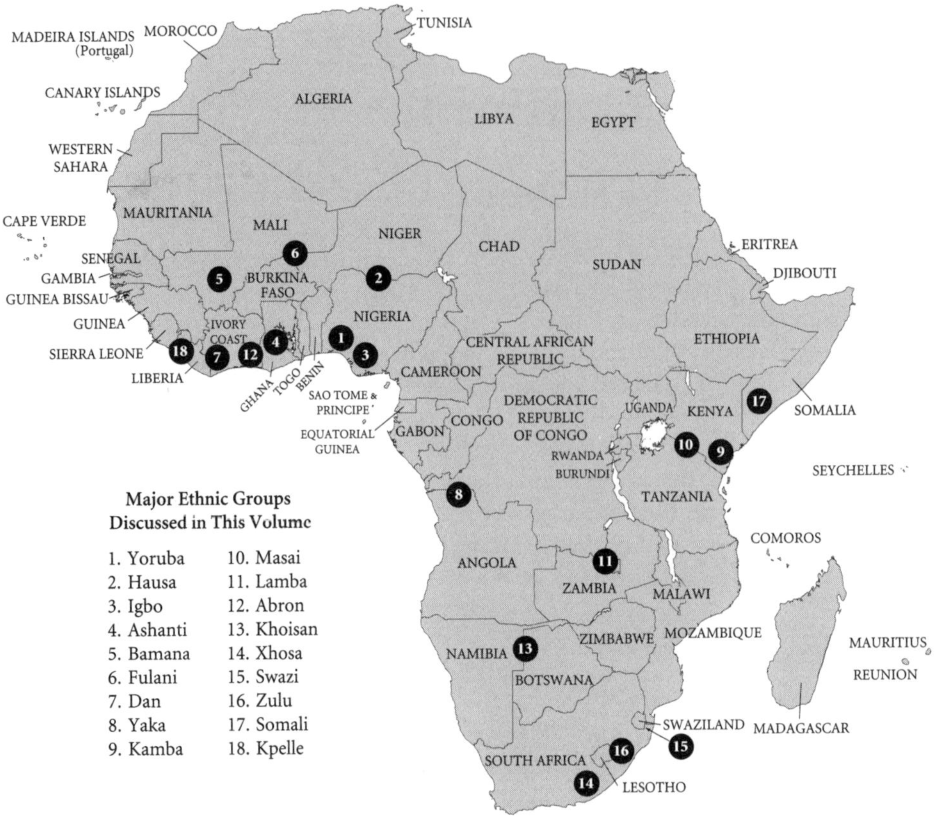

Figure 1-1. Political map of Africa and location of major ethnic groups discussed in this work.

emerges through Somalia near the coastal town of Giamme. In Southern Africa, the Tropic of Capricorn cuts through Namibia just south of Walvis Bay in the west, crosses through the Kalahari desert in Botswana and the Northern Province of South Africa, to emerge on Africa's east coast just north of Inhambane in Mozambique. Africa's southernmost point, Cape Agulhas, near the Cape of Good Hope, lies at 35 degrees S.

In the northern hemisphere, the Tropic of Cancer crosses Africa from the Western Saharan province of Morocco, traverses the Sahara in Mauritania, northern Mali, southern Algeria, and southern Libya and emerges in Egypt at Lake Nasser. The northern most point of Africa lies on the coast of Tunisia between the Straits of Gibraltar and Tunis at 35–37 degrees N.

The equator crosses the continent roughly at the center of the landmass and ten degrees to either side of it lies a forested tropical belt that produces broad-leafed evergreen trees. This humid tropical rainforest belt represents only about 10% of the African landmass. Indeed, most of Africa is not jungle, but grassland, or grassland with trees, alternatively called veld, sudan, steppe, or savanna. It resembles in places the natural prairies now part of the great American farm belt, but with poorer soils, a higher, elevation, and a hotter drier climate.

With the exception of the northern and southern fringes (i.e., the northern coasts of Morocco, Algeria, Tunisia, Libya, and Egypt and the Cape area of South Africa), the entire continent of Africa has a tropical climate. As is typical for a tropical climate, the continent has only two seasons, wet and dry.

Africa's geography is a rather compact one. Its shoreline has few natural harbors or inlets. Of Africa's four major rivers, the Nile, the Niger, the Congo, and the Zambezi, only the Nile can be navigated directly from the sea. Africa is essentially a vast plateau with few coastal plains. And most of Africa's land rises dramatically within a few miles of its shoreline. This topography made the continent somewhat inaccessible to explorers where rivers ended in swamps or lagoons, or formed rapids as they drained down from Africa's rocky highlands.

Ethnic Groups/Languages

An amazing variety of peoples live in Africa's 54 countries, and they possess a startling array of ways of living. Differences in lifestyles come from profound differences in the environment, in the styles of governance, in the systems of kinship, and in the systems of beliefs of the peoples of Africa.

African peoples have often been described in terms of tribe. A tribe was understood to be a loose collection of people with common cultural and linguistic traits who purportedly share a common ancestor. Because of the association of the term tribe with the domination of African peoples by outsiders, the term holds a negative connotation. Indeed so-called tribal maps were produced in great profusion during the colonial era by ruling Europeans who were keen to establish and maintain boundaries around entities that were not altogether fixed, and to put ethnic or tribal labels on groups that were not altogether pure. Today, the term "ethnic group" is preferred. Certainly there have long been major ethnic differences on the African continent. We must be careful to realize that the borders of the territories of these ethnic groups have rarely been as fixed as ethnic group maps may suggest. Moreover, there are many places where two or more ethnic groups have lived side by side in interdependent relationships with one another.

Given these difficulties, it has become more fashionable to discuss ethnic variability in terms of language groups. There are more than 1,000 languages spoken on the African continent by its 700 million people. These languages vary as widely from one another as Finnish does to Turkish, for example. It is possible to approximate ethnicity through identification of the mother tongue.

Linguist J. H. Greenberg has divided the continent into four major language families. The first is the Niger-Congo family of languages, which is considered the ancestor group of the most modern Negroid people of Africa, and which consists of six sub-divisions. These are 1) the Zande family of languages; 2) the Bantu family of languages; 3) the West African family; 4) the Kwa family; 5) the

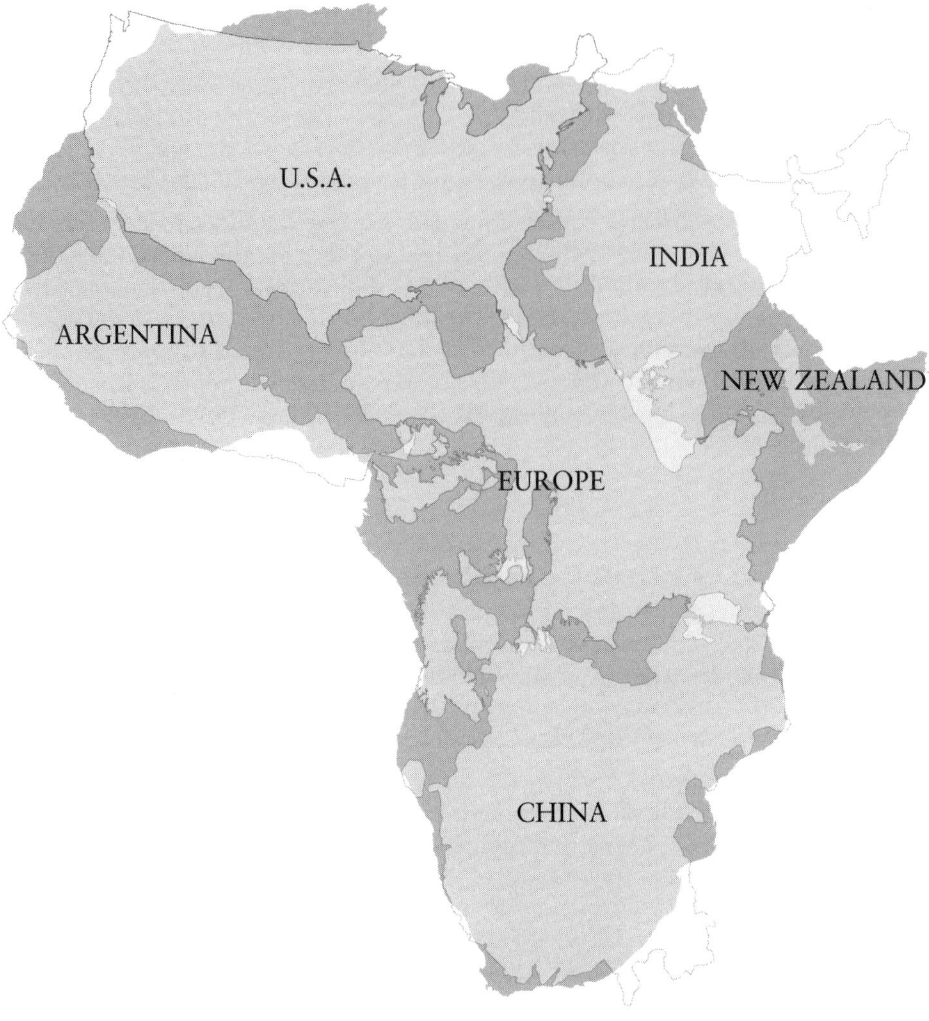

Figure 1-2. Africa in perspective.

Voltaic speaking group; and 6) the Mande, the latter of which are found in Mali and parts of Cote d'Ivoire and Guinea. The language of Swahili, spoken widely in East Africa, is also classified as a Bantu language.

The second major group of languages is the Sudanic group which includes many of the languages of the Nilotic peoples of East Africa, such as the Nuer of Sudan and the Masai and Luo of Kenya. Some languages spoken in Central Sahara and around the Niger bend, (particularly Songhai) fall into the Sudanic group. The third major language group is the Afro-Asian group. Related to the Semitic language groups spoken by a variety of peoples of the Middle East (including the ancient Hebrews), the Afro-Asian group also includes Hausa which is widely spoken in parts of West Africa as a market language. Finally, the fourth major group of languages is the Click language group, spoken by groups very ancient to Africa, such as the San of the Kalahari (McEvedy, 1985, p. 32). It is important to understand that the great variety of languages in Africa suggests the migrations of peoples at very different times in history.

Besides their distinct mother tongue, many Africans often speak a *lingua franca*, a vehicular language that serves as a bridge across many ethnic groups. *Lingua franca* are useful in markets, lorry parks and taxi/bus stations, at border crossings and any other points where large and varied groups of people mingle. These languages usually have, at their base, a genuine African language, such as Swahili in East Africa or Hausa and Mandingo in West Africa. Typically though, non-native speakers have simplified the grammar and vocabulary of a given vehicular tongue. In some parts of the continent, the *lingua franca* may be a simplified colonial language. In Coastal West Africa in the former British colonies, for example, people speak a colorful variety of Pidgin English. Pidginized French can be heard in the markets of Abidjan, Cote d'Ivoire and a "Kitchen Dutch" served in many parts of South Africa as a means through which the indigenous and the Caucasian populations communicated.

Many of the peoples of Africa also speak the official languages of their countries. These tend to be the European languages of the colonizers, notably English, French, and Portuguese. These official languages tend to be the media of instruction for school children, though there has always been debate about the difficulties of schooling children in a language other than their mother tongue. These languages are generally the languages in which the national laws of the land are written, the courts are conducted, and which much of the mass media are produced. The educated classes tend to be proficient in these languages, the masses much less so. To understand this state of affairs, it is first necessary to explore some of the history of European contact. Before doing so, however, it is useful to examine the pre-colonial world of Africa.

European Contact with Africa and the Slave Trade

Evidence of contact between Africa and Europe dates from ancient times. The Greek historian Herodotus traveled through North Africa as far west as modern day Morocco in the 5th century BC. And in the 4th Century BC, Pliny traveled from Mauritania westward to Libya, southern Egypt and Ethiopia. Indeed contact of Greeks with Africa is evident in shards of Greek pottery found in collections of Greek artifacts. The Romans established numerous colonies along the North African coast. After the fall of Rome in the 5th century AD European contact with Africa was made through Arab intermediaries. From about 750 AD, the Arabs, then settled in modern day Morocco, had successfully negotiated a trade route across the Sahara with the aid of the nomadic Sanhaja Berbers. Through the several caravan routes that developed until the end of the European Middle ages, West African forest and savanna regions were in contact with the North African coast.

Until the late 14th century, as noted above, Africa's contact with Europe came mainly across the Mediterranean Sea and through Arab intermediaries in North Africa. But then the Portuguese under Prince Henry made advances in

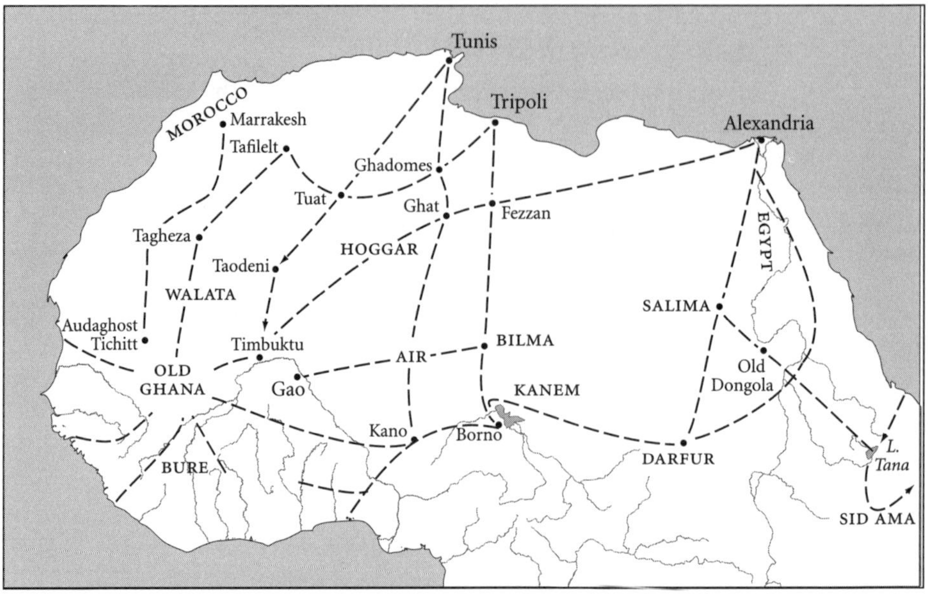

Figure 1-3. Map of Caravan routes across Sahara, 11th to 14th centuries. Fage 1969.

navigational technology and began to trade directly with the great civilizations of Africa and ultimately with the Orient. A series of Portuguese explorer ships set out from Portugal and traveled down the Guinea coast of Africa each one navigating farther than the last. They reached Cape Verde in 1460, the Gold Coast in 1471, and Kongo in1483. By 1488 they had reached the Cape of Good Hope (now known as Cape Town), so named because it offered the hope that ships would soon be able to navigate to India. This was accomplished with the next voyage, undertaken by Vasco da Gama in 1497.

Da Gama's successful voyage in 1497 paved the way for Portuguese trade with India, where the Portuguese concentrated most of their activity. During the 1500s, as the might of the English, French, and Dutch grew, they began to explore the high seas and to develop navigational routes initiated by the Portuguese. By the late 1500s, the French, Dutch, and English also began to develop plantations in the Western Hemisphere. The plantations needed manpower for which local populations proved unsuitable. Either they succumbed to European diseases or they resisted forced labor and escaped into the forests. Africans, who were somewhat resistant to European diseases and well able to sustain tropical heat, proved a suitable labor substitute. Soon business partnerships were forged between African middlemen and European coastal agents stopping at old coastal Portuguese forts and the slave trade was on.

The centuries of African slave trade from the early sixteenth through the early nineteenth centuries helped to alter irrevocably the course of African history. Millions of lives were disrupted as slavers created disputes and raided neighbors in search of human captives to be taken to the coast. Though estimates vary widely, it seems that somewhere between 10 and 13 million people survived the perilous shackled journey across the Atlantic. Another five to eight million more died in African slave raids; in the pre-transatlantic phase of their departure; or in the crossing. Fresh supplies of human cargo were in constant demand because the average slave did not live more than ten years in the New World (Keim, 1995, p. 116). Eventually this forced migration would lead to a population of 100 million people of Negroid origin in the New World today (McEvedy, 1985, p. 90).

Needless to say, this history of slaving had profound effects on the African states of the era. The kingdoms of Dahomey (in modern-day Benin) and Ashanti (in modern-day Ghana), among others grew more powerful in the 18th and 19th centuries as a direct result of their trade in human slaves.

Europeans also grew enormously wealthy with the slave trade, though by the late 1700s some Europeans, particularly some English, began to campaign against it. Some historians have argued that it was Enlightenment thinking in Europe that led to the campaigns against slavery. It should be recalled that the American and French Revolutions were eighteenth century wars fought over ideas of freedom and equality. Others take a more materialist view and argue that slavery ended because industrial power in England was growing in the late 18th and early 19th centuries and that human labor needs were on the decline.

As the slave trade declined at the end of the 18th century, Europeans began to establish trading colonies along the coastal areas of the continent. And explorers, spurred on by the curiosity of a scientific age, began to map the African interior. These colonies gave the Europeans a toehold on the continent, one that would culminate throughout the 19th century with the colonization of the continent. Missionaries followed closely on the heels of traders and coastal settlers, sometimes then pushing deep into the interior. Missionaries extended European influence, establishing schools, spreading European languages, translating the Bible, and establishing printing presses.

European technological progress in the 19th century led to improved transportation, medicine and firearms. Steamboats helped push Europeans into the interior, quinine reduced death from malaria, and rifle barreled breech-loading guns made the conquest of Africa a reality by the end of the 1800s. In 1885, European powers met in conference in Berlin to sign formal agreements detailing what was already a *fait accompli*, that African lands had been carved up and seized by the various European powers: France, Britain, Belgium, Germany, Italy, and Spain. The Conference of Berlin officially recognized the colonial period, a period that lasted until the 1960s.

The Colonial Era: A Clash with the Pre-Colonial Past

Although there had long been contact between Africa and Europe, not always harmonious, the European colonial adventure introduced cultural clashes on a whole new level. It is difficult to generalize about these vast geographical areas and vast sweeps of colonial policy. It is, however, necessary for the purposes of this book.

In the area of governance for example, pre-colonial polities represented a broad range of socio-political arrangements, from simple hunting and gathering bands to empires controlling multi-ethnic states. Pre-colonial leaders of small (as well as large) agglomerations of given African polities were considered by their people as living testimonies of their entire lineage groups. As anthropologist Evans Pritchard pointed out, the African ruler "was the axis of their political relations, the symbol of their unity and exclusiveness and the embodiment of their essential values" (1940, p. 17 quoted in Arens and Karp, 1989, p. xvii).

European colonies replaced local arrangements with their own alien systems of governance. In some places European created chiefdoms where there had been no chiefs. In others they replaced traditional heads with choices of their own. In so doing, the colonizers not only disturbed the temporal order of power, but altered the symbolic and spiritual order as well. The colonies, moreover, amalgamated ethnic groups with little or no desire for co-operation, combining peoples who would never choose to affiliate of their own free will.

Colonialism also severely disrupted established patterns of kinship relations. A complicated web of kinship and lineage obligations heretofore had regulated African society. Most African cultivator and pastoral groups had been organized socially into gender-specific age grades. The system of age grades had provided members of society with both a clear set of guidelines to expected behavior needed for social survival, and a strong network of friendships necessary for psychological well being. Indeed each age-grade member knew his or her place in the social order and acted accordingly. Married men, for example, were often responsible for the maintenance of roads and bridges; married women, for the performance of certain death rituals. The colonial enterprise interrupted the normal ebb and flow of age grade ascendance and other aspects of rural life by introducing schools for youth, paid labor, frequent seasonal migration for adult males, and alternative routes of accession to power.

The colonial enterprise was essentially a search for raw materials and new markets. As such the colonial powers or the interests they supported created mining and other extractive industries; plantations and nascent agribusiness. These ventures would prove profitable for the owners, and would provide jobs for African peoples in need of cash in the new cash economy. Cash was attractive to many an African who sought the means to pay for new imports flooding the markets from Europe. It was also needed to pay taxes newly imposed on the African peoples by colonial masters.

When the colonial era ended the economic structures created by the colonizers, the cash system, the export trade with Europe and the world, and the domestic "taxation without representation" was rather firmly installed. The fifty-odd African national economies were tethered to outside capital and outside expertise but had few ties with one another. Small wonder there are now massive economic problems on this huge but largely disconnected continent.

Colonialism in Africa gave a very grand push to trends toward urbanization that had begun during the era of slavery. Urban centers sprang up along African coastal towns where trading was especially heavy: Mombasa, (Kenya) and Dar es Salaam (Tanzania) in East Africa; Durban in South Africa; Douala (Cameroon) and Brazzaville (Congo) in Central Africa; and Lagos (Nigeria) and Dakar (Senegal) in West Africa. Trading grew around centers of extractive industries: notably in the Copperbelt of then Northern Rhodesia (Zambia); and around the diamond and gold fields of Kimberly and Johannesburg in South Africa. These trends have continued into the 21st century. Indeed rates of urbanization in Africa are growing at about 5% per year and it is estimated that 50% of Africa's population will be urban based early in the 21st century (Stock, 1995, p. 113).

Colonialism, as we shall see, was also about changing consciousness. It has already been noted that missionaries introduced Christianity to the African continent. The first missionaries, the Moravian Brethren, arrived in what later became South Africa as early as 1737, though the real thrust of missionary activity came during the 19th and early 20th centuries. Most of the major Christian denominations were among the missionary groups. In the 20th century, this has included representatives of Pentecostal and Holiness sects and neo-Pentecostal movements.

Some of the teachings of the missionaries dovetailed nicely with African belief systems. The concept of a single godhead as creator of the universe tended to mirror African beliefs. And notions of patriarchy embedded in Christianity tended to resonate well in a largely patriarchal continent. Although both missionaries and Africans supported belief in the afterlife, their approach was radically different. But the missionaries tended to discourage rituals to the African ancestors, and to lesser deities. They also discouraged African participation in many of the secret rituals associated with kin and lineage membership. And the missionaries forbade polygamy. A man who was baptized a Christian was required to give up extra wives, however disruptive this was to family and social life.

Changing consciousness was also about education. Missionaries created the first schools, some as early as the early 1800s. After World War I, the British and the French systematically began to create schools in their colonies so as to produce a cadre of literate clerks and other junior level administrators for the colonies. The medium of instruction in these schools was the national language of the colonizers. Pupils were discouraged from speaking their mother tongue at school; sometimes they were beaten. Many of the schools operated by both missionaries and by colonial governments were boarding schools, particularly at the post-primary level. Students attending these schools left their home villages for long periods of time, and lived in an alien Western environment learning the ways of the European overlords. Sometimes by the time they returned to their villages during school holidays, these African pupils had already missed important age-grade rituals. In any case, so much traditional pre-colonial education had been of the informal type: quiet observation of village life and attentive reception to village lore—all gradually giving way over a lifetime to a wealth of acquired knowledge. For many an African living under colonialism, the acquisition of a Western education came to mean sacrificing a traditional one.

One of the most significant aspects of Western education was the introduction of literacy. Literacy has been implicated in the development of individuality, because the act of reading is independent of group activity. Moreover, the act of reading and writing creates an imaginary context, in which individual readers psychically travel out of their customary milieu, into a temporary and fictitious one. And reading aids the mind to be dispassionate about the facts or ideas presented in the text. The experience of reading is very unlike that of listening to a speech.

In the latter case, the social context of the speech, the non-verbals of the speaker, and the reactions of other listeners all affects its reception by a given listener.

Post-Colonial Periods

Colonialism in much of Africa began to wind down at the end of World War II, in 1945. Indigenous political forces developed around the former soldiers returning from the European war front. Having defended their masters against the German war machine, they could no longer accept subjugation at home. Africa's major colonizers, France and Great Britain, moreover, found they lacked the resolve to continue to govern overseas territories. Their coffers were empty, their populations were dissipated and their armies were exhausted from the great struggle against the Nazis. Throughout the African colonies indigenous governments were hastily organized to take over the governance of the colonies.

The first country to gain its independence was the Gold Coast, which became Ghana in 1957. Most of the African colonies of Great Britain and France quickly followed suit. Through the early 1960s, one former African colony after another became independent. Young, idealistic heads of states, many who had been active in struggles to overthrow the colonialists, were now in charge of these new nations. Worldwide these were heady optimistic times. A very young president John Kennedy was in the White House; an African-American named Martin Luther King was leading a U.S. fight for civil rights.

But optimism was no substitute for experience. And the struggle to overthrow the colonialists had not included a rejection of the economic system the colonialists had installed. Soon after independence, Africans found themselves where Africa had always been, firmly positioned at the periphery of the world's capitalistic system (Amin, 1990, p. 70). This meant they had little real control over the purse strings of their economies. Rather quickly, the optimism of the independence celebrations gave way to bitter disappointment as people realized their lives had not changed a great deal with the new African governments. So the African continent witnessed a series of coups in the late 1960s and early 1970s. In one African country after another a new group of military adventurers took charge.

It has often been argued that the nations of Africa created by the colonists are not viable. Some contain artificial borders that divide similar peoples between two countries. The Hausa peoples live both in Niger, once a French colony, and Nigeria, a former British colony and the Yoruba people live on both sides of the Benin-Nigeria border. Owing to their different colonial histories, the former speak French and the latter speak English while both share a common mother tongue, the Yoruba language. Other countries it is said contain peoples who have ancient hatreds for one another. Rwanda and Burundi both have Hutu's and Tutsis among whom violence has flared up periodically over the years; and ethnic violence has long been a threat to Nigerian stability.

Most African nations lack an economy based on more than a few agricultural and industrial products. Others, such as Burkina Faso and Mali in West

Africa or Lesotho and Zambia in Southern Africa, are completely landlocked and must pay heavy transport costs and sometimes customs fees in order to ship their exports out by land or river.[2] Most lacked roads and communication infrastructures to all parts of their nations. These and other economic inadequacies have plagued Africa since independence.

During the 1970s and 1980s military rulers coped with their inadequate economic bases by aligning themselves with powerful external patrons. These patrons provided aid and facilitated capital investment to well-needing coffers. In exchange, the patrons demanded loyalty of the client states. In particular, they expected client states to vote with their patrons on key issues in the General Assembly of the United Nations. Africa's chief patrons during the 1970s and 1980s were the United States and the former Soviet Union. These two superpowers alternately supported both sides in Ethiopia and Somalia, helping to sew decades of future disorder and chaos. Another important African patron was France who continued heavy economic, political, and sometimes military involvement in her former colonies after their independence.

Corruption and mismanagement marked many of the African regimes of the 1970s and 1980s. Not elected by their own people, one-party regimes used patronage to shore up their own power. They appointed friends to high office; they persecuted their critics; they bought supporters with government contracts; and they funneled chunks of the national treasury into their own bank accounts. As the global recession touched Africa, economic conditions continued to worsen in the 1980s and human rights violations multiplied.

As the Cold War faded into history in the late 1980s, pressure mounted for changes in the power structures of many nations from both within and outside the continent. With access to new communication technologies, pro-democracy and human rights groups were able to gain support and assistance in their struggles from outside the borders of their own countries. The freeing of Nelson Mandela in February 1990, coupled with the prospect of eventual reform in South Africa, had ripple effects on the African continent, as did the independence of Namibia the following month.[3] One country after another clamored for multiparty elections.

The political history of the 1990s was a history of the struggles to secure multiparty elections in many countries. It was also a story of the difficulties new and freely elected governments have had to face in order to contain the contradictions of the countries they were elected to govern. Benin in West Africa overthrew 20 years of iron-fisted rule of Matthew Kérékou, replaced him with Nécéphore Soglo in 1991, only to democratically elect Kérékou again in 1996. Zambia in Southern Africa elected Frederick Chiluba in 1992, and reelected him in 1996. Chiluba had stood against Kenneth Kaunda's 27-year grip on the country. But by 1997, with a

2. Landlocked countries include Mali, Burkina Faso and Niger in West Africa; Chad and Central African Republic in Central Africa; Ethiopia, Uganda, Rwanda and Burundi in East Africa, and Zambia, Zimbabwe, Malawi, Botswana, and Lesotho in Southern Africa.

3. Once known as Southwest Africa, Namibia was a German colony from 1884–1917. After World War I the administration of the colony was ceded to the Union of South Africa. Namibia was finally granted independence in 1990.

coup plot in the offing, then President Chiluba declared a State of Emergency in Zambia. Zambians found Chiluba repeating some of the same political actions he so decried in his predecessor! Congo Brazzaville elected Pascal Lissouba in 1992 after a "national conference" in 1991 stripped Dennis Sassou-Nguesso, the former presidential strongman, of all but ceremonial power. Lissouba was reelected in 1995 but toppled by Sassou-Nguesso in 1997. Dennis Sassou-Nguesso has ruled Congo from 1979 to 1992 and from 1997 to the present.

The Troubled Present

Fate has not been kind to Africa during the last decade of the twentieth century. And problems seem to mount. The economic downturn of the 1980s led the World Bank and the International Monetary Fund, major multi-lateral lending agents, to propose economic overhauls of national economies, known as Structural Adjustments. The program of Structural Adjustment argued that the economies of most African nations were structurally flawed. African countries were invited to remedy these flaws as a contingency for receiving further aid or loans. The structural difficulties identified by the multi-lateral lending institutions were numerous. They included such internal factors as history, politics, geography, and climate. For example the banks recognized that the young age of the countries combined with the fact that they'd originated in colonialism was economically disadvantageous. They recognized that the African countries were young political entities with alien political systems inherited from the colonialists. They understood that many countries were cursed by geography, i.e., they were landlocked like Chad, or they contained vast tracts of impenetrable rainforest tracts as did Zaire (now Democratic Republic of the Congo) or the Central African Republic. And the lending agencies saw that many nations were cursed with inhospitable climates, such as Mauritania, which is mainly desert, or Lesotho which is comprised of the cold windswept peaks of the Drakensburg Mountains.

Structural Adjustment theory also recognized external factors, particularly Africa's general dependence on the trade terms set by the international marketplace, against whom Africa was usually unable to compete. Finally Structural Adjustment theory focussed on domestic fiscal and monetary policies of many African nations and argued that they were deficient. It questioned the role governments played in the economies of their nations. In so doing, it disputed agricultural policies set by governments that limited export of some crops and paid farmers below market value for their products. It criticized the size of the cadre of federal civil servants, including civil servants working in the health and education sectors. It objected to partial government ownership of companies known as parastatals, such as banks, airlines, mining corporations, and marketing and export boards. It objected to African governments' power to artificially inflate local currencies internally while limiting the people's access to hard currencies. The lending agencies said many of these policies had fostered mismanagement and corruption and contributed to kleptocracy of the elite classes. These agencies also believed these economic policies had contributed to Africa's growing indebtedness, which by the 1980's had ballooned almost beyond the size of many an African nation's Gross National Product (GNP).[4]

Although the IMF and World Bank recognized three sets of structural flaws, the remedies it proposed targeted only the last set of issues: domestic economic policies of the individual states. As a result of Structural Adjustment packages accepted by different African countries throughout the 1980s and 1990s, civil servants have been retrenched; parastatals have been sold off; currencies have been devalued and exchange controls have been lifted. Market reforms have encouraged the growth of exports in the agricultural sector and increases of food production in some places. Ironically, international lending agencies had little to say on military policies, the size of national armed forces, or on the military budgets of the individual nations they advised.

Africans were bitterly disappointed that so little attention was paid in the reform packages to the internal and external economic factors that have caused great economic distress and that so much attention was paid by lenders to African internal policy issues. And many (both within and outside the African community) have argued that structural adjustments were designed to make it easier for international investors to make profit in Africa rather than to facilitate the balancing of books and the feeding of people on the African continent.[5] Indeed, in this new millennium, the Structural Adjustment Programs of the 1980s and 1990s appear to have been linked with efforts to globalize the world's economic and technological systems, to form hemispheric trading blocks, and to lower trade barriers.

It is beyond the scope of this text to judge the soundness of the Structural Adjustment Initiative. At best what can be said is that the jury is undecided as to whether the individual Structural Adjustment Programs (SAPs) were beneficial or not. The results have caused considerable instability and have sometimes reversed democratic gains achieved in the political arena (as in the case of Benin). As Stryker and Ndegewa note, "The economic record is a mixed bag of positive growth and better macroeconomic policies for some countries, and continued decline and policy failure for others." (1995, p. 386). Stryker and Ndegewa point out that there will be no quick fixes for African economies, most of which are inherently unsound. They argue that "external factors (especially dependent economies, declining terms of trade, and growing debt) and structural factors (such as history, politics, geography, and climate)" need amending before many of these economies can make worthwhile gains (1995, p. 390).

In more recent years, African indebtedness has continued to soar, with the nations of Africa collectively owing hundreds of billions of dollars. Arguing there will be no development without debt relief, a group called Jubilee 2000 is calling for the cancellation of all Third World Debt. This obviously controversial approach to restructuring the world's economies has as many critics as it has supporters. Critics say debt forgiveness rewards those who have been profligate in

---

4. The Gross National Product is the market value of all final goods and services produced in an economy. This is typically measured annually.

5. See Economic Commission for Africa (ECA) 1989; UNICEF 1987; and Julius E. Nyangoro and Timothy Shaw, eds. 1991. See also Griesgraber 1997.

their spending or incompetent in their management and encourages future fiscal irresponsibility on the part of poor nations with better records. Supporters say the poor have been bled dry with debt repayment, and further squeezing of their economies will lead to more political instability, and an ever growing number of wars and refugees. They add, moreover, that debts incurred in many Third World countries were incurred by politicians neither elected nor supported by the majority of the peoples in those countries. Finally they note that much African indebtedness comes from White Elephant[6] development projects of the 1960s and 1970s, projects supported by foreign lenders including the multi-lateral lending institutions themselves.

Jubilee 2000 has been led by Christian churches in Europe and the United States and supported by the Vatican and the World Council of Churches. It is precipitated by a view of the world not from the perspective of multilateral lending organizations but from the world's poor. And from this perspective, life appears grim and seems to become bleaker with each passing year, largely as a result of national indebtedness. In some countries debt servicing has meant that the country can no longer provide free primary schools; in others that it cannot give out AIDS tests (Stryker and Ndegwa, 1995, p. 391). In 1997 Tanzania spent twice as much on external debt as it spent trying to provide safe water to its people. That same year Uganda spent $17.00 per person on debt servicing but only $3.00 per person on health care (Griesgraber, 1999, pp. 55, 58). Indeed, Sub-Saharan Africa owed 91% of her Gross National Product to lenders in the 1989–1990 period (Wacieni, 1997, p. 193)!

In many countries, debt servicing forces the destruction of irreplaceable ecosystems such as that of the island nation of Madagascar (Malagasy Republic) with its unique and precious biological heritage. For this reason, most conservation organizations active in Africa, in particular the Worldwide Fund for Nature, support swapping debt for guarantees of habitat protection. And Jubilee 2000 has been joined by Act-Up (AIDS Coalition to Unleash Power) and a Global Health Coalition to push for complete debt cancellation. These groups have recognized the terrible toll that African debt has taken on the health of her people and her environment!

Jubilee 2000's program to call attention to indebtedness in the Developing World has not been without success. In 1999, the G7 (wealthy nations) wrote off 100% of bi-lateral debts, i.e., debts owed directly to governments. And 23 of the world's poorest countries have qualified for debt relief on condition of adjustment of their economies. These countries have seen one third of their debt burdens cancelled (BBC World Service, 21 July, 2001).

Given the debt of 750 million dollars still owed by 23 of the world's most indebted countries and given the pressing needs for funds to save the environment and solve the AIDS problem, it seems likely that debt alleviation will be forth-

6. White Elephant projects are usually defined as high technology, high cost, large-scale industrialization projects, energy infrastructure or dam projects that are locally unsustainable because they depend upon heavy infusions of foreign capital, foreign maintenance contracts, and high technology spare parts. White Elephant projects have typically benefited a handful of multinational contractors who install these structures and local politicians who collect rents (kickbacks) from the foreign multinationals.

Figure 1-4. Africa's Debt

Region & Countries	Total external debt*	GNP at market prices*	Total debt service*	Total external debt as % of GNP
WEST AFRICA				
Benin	1,594	2,167	43	73.56%
Burkina Faso	1,294	2,527	49	51.21%
Cape Verde	211	419	6	50.36%
Cote d'Ivoire	19,713	9,795	1,347	201.26%
Gambia, The	452	-	29	
Ghana	6,202	6,203	470	99.98%
Guinea	3,240	3,785	114	85.60%
Guinea-Bissau	937	266	11	352.26%
Liberia	2,107	-	2	
Mali	3,020	2,597	116	116.29%
Mauritania	2,363	1,038	121	227.65%
Niger	1,557	1,958	57	79.52%
Nigeria	31,407	31,125	2,509	100.91%
Senegal	3,663	5,025	274	72.90%
Sierra Leone	1,167	922	59	126.57%
Togo	1,463	1,388	56	105.40%
WEST AFRICA	80,390	69,216	5,260	116.14%
CENTRAL AFRICA				
Burundi	1,127	1,123	31	100.36%
Cameroon	9,515	8,437	528	112.78%
Central African Republic	928	1,038	13	89.40%
Chad	997	1,133	30	88.00%
Congo, Dem. Rep.	12,826	6,050	48	212.00%
Congo, Rep.	5,240	1,878	339	279.02%
Equatorial Guinea	283	242	5	116.94%
Gabon	4,213	4,823	378	87.35%
Rwanda	1,034	1,317	19	78.51%
Sao Tome and Principe	261	-	3	
CENTRAL AFRICA	36,424	26,041	1,392	139.87%
EAST AFRICA				
Comoros	206	230	2	89.57%
Djibouti	241	-	11	
Eritrea	46	-	-	
Ethiopia	10,077	5,950	348	169.36%
Kenya	6,893	8,966	840	76.88%
Madagascar	4,175	3,986	76	104.74%
Seychelles	148	514	15	28.79%
Somalia	2,643	-	4	
Sudan	16,972	-	48	
Ugands	3,674	6,069	150	60.54%
EAST AFRICA	45,075	25,715	1,492	175.29%
SOUTHERN AFRICA				
Angola	10,612	3,454	694	307.24%
Botswana	613	4,760	150	12.88%
Lesotho	654	1,235	36	52.96%
Malawi	2,312	2,157	89	107.19%
Maturitius	1,818	4,241	198	42.87%
Mozambique	5,842	1,543	175	378.61%
Namibia	-	3,327	-	
South Africa	23,590	123,431	3,782	19.11%
Swaziland	220	1,037	33	21.22%
Tanzania	7,412	5,714	258	129.72%
Zambia	7,113	3,294	324	215.94%
Zimbabwe	5,005	7,227	664	69.25%
SOUTHERN AFRICA	65,189	161,421	6,403	40.38%
SOUTHERN AFRICA (without South Africa)	41,599	34,662	2,621	120.01%
NORTH AFRICA				
Algeria	33,260	43,349	4,215	76.73%
Egypt, Arab. Rep.	31,407	67,850	2,309	46.29%
Libya				
Morocco	21,767	35,609	3,174	61.13%
Tunisia	9,887	18,459	1,479	53.56%
NORTH AFRICA	96,320	165,267	11,177	58.28%
No data available for Libya, Western Sahara				
FOR COMPARISON				
Sub-Saharan Africa	227,078	282,393	14,548	80.41%
Sub-Saharan Africa (without South Africa)	230,488	158,962	10,766	145.00%
All Africa	323,398	447,660	25,724	72.24%
Russia	124,785	432,384	7,002	28.86%
Thailand	90,824	90,818	8,652	100.01%
Mexico	157,125	148,458	40,786	105.84%

* current US$, in millions

Adapted from Africa Information Policy Center, Africa's Debt in Numbers, 1998, pp. 4–5.

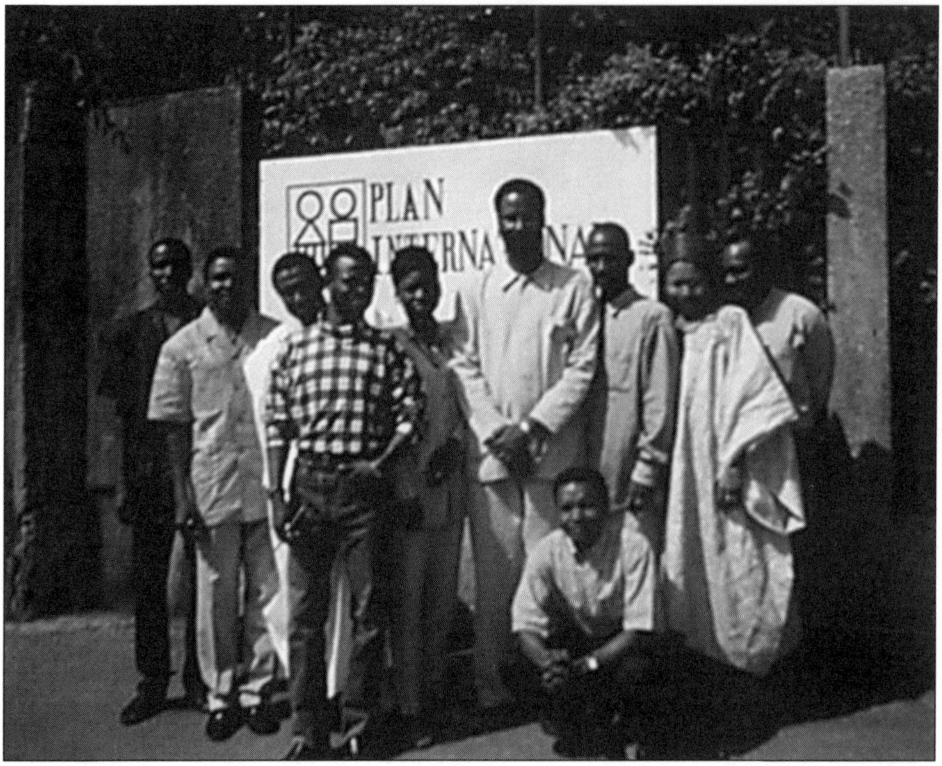

Figure 1-5. The Headquarters of Plan International in Bamako, Mali. Plan International is a major INGO tackling the issue of HIV/AIDS. Photo courtsey of Ann McGuigan, Childreach/Plan International.

coming during the present decade. If bankruptcy court can save individuals from out and out penury, then there should be some mechanism for countries to save their own citizens from abject misery and starvation. Indeed in many nations, there can be no development without debt relief.

Development

The term development as applied to Africa has generally implied a movement toward an improved standard of living for the citizenry of the country in question. It has meant the reduction of poverty and a decrease in rates of illiteracy. Development plans have proposed schemes for greater access to clean water and electricity for more citizens. And they have endorsed efforts for better nutrition and better health care. Development schemes have pushed for more access to the media of mass communication and for access to the personal media of books and computers. And development has implied better communication through paved roads, more telephone lines and other telecommunication infrastructures.

Since U.S. President Harry Truman first used the term "under-development" in the late 1940s, the best means of promoting development in the developing world have been hotly debated. For a long time, economists argued that a country's development could be measured by simple increases in the Gross National Product, the GNP of a country. This position assumed that increases in some sectors of a nation's economy would lead to improvements in the lives of all or most people. It did not anticipate export of capital out of the country in question; nor did it foresee the failure of those in power to otherwise redistribute economic benefits. Development schemes of the 1940s, 1950s, and 1960s applied the theory of "trickle down" economics to the developing world. The trickle down approach to development was well suited to the practice of granting foreign aid on a government to government basis, a bi-lateral basis.

In the 1980s large amounts of aid tended to move out of bi-lateral arrangements and into multilateral lending institutions such as the International Monetary Fund, the World Bank, and the African Development Bank. And a good deal of the remaining U.S. government aid as well as that of the other developed nations began to be funneled through organizations known as INGO, international non-governmental organizations.

International Non-Governmental Organizations represent a wide array of civic and religious groups dedicated to single or multiple issues that involve Africa and other parts of the developing world. Many of the INGOs are well known in the U.S. because they raise funds through television advertising. Such groups include Care, World Vision, and Oxfam, for example, and are involved in helping to coordinate grassroots community projects in a wide-range of African countries. Others such as *Médecins sans Frontières* (Doctors Without Borders) give special emergency medical assistance in wars or natural disasters.

While many INGOs are new, some of them represent an earlier genre of the nonprofit organization, the religiously affiliated philanthropic group. Lutheran World Services would fall into this category, as would the YMCA. INGOs, especially church and other well-established philanthropic groups, have long been recognized as some of the most cost-effective distributors of foreign aid. Moreover, INGOs have become well established in many rural areas, facilitating the distribution of aid directly to the rural poor rather than to urban intermediaries with government connections. And INGO operatives have tended to be idealistic and hard working, two virtues sometimes lacking in both foreign aid personnel and in recipient country civil servants. As early as 1983, INGOs controlled one-tenth of all bilateral aid funds (Staudt, 1991, p. 183). USAID, the United States Agency for International Development, is fond of using non-governmental organizations to disburse its funds for development. Almost 70% of its AIDS funds, for example, are funneled through NGOs (Dramatic Increases in AIDS Orphans, 2001, ¶7).

The growth of INGO power stems from several factors. Typically, INGOs operate by partnering with local organizations whose work they then coordinate. The use of INGOs in development has been beneficial for promoting local partnerships with indigenous groups. Indeed most INGOs will not work directly with the local people. Instead they demand partnerships with local NGOs before they will implement projects.

Indigenous groups, for their part, have benefited their societies not only with regard to the projects they undertake, but also from the way civic organization

Figure 1-6. The Progression of the epidemic of HIV/AIDS over time in sub-Saharan Africa. Courtesy of UNAIDS.

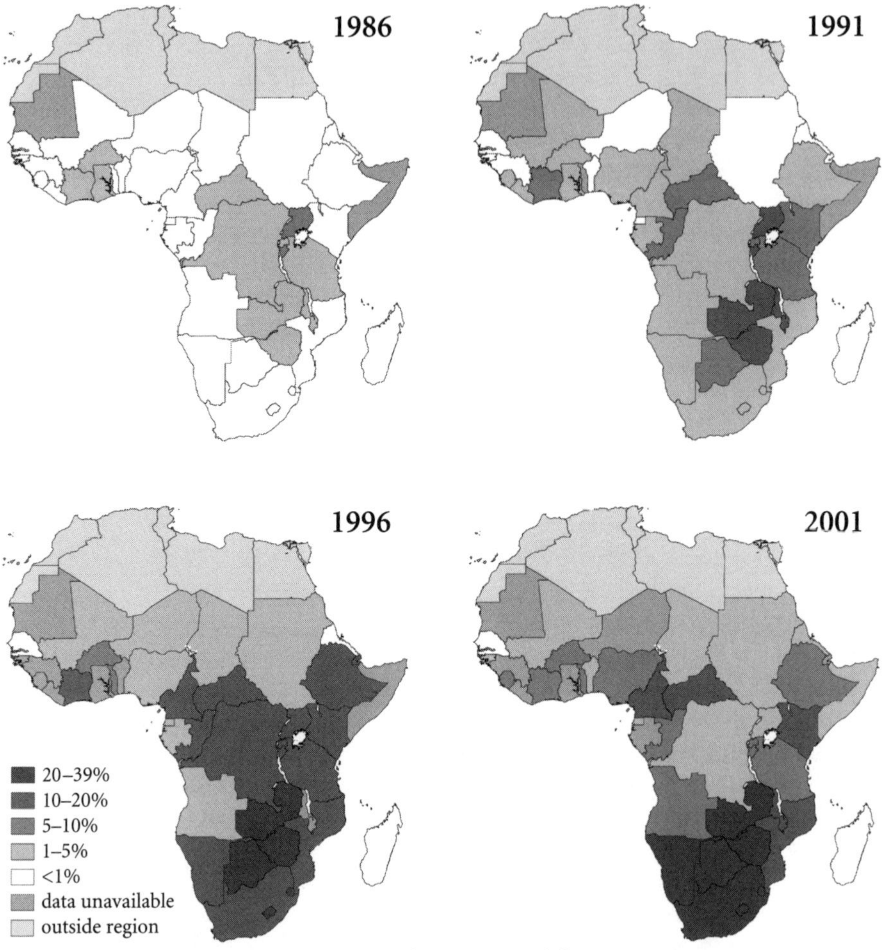

HIV prevalence rate in adults 15–49, sub-Saharan Africa, end 2001

Angola	5.5	Lesotho	31.0
Benin	3.6	Liberia	...
Botswana	38.8	Madagascar	0.3
Burkina Faso	6.5	Malawi	15.0
Burundi	8.3	Mali	1.7
Cameroon	11.8	Mauritania	...
Central African Rep.	12.9	Mauritius	0.1
Chad	3.6	Mozambique	13.0
Comoros	...	Namibia	22.5
Congo	7.2	Niger	...
Côte d'Ivoire	9.7	Nigeria	5.8
Dem. Rep. of Congo	4.9	Rwanda	8.9
Djibouti	...	Senegal	0.5
Equatorial Guinea	3.4	Sierra Leone	7.0
Eritrea	2.8	Somalia	1.0
Ethiopia	6.4	South Africa	20.1
Gabon	...	Swaziland	33.4
Gambia	1.6	Togo	6.0
Ghana	3.0	Uganda	5.0
Guinea	...	United Rep. of Tanzania	7.8
Guinea-Bissau	2.8	Zambia	21.5
Kenya	15.0	Zimbabwe	33.7

building strengthens societies. From this perspective many African societies seem very healthy indeed. For in the era of multi-party politics of the early 1990s, the flowering of democracy meant the flowering of civic groups, some with overtly political ends, others with more philanthropic interests. Many African scholars point to the growth of a vibrant civil society as the most optimistic sign on Africa' s grim horizon (Stryker and Ndegwa, 1995, p. 392).

Studies of the development projects of the post-colonial period have been the subject of much literature. Analysts have been particularly keen to determine why so many projects have failed. The reasons are as complex as they are numerous, but a few obvious causes of difficulty are readily apparent. First, too many projects designed for rural areas of Africa have been conceived by urban dwellers, both local and expatriate. Such projects have denied participation in planning to the targets of development efforts, the rural African populace. And secondly, a host of projects have failed because the communication components of the projects were inadequate. Indeed projects implemented with poorly planned communication are bound to fail, at the simplest level because those intending to benefit from the project are unaware of its existence or its benefits.

Today's development projects, particularly those entrusted to NGOs, tend to focus on empowerment of the most disadvantaged sectors of society. Sensitive to the communicative failings of earlier generations of projects, many projects today use indigenous communication forms to propagate their development information. Attuned to the issues of message acceptability, projects employ members of target populations in the design and production of development materials.

The AIDS epidemic seems to be the latest impediment to development to befall the African continent, a continent that has already seen its share of war, natural disasters, and crop and human pestilence. Unlike other epidemics, AIDS does not attack the very young and the very old, but rather it targets teens and young adults in their sexually active and economically reproductive years. In some parts of the continent entire generations are being wiped out, leaving only the very old to care for the very young. Officials at the US Center for Disease Control (CDC) believe that AIDS will have as deleterious an effect on the African economic and social development in the present century as slavery did in the last (AIDS Analysis Africa, 2000, p. 9).

With little prospect for an AIDS vaccine, African nations have embarked to the best of their abilities on programs of HIV/AIDS prevention through education. But providing effective information on possibly the two most sensitive of human topics—sex and death—continues to challenge the sciences and the arts of communication. Chapter 2 will discuss the AIDS epidemic in detail. Chapter 3 will examine efforts to stem the tide of AIDS and South Africa and Mali. Subsequent chapters in this volume will document and explore multiple uses of performance in the struggle against the spread of HIV/AIDS.

Review Questions

1. What are Structural Adjustment Programs and what impact have they had on most African economies?

2. What was the nature of European colonialism in Africa and what effects did colonialism have on the continent of Africa?
3. What is meant by the term "development" as it has been applied to African countries? In which ways are today's development projects different from the projects of the mid-20th century?

Chapter 2

Human Immunodeficiency Virus and Acquired Immunodeficiency Syndrome in Africa

By 2002, after a 20 year history, AIDS had become the number one killer in the world surpassing malaria, diarrheal diseases and other deadly tropical diseases. Sixty five million people will have been infected with AIDS-related illnesses by the end of 2002. Unlike most other diseases, AIDS typically affects people who are in their sexually reproductive and economically productive years leaving behind dependent children and the elderly. By 2020, HIV will have killed more humans than did all the wars of the 20th century. The AIDS pandemic is expected to peak sometime in the next decade. It will devastate those societies where it has a firm hold. Economic growth will falter, and educational and health gains will reverse themselves. Agricultural and industrial output will slow, and tax bases will shrink as life expectancies plummet and the death toll rises. The number of orphans will soar and the funeral business will continue to be a growth industry. Increasing instability is expected where the professional and political classes either flee or succumb to AIDS and hoards of orphaned and infected street gangs avail themselves of the abundant light weapons available in much of the developing world.

History of AIDS

In the late 1970s, doctors began to recognize a new pattern of illnesses among gay men in the US and Sweden and among heterosexuals in Tanzania and Haiti. In 1981, doctors identified these symptoms as a syndrome, that is, a group of illnesses generated from a common cause.

In 1982, the United States Center for Disease Control (CDC) linked the new disease to blood and began using the term AIDS, Acquired Immundeficiency Syndrome for its designation. In 1983, Dr. Luc Montaigner and his team in France and Dr. Robert Gallo and his team in the U.S. identified the underlying causative virus. And in 1984 both teams of scientists had isolated it. By that year, there were 11,055 cases of AIDS in the US and 5,620 AIDS deaths had been recorded (Newsday, 2001, ¶7). At the turn of the millennium, some seventeen years after the identification of the virus, an estimated 34.3 million people worldwide were living with HIV/AIDS. By mid-2002, that number had increased to 40 million HIV/AIDS cases worldwide. Twenty-eight and a half million of these (around 70%), were in sub-Saharan Africa. (UNAIDS, Report on the Global HIV/AIDS

Epidemic, 2002 July, data tables). As we shall see below, these figures have continued to climb in the new millennium.

What Is AIDS?

The acronym AIDS stands for Acquired Immunodeficiency Syndrome. The syndrome, or group of related illnesses, is caused by a human immuno deficiency virus (HIV), which is a retrovirus (a virus that contains RNA rather than DNA). HIV is introduced into the body through the exchange of blood products or bodily fluids. The virus attacks the body's white blood cells (the T4 cell lymphocytes) that constitute a major part of the body's defenses. The HIV inserts it own genetic material into the T4 cell, duplicates itself and eventually destroys the host cell. Over time, the number of T-cells diminishes and the body's immune system is compromised. Normally, the T4 cell count in the blood is **600+ per micro liter of blood.** When the body's T4 cell count is lower than 200 per micro liter, the carrier is said to have full-blown AIDS. The survival time for a person infected with HIV varies from a few months to more than fourteen years.

AIDS is caused by one of two types of retroviruses, HIV-1 or HIV-2. HIV-1 is responsible for most (99%) of the AIDS pandemic throughout the world, including Africa and the US. HIV-2 is less widespread but is common in West Africa and has spread to India and Europe. Both of these retroviruses are related to the simian immunodeficiency virus (SIV) that infects chimpanzees and several species of monkeys, but not humans. What has been learned about HIV-1 seems to apply to HIV-2, except that the latter appears less virulent and its rate of reproduction seems slower. It should be noted that 99% of the global AIDS cases are caused by HIV-1 (Stine, 2002, p. 197). Data in the present volume refer to both HIV-1 and HIV-2.

HIV-1 and HIV-2 are transmitted between partners during sexual contact, and from mother to child during gestation, birth, and sometimes through breast feeding. The virus is also spread through the use of objects contaminated with infected blood, such as razors, scissors, nail clippers and other blades or used syringes, or through transfusions with infected blood.

AIDS has no cure. Those infected with HIV fall victim to a host of so-called opportunistic infections including pneumocystis carinii pneumonia (PCP); toxoplasmosis; tuberculosis; herpes; candidiasis; cryptococcal meningitis; and aggressive Karposi's sarcoma. The AIDS patient eventually dies of a secondary infection. The cause of death in most AIDS patients is generally recorded as one (or more) of these opportunistic secondary infections.

Diagnosis of HIV/AIDS can be done three to six months after infection. The interval leading up to this time is called the window period, a dangerous few months when infected carriers are ignorant of their status.

HIV testing is done by screening the blood for HIV antibodies in a test known as the ELISA (enzyme linked immunosorbent assay), which is a highly sensitive test originally designed to safeguard blood supplies. If an ELISA test reports positive, a second test is performed for confirmation, either a Western Blot or a Fluorescent Antibody Technique.

In 1992, the Food and Drug Administration (FDA) conducted the first clinical trials of anti-AIDS drugs in the US. And in 1995, the first anti-HIV drug in the protease inhibitor class (a drug that slows the breakdown of DNA in the T4 cells) was approved for use in the US. Advances in viral therapy have considerably reduced the mortality of AIDS in the Western world. The main treatment for AIDS is a three drug combination therapy (referred to as a HAART or Highly Active Antiretroviral Therapy) designed to inhibit (slow down) the ability of HIV to make copies of itself. AIDS patients also often take prophylactic medications that help to reduce the risk of opportunistic infections arising in the wake of a weakened immune system. These include products to treat eye infections, yeast and other fungal infections, and pneumonia. Drug regimens available in the Western world since the mid-1990s have dramatically prolonged the lives of HIV+ patients and since 1997 have led to a downturn in the US AIDS death rate. But the cost of treatment, estimated at between $10,000 to $12,000 per annum in early 2000 (and even higher in the 1990s), is well beyond the means of most people (and most government health ministries) in the developing world. During this decade, political action by AIDS activists, the UN, and governments in the developing world, have led to a steady decrease in the cost of drug treatment. By December 2001, the cost of some combinations of AIDS medicines was down to $350.00 per annum. (See below). The 14th World AIDS Conference held in Barcelona, Spain in July 2002 called for renewed worldwide efforts to treat those infected with HIV/AIDS.

Figures 2-1 and 2-2 provide illustrations of the epidemic over time and by region.

AIDS in Africa

The UNAIDS Programme groups the North African countries of Morocco, Algeria, Libya, Egypt, Sudan, and Tunisia in the Middle Eastern region. All subsequent discussion of the African AIDS epidemic found in this chapter refers to the 48 countries that make up the region of sub-Saharan Africa.

An examination of the 2001 statistics documenting the AIDS epidemic in Africa makes for depressing reading. Africa is dying. In 2001, Africa witnessed more than 6,000 funerals per day due to HIV/AIDS (UNAIDS, 2002, July, table). At the end of the year 2001, the UNAIDS program reported alarming new statistics for the African region. The adult HIV seropositivity rate for sub-Saharan Africa had increased from 8.8% to 9%. New total case figures showed there were 28.5 million persons living with HIV or AIDS in Africa out of the world's new total of 40 million cases. Africa's percentage of the world's total number of AIDS cases still stood at around 70% (Whiteside, 2001, p. 1). There were also 3.5 million new cases of HIV/AIDS in Africa in 2001 and 2.2 million AIDS related deaths (UNAIDS, 2002, July, table). These deaths in Africa represented about 73% of the world's death from AIDS in 2001.

Four nations, all in Southern Africa, had the world's highest rates of HIV/AIDS in 2001. These were Botswana, with an adult prevalence of 38.8%; Lesotho, with a rate of 33.7%; Swaziland, with a rate of 33.4%; and Zimbabwe, with a rate of 31%. South Africa's adult HIV seropositivity rate was recorded at 20.1% (UN-

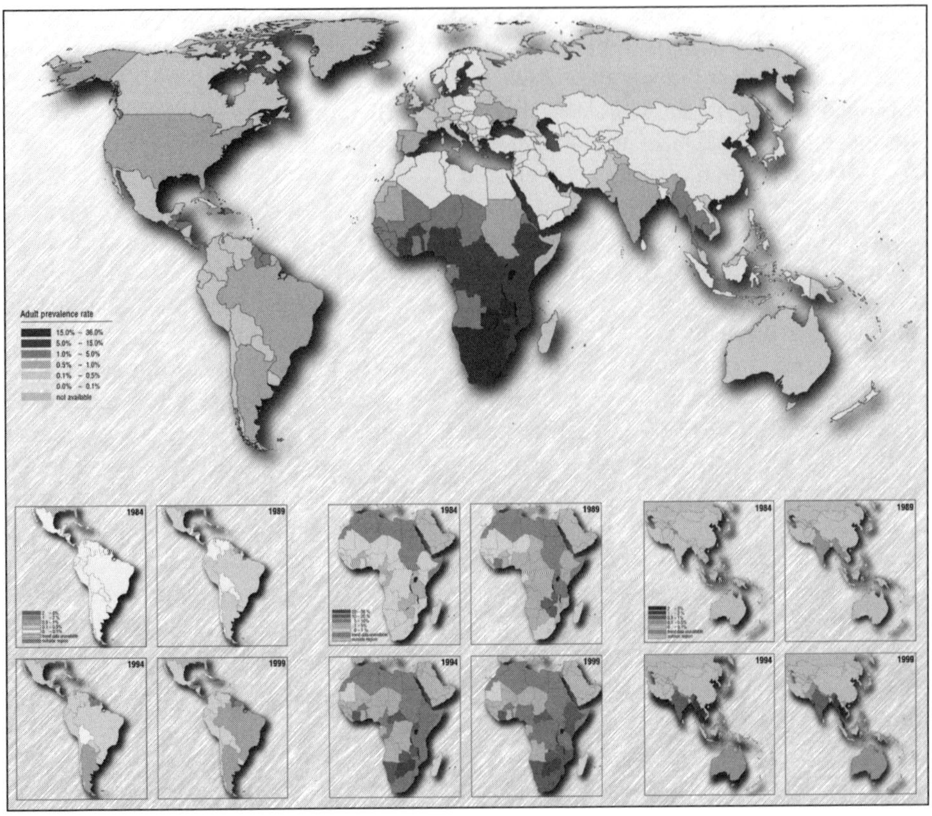

Figure 2-1. Global view of HIV/AIDS infection at the end of 2001. Courtesy of UNAIDS.

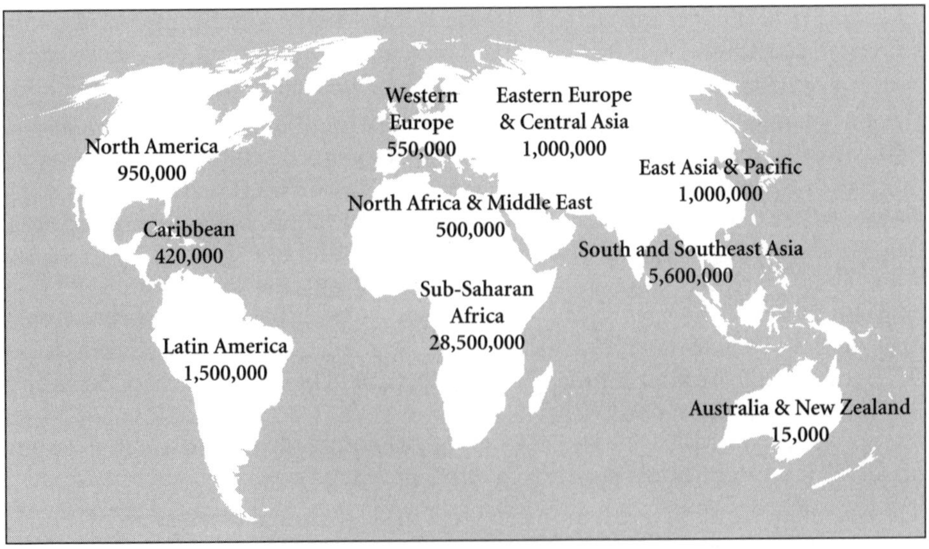

Figure 2-2. Global estimates of HIV/AIDS epidemic (by regions) at the end of 2001. Courtesy of UNAIDS.

AIDS, 2002, July, table). Botswana's epidemic is so alarming that the government has adopted a policy of providing anti-retroviral drugs to any Batswana needing them (*AIDS Analysis Africa*, 2001b, p. 9). Botswana's program of universal treatment for HIV/AIDS sufferers was still in the experimental and planning stages when I visited Botswana in June 2002.

In certain parts of Africa the epidemic is growing so rapidly that it is impossible to record accurate figures. I first prepared this material for publication in July 2001. One year later, in time for the Barcelona World AIDS Conference, UNAIDS released the 2001 epidemiological data. In response, I updated the statistics presented here in this volume. But the rate of growth of this epidemic is such that the epidemiological numbers will inevitably be out of date when *Playing for Life* goes to press. The South African Department of Health reports adult HIV seropositivity rates for individual provinces. South Africa's KwaZulu-Natal province ranked highest in levels of infection in 2001 with an adult rate of 35 to 45%. This rate is among the highest recorded anywhere in Africa. KwaZulu-Natal province, the source of many of the South African AIDS interventions presented in this volume, is the epicenter of the AIDS epidemic in South Africa. When the South African field-work was conducted for this volume (July–November 1999), the HIV+ rate for the province was at 32.5% for adults, a continent-wide record at that time as well.

National HIV+ rates reported by the joint United Nations Programme on AIDS (UNAIDS) are gathered by the national AIDS programs in the individual nations upon the advice of the UNAIDS Programme. In developing nations, where record keeping may be poor, births, deaths, and illnesses often go unrecorded. In most African countries, HIV surveillance has been conducted in pre-natal clinics selected as sentinel sites. Tests are run anonymously on blood samples derived from women seeking pre-natal care. In countries where heterosexual transmission is high, pregnant women are felt to provide a good representation of the adult population between the ages 15–49. Even in the poorest of countries, they argue, some modicum of pre-natal care generally is provided.

These statistics are complemented with comparative figures gathered from more general samples in selected sites. And the UNAIDS Programme claims these comparative figures have generally confirmed the reliability of antenatal sentinel site reports (UNAIDS, 2000, p. 117). Some countries also gather HIV screening results from adult men presenting themselves for treatment for sexually transmitted diseases or for donating blood. Estimates of new infections are based upon infection rates detected in the previous year. In countries with little or no life-prolonging therapies, death rates are calculated as a function of the known course of HIV infection. The disparity in AIDS statistics reporting arises from the way in which the figures are gathered.

Many African countries have been engaged in HIV monitoring since the late 1980s. This has helped their AIDS control programs to closely track the contours of the epidemic. These and other reports have shown that Africa is the continent where infected women (58%) most greatly outnumber infected men (42%). Other studies show that deaths from AIDS in African women tend to occur at a younger age than in men. For African women, the average death from AIDS is between 20 and 39 years of age; for men, it is between 40–59 years (Kamuzora, 2000/2001, p. 14). And figures released at the 2002 Barcelona World AIDS Con-

Figure 2-3. "Regional HIV/AIDS statistics and features, end of 2001"

Region	Epidemic Started	Adults & children living with HIV/AIDS	Adults & children newly infected with HIV (last 2 years)	Adult prevalence rate[9]	Percent of HIV-positive adults who are women	Main Model(s) of transmission[10] for adults living with HIV/AIDS
Sub-Saharan Africa	Late '70s–Early '80s	28.5 million	3.5 million	9.0%	58.0%	Hetero
North Africa & Middle East	Late'80s	500,000	80,000	0.3%	54.0%	IDU, Hetero
South & South-east Asia	Late'80s	5.6 million	700,000	0.6%	37.0%	Hetero, IDU
East Asia & Pacific	Late'80s	1 million	270,000	0.1%	24.0%	IDU, Hetero, MSM
Latin America	Late '70s–Early '80s	1.5 million	140,000	0.5%	31.0%	MSM, IDU, Hetero
Caribbean	Late '70s–Early '80s	420,000	60,000	2.3%	50.0%	Hetero, MSM
Eastern Europe & Central Asia	Early '90s	1 million	580,000	0.5%	26.0%	IDU
Western Europe	Late '70s–Early '80s	550,000	30,000	0.3%	26.0%	MSM, IDU
North America	Late '70s–Early '80s	950,000	45,000	0.6%	20.0%	MSM, IDU, Hetero
Australia & New Zealand	Late '70s–Early '80s	15,000	500	0.1%	7.0%	MSM
Total		**40 million**	**5 million**	**1.2%**	**50.0%**	

"[9] The proportion of adults (15 to 49 years of age) living with HIV/AIDS in 2001, using 2001 population numbers."
"[10] MSM (sexual transmission among men who have sex with men), IDU (transmission through injecting drug use), Hetero (heterosexual transmission)."
Courtesy of UNAIDS.

ference show the epidemic has become a ghastly assault on girls. Sixty-seven percent (67%) of persons infected between the ages of 15–24 are young women. In several countries, teenaged girls have an infection rate 5 times that of boys (Africa Action, 2002, July 6, ¶10).

The UNAIDS monitors the world epidemic and defends the statistics it presents. But AIDS activists, health professionals, and scholars generally urge caution. The latter groups argue that sentinel site samples may not be as representative as hoped. And they suspect that the number of cases appearing in official figures is badly underreported. Patients with no access to health care are never detected; and patients fearing an AIDS diagnosis may eschew testing altogether. AIDS experts point out that African governments, moreover, may wish to conceal the extent to the epidemic as alarmingly high rates of infection tend to discourage investment and tourism (Kalipeni, 2000, p. 966; McGeary, 2001, p. 207).

Because of the AIDS epidemic, average life expectancies in sub-Saharan Africa have fallen from 62 to 47 years of age, a mean drop of 15 years. AIDS Analysis Africa, a South African publication, reports life expectancies with and without AIDS. The numbers are startling. Botswana's life expectancy without AIDS in 1999 was 70.5 years, with AIDS included, 39.3 years. Ethiopia, without AIDS enjoyed a life expectancy of 56.1 years, but with AIDS, that number fell to 45.2 years. Kenya's life expectancy without AIDS was 64.9 years; with the disease, it fell to 48 years. Projections from this report were even more grim for 2010 where life expectancies in some African countries could drop by thirty or more years. At the end of this decade, South Africa's life expectancy without AIDS is expected to be 68.3 years, with AIDS 35.5 years. In a world without AIDS, Swazis could expect to live up to age 61.5; with AIDS, their life expectancy will drop to 29 years. And without the AIDS epidemic Botswanans could expect to live to age 73.2 in 2010; whereas with the disease, their life expectancy is projected to drop by 44 years to 29 years of age (Whiteside, 2000, p. 1)!

Because of the enormous demographic impact, plans must be made to help young people cope with the breakdown of extended families. And politicians should envision the need for strong leadership, one that would prevent widespread panic (Whiteside, 2000, p. 1).

AIDS Impact on Children

The impact of the AIDS epidemic on children in Africa is horrifying. At the end of 1999, UNAIDS estimated there were one million children (under age 15) living with AIDS in sub-Saharan Africa. By 2001 that figure had more than doubled to 2.6 million children. Of these, 250,000 were South African; and 13,000 were Malian. Because of the AIDS epidemic, it is estimated that one out of two children in South Africa will die before the age of 15 (Hunter & Williamson 2000). In some African countries UNAIDS estimates that between 50% and 82% of teens alive today will die of AIDS (Stine, 2002, p. 366).

UNAIDS defines AIDS orphans as the number of children under the age of 15 who have lost either their mother or both parents to AIDS. The number of

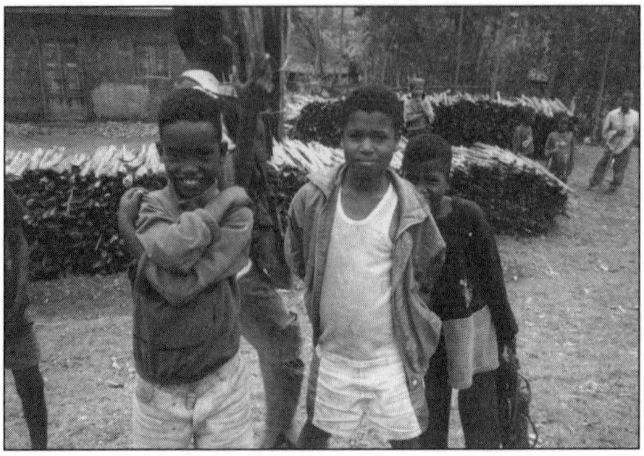

Figure 2-4. In 2001, Africa was home to 11 million AIDS orphans. Photo courtesy of David Schein, Awassa Children's Project.

AIDS orphans is staggering. UNAIDS estimates that the world total of living AIDS orphans is 14 million. Eleven million of these live in sub-Saharan Africa. In ten African countries, 15% of all children are orphans. Before the epidemic, the average percentage of orphaned children in the developing world was about 2% (Smart, 2000, p. 8). In 1990, AIDS accounted to 16.4% of parental deaths in Africa creating orphans. By 2010, USAID estimates that AIDS will be responsible for 68.4% of Africa's projected orphan total of some 42 million (Ramsay, 2001, p. 7; Hunter & Williamson, 2000, p. 46; UNICEF, 2002, p. 6). In some of the most-hard hit countries in Southern Africa, one in three children will be an orphan by 2005 (Stine, 2002, p. 359).

Uganda and Senegal, Bright Spots on a Blighted Continent

Uganda's struggle with the AIDS epidemic is considered an upbeat note on an otherwise somber continental story. Uganda's epidemic was first diagnosed as early as 1986, when Ugandan troops, sent to Cuba for military training, were diagnosed with HIV. In the early 1990s, Uganda's epidemic appears to have peaked at about a 14% adult seropositivity rate. Then the rates began to drop. By the end of the 1990s, HIV+ rates had dropped 40% among pregnant women (UNAIDS, 2000, p. 9). And early in the new millennium Uganda was enjoying a low rate of adult HIV incidence of about 8% (Whiteside, 2001, p. 2). By the end of 2001, UNAIDS reported that the Ugandan HIV adult rate had dropped to 5% (UNAIDS, 2002, July, table).

A group of researchers who have studied Uganda's so-called miracle have concluded that "openness" was a key to Uganda's almost unprecedented success in lowering HIV rates. The book, *Open Secret: People Facing Up to HIV and AIDS in Uganda* (Kaleeba, Kadowe, Kalinki, and Williams 2000) shows how Uganda's government was long engaged in an overt policy of destigmatizing the disease. President Yoweri Museveni, the first African president to acknowledge the problem, did so in 1986. These authors credit Museveni with the courage to pursue a policy of openness and to have fostered its trickle-down, that is, a sense of openness diffused to all levels of Ugandan society. Openness about the epidemic is extremely important in the fight against HIV/AIDS because it decreases the amount of individual and societal denial of the disease. Openness also helps to curb the development and spread of rumors and myths that emerge in the context of an information vacuum (*Aids Analysis Africa*, 2001a, p. 2). (See below).

"Openness" claim authors in their ACTIONAID publication, helped Ugandan communities to provide support and care for the ill. Openness led to broad reaching efforts across many sectors of Ugandan society, all supported by the government. And openness, they argue, led to behavior change, a decrease in the number of sexually active school age children and a rise in the age of first intercourse (Kaleeba *et al.*, 2000, p. 2). Some demographers are less sanguine than the authors of *Open Secret*. They argue that seroprevalence begins to level off naturally in the 11th to 13th year of the epidemic when adult HIV+ rates are between 13 and 15% (Kamuzora, 2000/ 2001, p. 8). Expressed more bluntly, these analysts say that Uganda's AIDS crisis has now passed because so many Ugandans have already perished!

The case of Senegal also appears to provide a useful model of HIV prevention with its admirable rate of less than one percent (0.5%) adult seropositivity. Senegal's health officials can also be commended for early public acknowledgement the illness. Indeed the Senegalese government began its battle against AIDS in 1986, when there were only six cases in the entire country! It solicited the help of organizations active in health education. These included the very politically significant Islamic brotherhoods as well as Roman Catholic-based social service groups among others. These groups worked together to launch information campaigns, campaigns that would refrain from speaking out against condom use.[1] The government of Senegal also enlisted the help of traditional healers. And as early as 1988, two individuals who were HIV+ went on TV to speak about their status. Senegal's openness policy has also kept the stigma of HIV in Senegal to a minimum and that has kept the disease from going underground. Openness appears to apply to prostitution as well. Senegal is one of the few countries in Africa with commercial sex regulation. Commercial sex workers are required by law to undergo periodic medical examinations. This practice has kept STDs under control and facilitated the condom adoption rate, at more than 90% among commercial sex workers (Diop, 2000, p. 14). Such openness seems to mitigate the stigma of HIV/AIDS and is an important factor in controlling the AIDS epidemic.

Uganda and Senegal are Africa's bright lights in the AIDS epidemic, but there are also some dim bulbs. Zimbabwe's AIDS initiatives have received mixed support at the presidential level. President Robert Mugabe is, at best, ambivalent about the crisis, having failed to publicly acknowledge it until 1999. Zimbabwe's ruling party has levied a controversial AIDS tax on all salaries so as to raise funds to purchase AIDS drugs and to care for AIDS orphans. Critics in the oppo-

1. The Catholic Church has often spoken out against condom use in Africa even during the course of the AIDS epidemic. The attitude of various Islamic groups has been decidedly mixed.

sition say funds for AIDS should be derived from direct government allocation. And they says the funds could come from redirecting monies spent to pay for Zimbabwe's costly participation in civil war in the Democratic Republic of the Congo (Machipisa, 2000, ¶5).

And the South African leadership has been mixed. While the stately Nelson Mandela rallied the South African public against AIDS soon after taking office, current President Thabo Mbeki has blundered badly on the AIDS issue. President Mbeki long denied that the HIV virus causes AIDS. In so doing, he had teamed up with a fringe group in the AIDS medical establishment. His views have been very controversial and have generated widespread condemnation among AIDS activists, as well as medical and social science researchers (Crewe, 2000, pp. 10–11. See also AFP 2000). Scholars who defend his position suggest Mbeki merely wished to highlight poverty as an important co-variable in the epidemic (Stillwaggon, 2001, p. 22). Others argue that Mbeki's position is political window dressing that makes it easier to preference other governmental expenses over costly treatment in the country with the world's worst AIDS epidemic (Stine, 2002, p. 37). But pressure on Mbeki finally caused him to soften his position. The executive committee of his African National Congress party averred in 2002 that it is acceptable to assume HIV causes AIDS, but that it is only an "assumption" (Africa Action, 2002, March 27, ¶33). Mbeki has generated further controversy because his government has refused to provide a course of retroviral treatment for pregnant women. These treatments have been dramatically effective in decreasing the rate of mother to child infection. South Africa's Treatment Action Coalition (TAC) took the Mbeki government to court and won a suit in 2002 that forces the government to provide this service for pregnant HIV+ women in all government-run clinics. Mbeki's government has said it lacks the funds to treat 70,000 or so women per year. Mbeki has argued that South Africa lacks the infrastructure needed to monitor the administration of the anti-retroviral Nevirapine, the drug that would be used to combat mother-to-child transmission of HIV. Others in South Africa disagree. Some suspect that Mbeki prefers to allow these children to die rather than add them to the staggering number of AIDS orphans, already predicted to reach 10 million in South Africa by 2010 (McGeary, 2001, p. 212).

Factors that Fuel the HIV/AIDS Epidemic in Africa

Sub-Saharan Africa possesses a cauldron of conditions bubbling over with opportunities for AIDS transmission. These include ecological factors, economic factors, migration patterns, conflict, as well as issues of gender and demography.

Ecological Factors

The continent of Africa is as physically and ecologically varied as are its human populations. A broad spectrum of climatic conditions, vegetation, landscape, and bio-geography help to explain the prevalence of a host of disease causing organisms:

viruses, bacteria, protozoa, and worms. Chronic conditions such as malaria and schistosomiasis,[2] together with diarrheal and other tropical diseases, generally serve to weaken the immune system and increase the likelihood of susceptibility to HIV infection. High heat and humidity in tropical zones favor the development and rapid spread of infections in general, including Sexually Transmitted Diseases (STDs). Untreated, these STDs (also known in the literature as STIs or Sexually Transmitted Infections) are important sites for the transmission of the HIV virus (See Grosskurth *et al.*, 1995; Alder, Foster, Grosskurth, Richens, and Slavin 1998; and Nicoll 1998).

Poverty

The combined Gross National Product (GNP) of all sub-Saharan African countries excepting South Africa is less than $150 billion dollars or 1.2% of the global Gross National Product. This figure is equal to the GNP of Belgium, a country with a population of 10 million as compared to the 500 million who live in sub-Saharan Africa (Ramsay, 2001, p. 5).

Nutritional standards in much of Africa have been in decline since the 1970s. Between 1970 and 1997 protein supply per capita fell by more than 15%. There were also 22 famines on the African continent during the 1980s and 30% of the entire continent was reported to be malnourished. General protein and calorie deficiency together with vitamin or other mineral imbalances can cause serious weakening of the immune system and damage to the skin and mucus membranes. The latter two are especially implicated in the transmission of HIV (Stillwaggon, 2001, p. 22).

The majority of countries ranking lowest on the UNDP's Development Index and highest in the Human Poverty Index are in sub-Saharan Africa. The figures are grim. Thirty four percent of sub-Saharan Africa's people are not expected to survive to their fortieth birthday. Fifty percent are without access to a safe water supply. Fifty percent are illiterate (UNDP 1999). Less than half the people of sub-Saharan Africa have access to health care (Bread for the World Institute, 1994, p. 117). Africa cannot afford to fund its own AIDS struggle. In 1997, for example, $150 million went into the AIDS struggle in Africa. Only $15 million, or 10% of those funds came from Africa (Machipisa, 2000, ¶ 13).

Structural Adjustment Programs mandated by the World Bank in the 1980s and early 1990s had a deleterious effect on African public health care systems. Governments were forced to reduce their staff in government-operated public health clinics. And many introduced user fees that have led to a decrease in clinic use. Zimbabwe's pubic health system, which made steady advances throughout the 1980s, for example, was forced by the SAP to decrease its public expenditure on health by 35% between 1991 and 1994 (Chisvo and Monro 1995). Indeed Structural Adjustment throughout Southern Africa has caused the resurgence of a number of diseases (TB and sleeping sickness, for example) once under control (McPake 1993).

---

2. Schistosomiasis or bilharzia is a water borne parasitic disease that is contracted by humans who walk or work in lakes and streams. The schistosome larvae enter human skin, travel through blood vessels, and develop into worms that live in the human liver, bladder, and intestines.

Programs of currency devaluation in many African countries also accompanied Structural Adjustment. This has put Western medicine beyond the reach of many consumers. It has also contributed in many cases to the aforementioned decrease in protein intake.

Inadequate access to health care means that many people live with low levels of disease at any given time. Chronic levels of intestinal parasites, malaria, and STDs are very common throughout sub-Saharan Africa. These conditions often go untreated because clinics, the drugs themselves, or the funds to pay for them are unavailable.

Migration

Since colonial times, economic activity on the African continent has been concentrated in the coastal areas. Today, these coasts, along with strategic industries along the way, are focal points for economic migration. In West Africa these are the main auto and truck routes between Abidjan, Cote d'Ivoire and Senegal on the westerly axis of the region; from Abidjan through Burkina Faso to Niamey on the central axis; and from Abidjan to Lagos, Nigeria along the coastal route fringing the Gulf of Guinea (See Figure 2-5). Agro-industrial workers also follow these routes so as to work seasonally in plantations of the coastal portions of West Africa.

In the southern portion of the continent, South Africa draws migrants from all countries in the region. A particularly dangerous axis for HIV is the coastal route from Tanzania through Mozambique and onto the Indian Ocean ports of South Africa. Of these, Durban, in KwaZulu-Natal province in South Africa boasts one of the busiest ports on the African continent and probably the highest HIV+ rate of any African city (AIDS Analysis Africa, 2001d, p. 6). Another is the Lusaka (Zambia)-Durban (South Africa) highway that connects Zambia, Zimbabwe, and South Africa.

Migration creates conditions particularly suitable to risk-taking behavior. Men engaged in long distance hauling are separated from their families for long periods of time. They endure long hot days, and lonely and sometimes dangerous nights on the road. They tend to have an overall increased number of sex partners, and they tend to engage in other risk-increasing behaviors such as alcohol and drug use. The movements of sex-professionals have been closely tied to both seasonal migration and Africa's long haul transport industries (Sakho, 2001, p. 11). Sex professionals ply their trade on truck routes, at border bars, and in hotels patronized by truckers. Seropositivity rates for adults in border towns often reach a rate of 50%. One small sample of long distance truckers in Johannesburg, truckers who plied the Lusaka-Durban road, revealed that 79% were HIV+ (Family Health International, 2000, p.17).

Migrant populations are considered at greater risk for spreading HIV. For this reason Africa's numerous corridors of migration are the sites for special research and AIDS intervention projects. These include, among others, the USAID "Corridors of Hope Initiative" in Southern Africa, and the *Projets SIDA* 2 & 3, seven country West African initiatives funded by the Canadian government and many other partners.

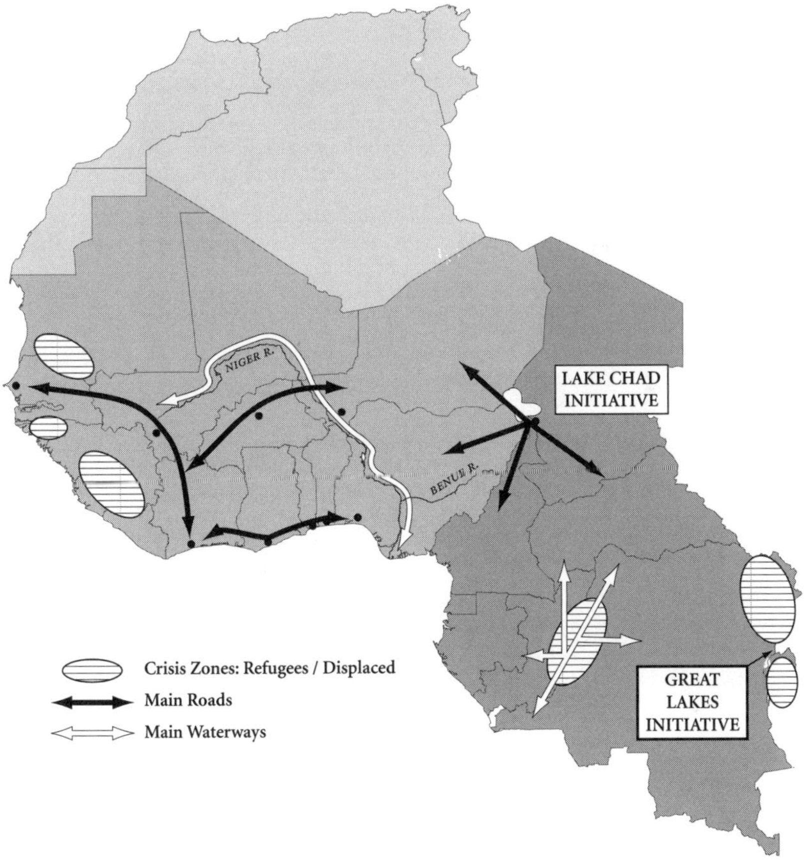

Figure 2-5. Migration and Mobility in West and Central Africa. Courtesy of UNAIDS Inter-Country Team/West and Central Africa.

Mining on the African continent, particularly in Southern Africa, often involves migration. And pathological behaviors surrounding mining in Southern Africa are almost legendary. Campbell and Williams have shown how daring sexual behavior may constitute for many miners what it means to be male. These authors have observed that the risks of unprotected sex may pale in comparison to dangerous work in the mines (Campbell and Williams 1995; and Campbell 1997). Gould (1993) who studied Malawian miners who migrate to South African mines, estimated that nearly half returned to rural areas in their own country, infected with HIV and passed that infection onto their wives and other women.

Conflict

Much of the African continent is embroiled in conflict. Chad, Eritrea, Ethiopia, Mozambique, and Uganda were engulfed in conflict in the 1990s. Conflicts continue in Liberia, a country that spent most of the 1990s embroiled in civil war. The Liberian altercation has spilled over into Sierra Leone and Guinea

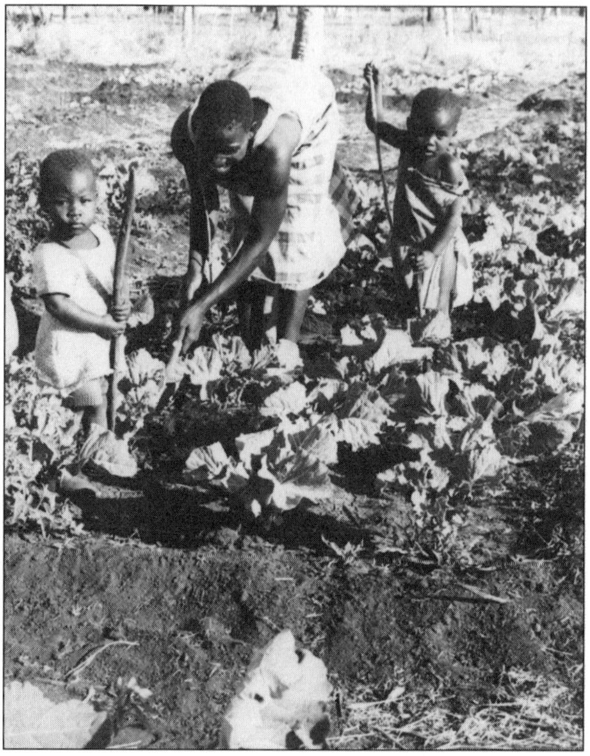

Figure 2-6. African women are responsible for 60–80 percent of Africa's agricultural production. Photo courtesy of Ann McGuigan, Childreach/Plan International.

in the new century. Civil war also continues in Angola, Djibouti, Rwanda, Sudan, Democratic Republic of the Congo (former Zaire) and Somalia. Meanwhile there is considerable political strife in Zimbabwe and in Nigeria early in the third millennium.

In the last three decades, internal and external conflict has pushed millions of refugees into crowded and dirty camps where food, shelter, and sanitation have been scarce. Refugees put burdens on those communities or countries housing them, and the tensions they cause leaves their most vulnerable at risk of violence. And armed conflicts are ripe with possibility for the transmission of HIV. Unaccompanied armed males engaged in high-risk military work encounter vulnerable women and children displaced by war, potential participants in the sex trade and potential targets for sexual violence ("Abuse of Women Escalates" 2001, ¶2; Nafo, 2001, p. 6). Prolonged decades of civil war, moreover, have destroyed much of the existing health infrastructure.

Gender Disparities

In Sub-Saharan Africa 58% of the HIV positive cases are women. This is the region of the world in which women are most at risk for contracting HIV/AIDS.

For physiological reasons, women are two to ten times as likely to contract HIV from men than men are from women (Doupe, 2001, p. 6; Stine, 2002, p. 340). The vagina presents a much broader area of vulnerable tissue (and hence exposure to HIV) than does the penis. And HIV exists in higher concentrations in semen than in female genital secretions.

In Africa, sheer physiological facts combine with macro political and economic realities to make the risk of contracting HIV/AIDs very high for African women. Women constitute the vast majority of commercial sex workers, and many are forced by circumstances into these occupations before they reach the age of 15. Gender norms in sub-Saharan Africa tend to stress female compliance with male desires. On average, the gender gap between age at first marriage (20.7 years for women and 26.5 for men), is the highest anywhere in the world (United Nations, 1995, p. 7). In matters relating to sexuality, the value of female circumspection is much admired. Paradoxically perhaps, fertility is highly prized and female achievement of personhood is very often tied to reproduction, further aggravating female risk.[3]

On the African continent gender disparities that exist worldwide are particularly glaring. Men have access to the best jobs and the highest paying salaries. Men's work is recognized and remunerated while women often go unpaid or unnoticed. In Southern Africa where 70% of full-time small holder farmers are women, for example, most are by-passed by agricultural development schemes (World Bank 1992). And although the new South African government is busy with legislation and policy initiatives designed to tackle gender discrimination, most South African women would agree the country still has a long way to go.

Structural Adjustment Programs have further exacerbated disparities between men and women by programs emphasizing cash crops above small family subsistence plots. Cash cropping has long given men more discretionary income, funds not necessarily shared in the family. The production of cash crops, it should be recalled, was greatly intensified during the colonial era, as was the system of migrancy that persists into this new century. As noted above, migratory work patterns take chiefly male members of the work force out of rural areas leaving women behind for long periods of time. Rural women, often overburdened with both the cares of children and elderly relatives, are left to tend to women's as well as men's agricultural activities. Impoverished rural women must wait for support from migrating spouses who may have already set up "alternate households" in their place or places of paid remuneration. Oftentimes this support is meager. Sometimes it never comes. And very often these days, the migrating husband comes home after his urban adventures only to give his wife AIDS. And rural areas, disproportionately home to more women than men, are less well served by health facilities (Kalipeni, 2000. p. 969). It is not surprising that young women have also begun to migrate to the city in search of opportunity.

3. Brand shows that among the Mande, social relations take precedence over individuality. A person must grow up, get married, and reproduce in order to achieve full personhood. This is especially true for women. See Brand, 2001, pp. 15-23.

But for young African women who move to urban areas in search of paid employment, life can be precarious indeed. Those fortunate enough to find paid employment are likely to be less well paid than their male counterparts. They may suffer sexual harassment, sexual violence and other forms of discrimination. Many drift into prostitution, an occupation that ebbs and flows seasonally, as noted above, in direct relation to the patterns of agricultural migration.

For many young women migrants, work as domestics or as prostitutes is sometimes the only steady paid remuneration (Kalipeni, 2000, p. 967.). And because domestic and other employment in many African countries is poorly regulated, maids tend to be underpaid. Moreover, they may be forced or feel compelled to grant sexual favors to male employers. Indeed, the phenomenon of "clientism" is alive and well among young urban women who may seek protection from an older, more wealthy male.[4] Should a young women become pregnant, her situation will become even more desperate as she seeks to support one or more children.

Women everywhere are saddled with triple burdens of household chores, pregnancy, and child rearing. And throughout sub-Saharan Africa, women tend to eat less and to eat less well than men (Svedberg 1990). The physical stress of multiple pregnancies and births takes its toll on women's health. Women moreover must bear the burden of caring for others in the family, including those hungry or ill.

Throughout the African continent, norms governing sexuality invite men to spread the disease and encourage women to be vulnerable. In many parts of Africa polygyny was once the norm and successful men were expected to take multiple wives. In theory, faithful polygamy could be as effective as faithful monogamy in containing AIDS. Today, though modern economics or religion have suppressed polygyny, male sexual mobility is often widely tolerated (by both men and women) if not openly admired. And men seem particularly eager to display their "young mistresses." For these serve as testimony to their sexual, as well as their economic prowess. For their part young urban women seek out rich men to serve as their "grotos," or their "sugar daddies." These men may pay their mistresses' rent, their tuition fees, their clothing, or other expenses, or to help them support their children or other dependants (Byabarumwanzi, 2001, p. 7).

Despite the obvious contradictions, African women generally speaking are expected to display less interest and less knowledge of sex than their male counterparts. Repeated surveys of sexual behaviors show that men consistently report having more sexual partners than do women. Cultural norms, as well as economic conditions, though these vary widely across the African continent, generally put women at considerable disadvantage in negotiating the conditions in which sex takes place. These factors help explain why the alarming ratio of HIV+ young women to young men, a ratio of two females for every one male (Africa Action, 2002, July 6, ¶37).

4. Clientism or patron-client relations refers to a practice which is fairly widespread in Africa wherein an individual with political power or financial resources (or both) offers financial care or physical protection to a weaker individual.

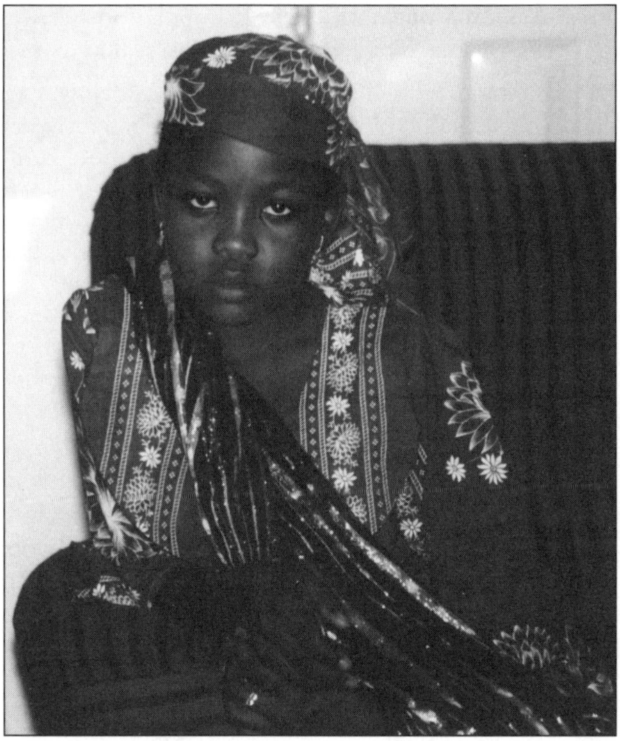

Figure 2-7. More than half of the women in West Africa are married between the ages of 15–19.

Urbanization and the Youth Bulge

Although Africa is the least urbanized of the world's continents,[5] it is the continent with the world's most rapid rates of urbanization. Rapid population growth caused by high fertility has sent legions of young people into urban areas. These trends are exacerbated by economic imbalances in the global economy. The urban growth rate for Africa for the 1990–97 period was 5.08% per annum as compared to a world rate of 2.43% per annum. Mali, which is already 28% urbanized, is increasing its city populations at a rate of 3.1% per annum. South Africa, which is presently 51.2% urbanized, has been urbanized since early in the 20th century, and its urban population is growing at 2.9% per annum (Africa in Figures 1998).

And the cities in Africa are disproportionately home to the young who themselves are over-represented on the continent. Indeed, almost half of sub-Saharan Africa's population is under 15 years of age. In Mali, 47.2% of Mali's popula-

5. 45.8% of the world's population is urbanized while only 35.6% of Africa's population is urbanized.

tion is under 15 and 32.5% of South Africa's population is represented by the under 15 group (Bread for the World Institute, 1994, p. 117).

Many of the pathological social problems described below, particularly those related to violence and sexual exploitation, are exacerbated by urban living and precarious economic conditions. In earlier times, and in more rural settings, gender violence and exploitation were mitigated by the presence of strong extended family systems, including males[6] who kept watch over their female kin. Increasingly with urbanization and migration, these systems have broken down, and have left society's most vulnerable people to their own devices.

Western Popular Culture

One of the products of urbanization is the adoption of Western norms of individualism and materialism, coupled with the gradual abandonment of rural communal values and folkways, mores and lifestyles that have governed African rural life for centuries. Here the role of Western mass media has been deeply implicated in this process (Bourgault, 1995, pp. 226–238). What is perhaps underappreciated in the literature on AIDS in Africa is the extent to which Western popular cultural media models of gender relations have been absorbed by modern young Africans (Mwikisa 2002). The 1990s have seen an explosion in the availability of media outlets. In the cities, satellite-supplied television brings an unprecedented amount of popular Western television fare to Africa. This programming has supplemented the material that became available in the 1980s resulting from the videotape boom. The 1990s have also seen the opening up of the airwaves to deregulated radio and the proliferation of community and private radio stations. Through much of these new media channels has come little more than a relentless stream of commercial Western media images and values, replete with gendered images of Western women designed by male-centered multi-national media conglomerates. Western popular culture, especially that targeted at teens, is legendary for serving up a potent mix of commercialism, violence, irresponsible sexuality, and commodified female bodies eager for male domination (Dinozzi 1994; Jhally 1995; and Ericsson and Taireja 1999). In the United States, and in other Western countries where these images are produced, a feminist movement and the social changes it has spawned serve to mitigate some of sexism's most egregious effects. But on the African continent, with feminism struggling for a toehold, women have been encumbered with the double yoke of pre- and post-colonial imposed gender roles. In short, African notions of male privilege have been reinforced by Western mediated images of male superiority. This potent notion of male power has disastrous consequences for females as I will demonstrate below. Moreover many of the so-called African "cultural" practices that have been implicated in the literature on HIV/AIDS are related primarily to gender boundary maintenance.

---

6. This has not been the case in South Africa since the mid-19th century because labor patterns introduced in the region forced men to live apart from their women. It is also noteworthy that violence in that country has long been high.

Cultural Practices: Pro-Natalism, Levirate Marriages, Widow Cleansing, and so on

Africa has often been said to be "pro-natalist," as evidenced by having the world's highest fertility rates of 5.9 births per woman (Africa in Figures 1998). For Malian women the fertility rate is a high 6.7 children per woman, one of the highest on the continent. What is sometimes not appreciated from a distance is the extent to which fertility, particularly a woman's fertility is bound up in her status as a person. On many parts of the continent, a woman who has not given birth to a child is barely considered an adult. Women's fertility is considered so important that many young women feel compelled to produce at least one child in order to make them marketable marriage partners (Brand 2001; Obbo, 1987, p. 80). In many societies, males also feel the need to prove their fertility. Anita Jacobson Widding has shown that among the Shona, a man cannot become an ancestor unless he has proven his potency (Komba-Malekela and Liljeström, 1994, p. 144).

In many parts of Africa, especially those with polygyny, the practices of levirate and sororate marriages are endorsed. In societies that practice levirate marriage, it is assumed that a widow, after a period of requisite mourning will become the wife of her husband's brother. In sororate marriage, it is assumed that a widower will take an unmarried sister of his deceased wife as bride. These social practices, while deeply humane in their origins, can put entire families at risk during these times of the AIDS pandemic. Many African countries, including Mali, where these arrangements are well established, are urging people to proceed with caution into any family situation that might inadvertently help transmit the HIV virus.

Across the African continent a range of culture-specific sexual practices have been found intermittently among different ethnic groups. One of these is the practice of "widow cleansing" in Zimbabwe, wherein a member of the dead husband's family expunges the soul of the deceased by having sex with his widow (McGeary, 2001, p. 210). Alternatively, the widow may be expected to undergo ritual sexual cleaning with a social outcast (such as an insane person) in order to expunge her husband's alleged curse (Sithole, 2002, p. 3). Other practices might include a once widespread tolerance for sexual experimentation among youths of both sexes as long as it did not lead to pregnancy. (See for example, Setel, 1999, p. 47 for a discussion of Chagga norms in Tanzania; see Ahlberg 1993 for a discussion of Kikuyu pre-colonial sexual mores; see von Kapff, 1997, p. 38 for a discussion of sexual mores among the Zulu).

I should like to call the reader's attention to certain qualifiers discussed below when considering the data presented on cultural practices. There has been a tendency in much writing on Africa to focus on perceived exotic sexual practices and the implicit suggestion of rampant sexuality on the continent (Gumisai 2001). But Stillwaggon, an AIDS researcher who has worked in Zimbabwe and Tanzania, urges caution. She notes that weakened immune systems caused by ill health and malnourishment account for a far greater percentage of HIV transmission than do any African behavioral patterns. She argues convincingly that sexual behavior alone could certainly fail to explain Botswana's rate of HIV/AIDS, 50 times than of the US and 1000 times that of Cuba (Stillwaggon, 2001, p. 22).

Gender Violence

Worldwide, gender violence against women crosses all cultural, religious and regional boundaries. The most pervasive form of gender-based violence is reported to be abuse by husband or intimate partner. Mali, a country that appears to be otherwise peaceful and tolerant, a country with seeming "Old-World manners," accepts wife beating as a husband's right. And South African statistics show that one in three women in that country has been assaulted by her male partner (Human Rights Watch/Africa, 1995, p. 45). And the South African Department of Justice reports that one in four South African women is a survivor of domestic violence (Soul City, 1999a, p. 10). Rape is a constant problem in South Africa where a conservative estimate suggests that one in three women is raped at least once within the course of her lifetime (Human Rights Watch/Africa, 1995, p. 45). More generous estimates put the rate at one in two women[7] (Soul City 1999a, quoting Vogelman, p. 17). In South Africa, township women are subject to all manner of violent crimes including gang rape (Soul City, 1999a, pp. 18, 23). Mali, which has no gang violence, does not recognize the concept of marital rape.

Women's powerlessness in sexual matters emerges quite clearly in the course of KAP (Knowledge, Attitude, and Practices) studies. In a KAP study conducted in Mali in 1998 by the CNIECS (*Centre Nationale d'Information, D'Education et de Communication sur la Santé),* almost 40% of young females responded that they had not consented to their first sexual encounter.[8] The study was conducted on youth in the 15–25 age range. And non-consent responses might have been higher if young married teenaged women did not assume marital/engagement status was tantamount to consent.[9] Female non-consent figures compare dismally with those of males, where less than 4% responded that they had not agreed to their first sexual encounter ("*Connaissances, attitudes, et comportements des jeunes,*" 1999, pp. 33–35).

The vast majority of South African teenaged girls surveyed on their attitudes toward sex responded with "no" or "don't know" to the question of whether or not they like sex (Kelly, 16 Sept., 1999, interview). And studies by a number of South African researchers show that 28–30% of the first sexual experiences for adolescent girls was a forced encounter (Soul City, 1999a, p. 17). A study of South African sexually active girls by the Kaiser Family Foundation found statistics on female lack of choice of even more concern. Sixty-one percent admitted having been forced to have sex. Thirty-three percent said they were afraid of saying no to sex; and 55% agreed that there were times they gave into sex against their will because their boyfriends insisted upon it (World Health Organization/UNAIDS 2002).

---

7. Note that the rate of attempted rape in the U.S. is one in four women. The rate of completed rape in the U.S. is one in five women.

8. 60% of American women who have had sex before the age of 15 report that it was non-consensual.

9. Note that the median age of marriage in Mali is 16 years for females and 25 years of age for males.

Forced sexual encounters promote the spread of the AIDS epidemic. Rape is likely to cause genital injury and vaginal injury increasing the risk of HIV/AIDS transmission particularly in young females. This is because the vaginal mucosal lining of young girls is tender and can easily break. This factor probably accounts for an HIV rate six times higher for girls than for women over 35. Girls are also far more likely than boys to be forced into sex by older persons, including husbands. This no doubt helps to explain the disparities of HIV rates in African teens where about one in four teenaged girls lives with HIV but only about one in 25 teenaged boys is infected ("Abuse of women escalates HIV infections in Africa," 2001, ¶13).

Gender violence is related to patriarchy. So is a woman's right to control the integrity of her own body and the right to enjoy pleasure from sex. These rights are severely abrogated by practices of female genital mutilation (FGM), widespread in Africa in 30 African countries.

Female genital mutilation (FGM), also known as female genital excision or female genital cutting (FGC) refers to a collection of practices reported widely in sections of Africa and West Asia where parts of the female genitalia are removed for non-therapeutic reasons. The World Health Organization classifies various forms of female genital cutting together with other mutilations carried out in Southern Africa that are designed to promote "dry sex" (World Health Organization, 2001, ¶1).

Female genital cutting procedures are often classified into three categories. The mildest form of female genital alteration is the *sunna,* a practice that alters or removes the prepuce of the clitoris. An intermediate form removes the clitoris and parts of the labia minora. The most extreme practice is the pharoanic circumcision that excises the clitoris, the labia minora, parts of the labia majora and then sutures together the remaining labia majora to form a bridge of scar tissue over the vagina (Lightfoot-Klein, 1989, pp. 32–33).

The origins of the practice are shrouded in mystery, veiled by a variety of cultural explanations, most having to do with perceived notions of body aesthetics. Islam is often used to justify female genital cutting but it seems more likely that the practice originated in Africa and was subsequently accepted by Islam (Hansen, 1972/73, p. 19). It is noteworthy that FGC is absent from most Islamic countries outside of Africa with the exception of Oman, Yemen, and Saudi Arabia (See Lightfoot-Klein, 1989, p. 41; see also Warraq, 1999, p. 97). Female genital cutting seems likely to have spread in conjunction with the rise of patriarchal society as a way of placing the control of women's sexuality (and hence her fertility) squarely in the hands of men.

Female genital cutting is practiced across the wide West African belt of sub-Saharan Africa, through the Central African countries of Chad, the Central African Republic (CAR) and the northern part of the Democratic Republic of the Congo (Zaire), and east through the horn of Africa. The practice also extends southward from the horn to much of Kenya and Tanzania (Lightfoot-Klein, 1989, p. 32). Ninety-two percent of Malian women have undergone some form of genital mutilation (USAID, 1999, p. 7).

Female genital cutting is deeply ingrained in cultural tradition and is often practiced in conjunction with rituals that prepare women for marriage and childbirth. In the last decades of the 20th century, the practice began to come under attack from coalitions of feminist groups both within and outside the countries where FGC is practiced. Some countries have outlawed the practice or tried to place it under the control and practice of proper medical authorities.

FGC is believed by its critics to cause deep trauma and psychological scars, to make women passive, listless, and pessimistic. Those who defend FGC insist that an uncut female suffers stigma, humiliation, and ultimate rejection and that these are far worse than the pain of the knife (D'Haem 1997, pp. 57–62; Cameron and Anderson, 1998, pp. 49–50). Certainly FGM teaches women how little control they have over their bodies and their lives. And it provides a painful lesson for the flesh as to how much a woman is expected to suffer for the purported benefit of her kinsmen. FGC no doubt prepares African women for a lifetime of toil and pain and is without question partly responsible for the seeming passivity often found in many of Africa's females. A woman's stoic resignation to her fate no doubt compounds female vulnerability to HIV/AIDS that I have already shown.

The transmission of HIV is also directly implicated in the non-sterile ways in which the FGC is carried out and the long-term anatomical and physiological effects of these practices. Controversies and secrecy surrounding FGC make it a difficult phenomenon to study in the relation to the AIDS epidemic. There are as of 2002 no definitive measures of the multiple risks associated with this practice in the context of the AIDS pandemic.

In the "best" of circumstances, trained physicians, in African hospitals, under sanitary conditions, practice FGC. With the colonial introduction of Western medical practices this tendency has grown in the 20th century. Genital cutting in any case, even in hospitals, may subject the patient to immediate and long-term risks. The World Health Organization strongly opposes the medicalization of all practices of Female Genital Cutting.

More low technology methods of FGC are far more common than clinical procedures. Typically older women or midwives who specialize in the practice handle the operation. Such specialists tend to operate in unsanitary conditions, using a razor blade, machete, a sharp piece of glass or other cutting instrument to perform the operation. The patient often suffers shock and severe blood loss and can die from this procedure. A reused "surgical implement" may also expose her to HIV. If she is already infected with HIV, then village midwives or excizers may pass on the virus to their next patient.

Women who have undergone FGC often suffer reproductive complications throughout their lives. Those who have been infibulated (about 15% of all women who have undergone a FGC procedure) must be "opened-up" for sex. In some cultures, it is considered a badge of honor if a man is able to enter his woman without resorting to the use of a sharp implement. However desirable, it is not always possible because a woman's vaginal scarring may be too tough. In such a case, a man will cut his bride on their wedding night in order to perform the sex act. Sex thereafter is likely to be painful and dangerous, opening and reopening wounds and inviting the transmission of HIV.

FGC presents its own special complications for childbirth. In order to deliver a baby, the infibulated women must be further cut. The scarred tissue lacks the elasticity of a normal vagina, prolongs labor, and increases blood loss and the chance of anemia. After the woman gives birth, she must be re-sewn or tightened in order to render sex more pleasurable for her husband. If a woman's husband insists, she may be forced to resume intercourse before her various wounds have healed.[10] All of these procedures and their resultant complications directly lower women's general immunity while exposing them through open wounds to HIV infection.

In many parts of Southern Africa, where female genital cutting is generally not practiced, women "dry and tighten" their vaginas through the use of corrosive substances. A dry and tight vagina is believed to enhance male pleasure during intercourse. Some young women also claim to use vaginal drying to mask alleged evidence of unfaithfulness to a given partner (Xaba, 1999, personal communication). Women insert herbs, tobacco or fertilizer into the vaginal cavity; or they douche with, or soak in basins of astringent products such as bleach, dettol (a cleaning product or disinfectant), or salt water. The treatments cause the vaginal membranes to swell up and dry out. These procedures kill naturally occurring defensive vaginal bacteria; lead to painful intercourse, vaginal lesions and bleeding; and generally facilitate the transmission of HIV. Many of the drying agents can also interfere with effective condom use.

Myths Surrounding the AIDS Epidemic

AIDS is a disease that leads in many societies to social rejection. Given the importance of group membership in African societies, social rejection means loss of identity. And given the unavailability of drugs, HIV+ status is (for all but a lucky few) a death sentence. The prospects for individuals and societies affected with the virus are so grim that a host of stories have been created around the virus, stories that in my view both aid in denial and simultaneously help people cope with tragic reality. These stories help divert people's attention from the horrible and frightening truth which is often too much to bear.

There are myths about the disease, i.e., that it does not exist, that it cannot be caught from a healthy looking person, that it cannot be transmitted during first intercourse, and so on. There are stories about the origins of the disease, i.e., that it comes from the West and that it's a ruse to keep Africans from reproducing or from enjoying sex; that it is a punishment from God; that it is caused by witchcraft; that it comes from cooking with Maggi Cubes,[11] and so on. There are myths about a cure for AIDS, i. e., that traditional healers can cure AIDS; that sex with a virgin can cure it; or that sex with a baby can cure the disease, and so on.

10. Traditional practices in many societies required post-partum abstinence from sex for a woman and her husband until the child was weaned. This could sometimes be for a period as long as three years. During this time, it was assumed men would seek sex from other women, notably their other wives. Today, with polygyny in decline, post-partum taboos against sex are falling away.

11. Swiss-made bouillon cubes widely sold in francophone Africa and used in the preparation of African soups and sauces. Maggi cubes are apparently symbolic of a widespread dependence on imported Western products and lifestyles.

Social stigma provides a particularly potent disincentive for people to have the test for HIV. And the stigma also serves to deter people from acting prudently in matters sexual. Adopting safe sex practices often subjects an ostensibly HIV- person to suspicion of being HIV+. The social stigma surrounding AIDS leads to a vicious cycle of denial which leads in turn to greater levels of infection.

Controversy over Generic Drugs

With anti-retroviral treatment expenses topping $12,000 per annum, all but palliative care is beyond the means of most African sufferers of HIV and AIDS. "Big Pharma," the major pharmaceutical corporations who have developed and patented these drugs, are accused by activists of making obscene profits from the wealthy few while pricing the drugs beyond the reach of 95% of AIDS patients worldwide ("HIV/AIDS: Drowning by Numbers," 2002, pp. 18–19). As the epidemic has raged into the 21st century, the cries for access to treatment for all have become more shrill. For it has been observed that access to treatment in the Western world has made HIV/AIDS a condition that can be managed and controlled, rather than the death sentence it was until 1996. The 13th World AIDS Conference, held in Durban, South Africa, in 2000, ended with a resolution to seek treatment for the millions suffering from HIV/AIDS.

Early in the 21st century controversy began brewing over plans by some nations in the developing world to import generic copies of AIDS drugs manufactured in India, Brazil, and Thailand, copies of drugs patented by wealthy pharmaceutical firms. Trade agreements signed by members of the World Trade Organization (WTO) prevented signatories from importing generic drug copies except in national emergencies. Faced with the world's greatest number of HIV/AIDS cases, the South African government decided to invoke the "national emergency" clause in the WTO agreements. This brought down all the muscle of 39 pharmaceutical industries that filed a lawsuit against South Africa. In response, *Médecins Sans Frontières* (Doctors Without Borders) and other groups mounted a "Drop the Case" petition that galvanized 140 groups and people from 130 countries to put pressure on this very profitable industry. Caught in a public relations nightmare, Big Pharma (as the major pharmaceutical corporations have come to be known by treatment activists and the media) was forced to drop its suit against the South African Ministry of Health (*Médecins Sans Frontières* 2001).

In the wake of treatment activism and lobbying for the United Nations, major pharmaceutical companies have begun to reduce the price of AIDS therapies (and other treatments for common tropical illnesses) to low and middle income countries. AIDS regimens in 2002 were available through Big Pharma or from generics for as low as $350 per annum (UNAIDS, 2002, July, Fact Sheet: Accelerating). This price is still very expensive for many developing countries and most African ones. Ironically, in 2002, the South African government, despite its victory against Big Pharma, was refusing to provide anti-retroviral treatment to AIDS patients in its government funded clinics (Stine, 2002, p. 38)!

In 2001, with controversies still raging over the cost of AIDS treatment, the United Nations created a global fund for AIDS and other infectious diseases. UN Secretary General Kofi Annan, who launched the fund, called for a war chest of $7–10 billion a year to fight the global epidemic. In mid 2002, $1.7 billion had been pledged, and a fraction of that raised. The Global Fund has five objectives: 1) containing the epidemic through education programs; 2) reducing mother-to-child (MTC) transmission of HIV; 3) advancing scientific breakthroughs so as to find a vaccine and a cure; 4) protecting AIDS orphans and those made vulnerable by the epidemic; and 5) ensuring that care and treatment is within the reach of all.

Providing care and treatment still remains controversial. Besides the cost, anti-retroviral regimens can be complex to administer. They are often ineffective and also have powerful and dangerous side effects. Moreover, because HIV can mutate rapidly, immunity to the drug cocktails can quickly develop. For these reasons, insiders avow that treatment and care programs will take a back seat to prevention and that most of the 40 million of the world's afflicted will remain untreated (Stine, 2002, p. 452). Nevertheless, the initiative of the United Nations to increase treatment access is important and ongoing. It continues to negotiate with pharmaceutical corporations to make drugs available and to work with countries to expand the medical infrastructure to deliver care, treatment, and support (UNAIDS, 2002, July, Fact Sheet: Accelerating).

Meanwhile, prevention and containment of HIV/AIDS through information, education, and communication (IEC) continues to be a cornerstone of the UNAIDS joint program since it was established in 1996.

AIDS Information, Education, and Communication Programs in Africa

Typically, the United Nations Joint Programme on AIDS (UNAIDS) and other groups have put enormous emphasis on information, education, and communication (IEC) programs in order to contain the epidemic. IEC efforts involve a range of HIV/AIDS educational interventions aimed at different target populations. These activities have generally included information about the risks of HIV/AIDS transmission; lessons concerning safer sex practices; and messages designed to reduce stigma against those ill with HIV/AIDS. Other activities have involved condom distribution through social marketing and information dissemination on condom availability and use. The effectiveness of these efforts is measured on a regular basis within target populations through KAP (Knowledge, Attitude and Practices) studies. KAP studies are designed to track the growth of public information about AIDS and other STDs; to detect shifts in attitudes regarding sexual practice; and to document reports of actual changes in sexual behaviors. For example, KAP studies measure individual knowledge concerning HIV transmission. And they investigate people's awareness of their own risk levels and their willingness to adopt safer sex practices. The studies also inquire about intimate practices, such as age at first sexual intercourse, the number of sexual partners within a recent time period, the level of condom use, and so on. Important target groups in Africa include commercial sex workers, migrant populations, and youth and young adults in their reproductive years.

UNAIDS and their partners see the provision of information, education, and communication (IEC) as crucial to attempts to stem the tide of the AIDS epidemic in Africa and worldwide. And these efforts have paid off in terms of information gains.

Twenty years into the epidemic, awareness of the existence HIV/AIDS in some parts of Africa is high. In South Africa, for example, it is well over 90%. In Mali, awareness is about 77% for females and 96% for males (*Plan Stratégique*, 1999, p. 11). But information gains across the African continent have been uneven. Figures released by UNAIDS in conjunction with the Barcelona World AIDS conference in 2002 show high levels of ignorance about sexual matters in several African countries, among them, Cameroon, Central African Republic, Equatorial Guinea, Lesotho, and Sierra Leone. And alarmingly, 95% of young women in Nigeria perceived their risks of contracting HIV/AIDS to be minimal or non-existent (Africa Action, 2002, July 6, ¶ 18). In any case, awareness of this disease has rarely translated into major shifts in behavior in the general public.[12] Indeed changing behavior through information, education, and communication about an epidemic that involves the twin taboo subjects of sex and of death, challenges the world's joint expertise in the science and the art of persuasion.

Trends in Post-Modern Epidemic Fighting

Today, AIDS awareness and information campaigns bear the clear marks of trends toward post-modernism and globalization in communication studies in the late 20th century. If this epidemic had happened in Africa in the 1960s or 1970s, AIDS information campaign designers from wealthy countries probably would have attacked the problem with techniques learned from mass mediated-propaganda. They might well have disseminated a few bold (and probably scary) AIDS awareness messages[13] blanketing whole populations with similar messages. It is more than likely that campaign planners would have measured the effectiveness of their efforts, learned of their failure, and returned home, the problem unsolved.

12. There are, however, shifts among certain groups. In Bamako, Mali, for example where commercial sex workers are organized and represented by an the NGO (*Danaya So*), condom use with customers is at 99% (*Plan Stratégique*, 1999, p. 8).

13. In the mid-1980s, the government of Australia launched an AIDS awareness campaign designed to target gay men and to encourage them to have an AIDS test. The campaign used scare iconography especially the figure of the medieval symbol of death, the Grim Reaper. The campaign generated little response in the gay community although it generated responses and calls for testing from the heterosexual population. The Grim Reaper campaign, symbolic of old style propaganda campaigns, is usually cited in the literature as an example of what not to do. The Grim Reaper campaign was blamed for further stigmatizing the HIV+ and by association, the gay community. It was blamed with further alienating the gay community, (Morlet, Guinan, Diefenthaler, and Gold 1988; Pegrum 1997).

This is because earlier operations in development communication[14] operated from a ***modern*** notion of what has been simplistically called a "Grand Narrative." The Grand Narrative is a belief in a universal truth, a truth that can be derived and known through the application of scientific principles, a truth that could be presented to whole populations. The "Grand Narrative" solution to AIDS communication would be to propound a few simple messages about HIV/AIDS transmission and assume audiences would respond to the logic of the perceived threat.

Today's ***post-modern*** approaches are less ambitious, preferring to work with bits or fragments of life or reality than to look for totality. They tend to seek out discrete segments of whole audiences as targets for messages. And post-modern approaches to communication also tend to focus on those aspects of communication long ignored by the modernists: play, namely entertainment in its various forms, and carnival (O'Sullivan, Hartley, Saunders, Montgomery and Fiske, 1994, p. 234). Most of the time, they appeal less to human cognitive sense and more to human emotion. The shift in focus (away from the "Grand Narrative" to "fragments of human experience") in communication studies (together with other fields) has been called a ***paradigm shift*** and it has profoundly affected the way we organize campaigns. The paradigm shift also comes in the wake of economic and cultural globalization.

Globalization theory in communication recognizes the growth and acceleration of economic and cultural links that operate on a worldwide basis. Because of globalization, national governments, national boundaries, and national institutions including media are far less important than they were in the third quarter of the twentieth century and earlier. In the southern hemisphere, especially in Africa in the 1980s and 1990s, the national media systems were de-regulated and private broadcasting was allowed. This paved the way for an unprecedented onslaught of foreign, mainly Western, mass media entertainment programming while it decreased the relative power of national African governments over their media. In the northern hemisphere, the power of national governments has also shrunk with the rise of multi-lateral trade organizations. Meanwhile national foreign aid from the developed northern hemisphere is channeled increasingly through international non-governmental organizations (INGOs,) rather than through governments. These organizations, CARE, OXFAM, *Médecins Sans Frontières* (Doctors without Borders), etc., enjoy bonds of common interest with their overseas partners in the South. And new technologies, especially those related to the internet, widely available by the late 20th century, have facilitated the linking of local partners in the developing world with those in the more developed world. In this way the Internet has fostered global INGO movements.

Within this context, the entertainment-education strategy (henceforth referred to as edutainment) has been applied to a range of development issues in Africa. These include environmental education, human rights promotion, democracy, but most consistently to HIV/AIDS prevention. "Entertainment-education is the process of designing and implementing an entertainment program to increase

14. Development Communication refers to a sub-field in Mass Communication or Communication Studies that seeks to understand and apply the ways media can be used to promote social change, especially in developing nations. For a review, see Bourgault, 1995, pp. 226–256.

audience members' knowledge about a social issue, create more favorable attitudes, and a change in their overt behaviors regarding the social issue" (Vaughan, Rogers, Singhal, and Swalehe, 2000, p. 82).

Edutainment and Participatory Methodologies

Edutainment strategies have been applied to the AIDS pandemic in the form of popular radio and television soap operas; talk shows; pop music and celebrity concerts; feature films; animation; and live events including fairs, bicycle rallies, sporting and gaming competitions, soccer matches, and even condom-blowing contests. The cumulative effect of these techniques has been to raise widespread general awareness of the dangers of HIV/AIDS on the African continent. And its proponents argue that entertainment-education strategies "have measurable effects on changing HIV prevention behavior" (Vaughan, Rogers, Singhal, and Swalehe, 2000, p. 82).

Edutainment strategies are grounded in theories of role modeling and para-social communication. They operate from the principle that audiences will view the media models who appear in the edutainment, identify with them, and then imitate their behavior. The methodologies also assume that edutainment promotes para-social involvement with story characters or the media phenomenon in which they are embedded. This involvement will lead to interpersonal communication with a viewer's family and community about story lines, story themes, and the problems of story characters. It may also lead to the participation of an audience member in contests or other program activities.

Edutainment methodologies recognize the importance of engaging audiences in interpersonal communication around the programs. Experts in development communication believe social interaction around the problem at hand is a key prelude to behavior change. Edutainment methodologies represent a break from older forms of development communication in that the stories, songs, plays, and other genres created for purposes of social change are generally made by and with representative members of the target culture and are resonant in the societies where they are promulgated.[15]

The edutainment methodology has been perfected and used extensively by the Johns Hopkins University's Center for Communication Programs. The technique implies the use of formative evaluation in the process of media development. This is to say materials are tested and re-tested in a sort of on-going loop on their intended audiences. Edutainment methodology recognizes the need for audience segmentation. This is to say that the creators understand that many messages, rather than one message, must be designed for many small, rather than

15. In earlier development projects, those of the 1960s and 1970s, it was not uncommon for a project to have European or North American project designers and producers creating media for social change for use in developing nations. Much of the media created in such projects had little resonance with target audiences.

one, large public. Edutainment methodology recognizes the importance of variety in creative techniques and uses a range of creative stratagies in campaign design. Creators understand the importance of using Big Media as a backdrop and a resonator for Small Media interventions. Big Media would be defined, for example, as a media product reaching broad swathes of the population, such as a major television series on a national network. Small Media would be defined as a medium that reaches only a limited target audience, a video recording about STDs available at a health clinic, or a comic book targeted at high school dropouts. Edutainment project planners also know the importance of using media celebrities and other public figures in order to engender role modeling among audience members.

Large aid donors tend to favor edutainment strategies. Many of these edutainment projects are radio or television series targeted at national populations. Some, like Soul City (see Chapter 8), are extremely slick in their production values. Typically, they have been developed and produced by international teams of communication experts, including local media professionals in the countries where they are shown. Several of these edutainment projects have been extensively researched and are the subject of voluminous social science literature (Singhal and Rogers 1999). As useful as is this research, edutainment methodologies have sometimes been faulted for research excess (Singhal and Rogers, 1999, pp. 198–199). Some critics say this zeal for research comes from a greater concern for the needs of project funders than for those of project recipients, i.e., target audiences (Dagron, 2001, pp. 12–13).

Closely related to edutainment methodologies are a group of communication strategies known collectively as participatory methodologies. Participatory methodologies are like edutainment, but they tend to be more grassroots in orientation. They tend to be less slick.

Participatory methodologies take edutainment methodologies to a deeper level of local involvement by enjoining even more fully, the recipients of the messages in the process of their own creation. Examples of participatory methodology media might include local community video, community or school theatre, school newspapers, community newsletters, low power radio broadcasts, and so on. Because media created through participatory methodology are small and less sophisticated, they are even more likely than edutainment to promote interpersonal communication around the desired change.

Participatory methodologies go to extreme lengths to ensure that recipients relate in a very personal way to messages, and have a direct sense of ownership over them (Tomaselli, 1997a, p. 1). Technically speaking, participatory communication need not always be entertaining, though a great deal of it is. A telephone conversation with an AIDS hotline worker would be an example of a participatory communication intervention that is not particularly "entertaining" in the strictest sense. So would a workshop or public lecture facilitated by member of the National Association of People with AIDS (NAPWA), a South African AIDS support group. And technically speaking, edutainment need not *necessarily* involve target audiences in its production, though most of it does. This is because edutainment media are unlikely to be ineffective in deeply engaging the audience and promoting behavior change if target audiences have been ignored in the production process. The major difference between edutainment and participatory methodology media is one of emphasis and scale. Media products classified as edutainment tend to be more technically sophisticated (and hence expensive) while media products classified as participatory methodology media tend to be more grassrooted in their orientation. Projects featuring edutainment tend to focus more on the ***media package***, whereas projects using participatory communication methodologies are more concerned with the ***process of message design*** than the end product.

Just as methods of presenting development communication content have evolved over the years, so too have the techniques of message evaluation. During the 1960s and 1970s development communications were measured in large-scale quantitative assessments. Research was designed to answer the question "Did this intervention succeed or fail?" In those days, researchers were obsessed with proving that media had any effect at all on audiences. Today we accept that media or other performance interventions affect people (Singhal and Rogers, 1999, p. 143). The questions we ask today tend to involve learning just what kind of media or what kinds of messages will be most effective (singly or in combination) with a given audience segment. This leads, at least theoretically, to a process of ongoing evaluation. Ongoing evaluation implies the testing and re-testing of informational materials along the way, throughout the course of an information intervention or campaign. Obviously, the smaller the project initiative, the more responsive it can be to testing or formative evaluation. Large-scale edutainment projects do engage in a good deal of pre-testing before they embark on a costly production commitment. But once a project is heavily invested, there can be little turning back. Participatory methodologies, generally smaller in scale, provide the flexibility of constant formative research.

Over the years this process of constant research has come to be called Action Research. Action research "involves an action collaboration between the researchers and persons from the community or section of study throughout the research process" (Parker, 1994, pp. 66–67). Action research involves a whole battery of tests and observations, all of which are made with the view to constantly upgrade the information campaign or information activity at hand. The action researcher is not testing an AIDS campaign to "see if it worked." Rather the action researcher is immersed in an ongoing struggle to find what ***must*** work.

Today, in this post-modern climate, even final or summative evaluations, designed to determine if campaigns have been successful, tend to lack finality. This is because post-modernism recognizes that meanings are constantly being created in any information environment, with any campaign. Thus, evaluations tend to be forward-looking rather than backward-looking. They tend to ask not so much "Has X campaign succeeded or failed?" but rather "What now needs to be done in order to achieve the goals we set out to achieve?" Thus, communication project evaluations tend be "process evaluations" because campaign organizers recognize that communications are inherently open-ended. And project reports tend to be summaries of "Best Practices," i.e., in-depth real-life accounts of workable health and social policies, and the media that promoted them. Such accounts of "Best Practices" describe projects in given communities, regions, or countries, and supply one or more lessons-learned in fighting the AIDS pandemic.

There is another important aspect to the ***paradigm shift***. It is the fact that development projects today are ***partnerships*** between rich and poor nations, between the North and the South. Today, with projects largely in the hands of INGOs and their local partners in the developing world, there is less of a tendency to see a project from the point of view of the northerner who comes to the southern hemisphere, imparts northern wisdom to the South, and goes home. For the southerners, at least, AIDS information campaigns are ***not experiments*** in information diffusion. They are part of an ongoing historical process that involves southern NGOs. And those from the South, in whose countries the intervention is happening, are there to stay. They therefore need to know periodically what they are doing right or wrong so that they can correct themselves and get back on track.

Today there is an increasing tendency for bi-lateral aid grants (government programs referred to domestically as "foreign aid") to be funneled through international non-governmental organizations (INGOs) and their local NGO (non-governmental organization) partners. The United States Agency for International Development (USAID) reports for example that nearly 70% of its AIDS interventions are funneled through small groups (USAID n.d.). The increased use of INGOs by government aid donors to distribute aid came gradually throughout the 1980s and 1990s. Aid organizations, such as the USAID or the Canadian International Development Agency (CIDA), for example, came to rely on INGOs and their counterparts in developing countries, known as NGOs. This is because NGOs are generally thought to be more in touch with the locals, with "the people" than are the urban-based government bureaucrats of so many developing countries. These latter civil servants, moreover, have sometimes been more interested in political gamesmanship and corruption than in development goals (Bourgault, 1995, pp. 232–238). INGOs, many of them religiously based, have long histories of project organization and fund disbursement in the developing world. And because their whole reason for being *(raison d'être)* is to do good work and to promote development, they seem ideally suited to organize aid on behalf of the North.

This volume takes the view that edutainment must continue to be an important component of projects designed to increase knowledge and shift the attitudes together with the social and sexual behaviors implicated in HIV/AIDS transmission. This is because edutainment products provide role modeling and para-social interaction surrounding edutainment media. This book also takes the view that *participatory methods of communication* are especially effective in promoting attitude and behavior change because they implicate audiences directly into performing the cure to their own problems. In so doing, they engage the proponents on a personal level in the struggle at hand. Participatory strategies are particularly suited to African societies because the latter have a strong community ethos fostered by an oral and a performative tradition.

Both edutainment and participatory methodologies call upon Africa's vast repertoire of performance in the creation of messages used in the struggle against AIDS. As we shall see, South Africa has been particularly keen on participatory methodologies. This is undoubtedly due to the particular history of South Africa and the coincidence of the AIDS epidemic with the emergence of Black rule in the country. But before examining performance in more depth in Chapter 4, the next chapter will present brief reviews of the nations of South Africa and Mali and together with the organization of their struggles against the AIDS pandemic.

Review Questions

1. What are the main factors that have helped to fuel the AIDS pandemic on the African continent? What role does gender inequality play in spreading the HIV/AIDS epidemic?
2. Which two African countries appear to have adopted policies that have helped to decrease the rate of infection from HIV/AIDS? How have these policies helped to arrest the spread of HIV/AIDS?
3. What challenges do campaign planners face in designing campaigns in Africa intended to impart information, education, and communication (IEC) surrounding HIV/AIDS? In which ways are edutainment and participatory communication methodologies expected to overcome some of the hurdles involved in educating diverse African publics about HIV/AIDS?

Chapter 3

Country Profiles: South Africa and Mali

The spread of AIDS in Africa is related to complex interactions of history and geography, as well as economic, political, and social realities. The contours of the epidemic vary from country to country as do the responses of governments and people. In order to examine the African AIDS epidemic in context, this chapter provides a look at two very different African countries: South Africa, a relatively prosperous nation on the southern tip of the continent; and Mali, a very poor landlocked nation located in the heart of the West African sahel.

Geography, Climate, and People of South Africa

The nation of South Africa lies at the tip of the African continent between roughly 25 and 35 degrees latitude, and falls mostly south of the Tropic of Capricorn.[1] The country is surrounded on the east and south by the warm currents of the Indian Ocean and on the southwest by the cooler Atlantic. South Africa borders with Namibia to the northwest,[2] and with Botswana and Zimbabwe to the north and northeast respectively. South Africa borders with Mozambique and Swaziland to the east. One country, Lesotho,[3] sits within South Africa's borders and is completely surrounded by South Africa. South Africa is a large country stretching about 1,935 kilometers (about 1200 miles) from the Limpopo River on its northernmost border to Cape Agulhas, its southernmost point. And the country stretches about 1,450 kilometers (nearly 900 miles) at its widest point between Port Nolloth in the west and Saint Lucia in the east. About twice the size of Texas, South Africa has a range of climates and three major natural regions: the central plateau, the mountains, and the

1. Sydney, Australia is on the same latitude as Cape Town, and Brisbane is on about the same latitude as Johannesburg.

2. South Africa held Namibia, then called Southwest Africa, in protectorate status until 1990.

3. In 1870, the Sotho who had already lost half of their territory to Afrikaners sought and obtained protection from the British against further incursions by Afrikaner settlers. The territory (then known as Basutholand) was administered separately from South Africa. Lesotho was governed by Britain until 1966 when it was granted its independence.

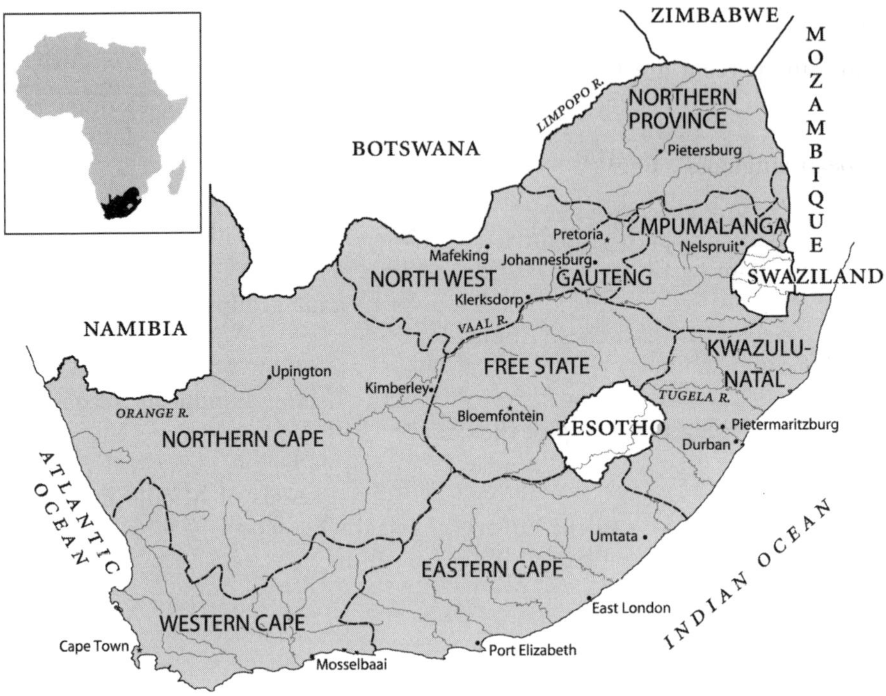

Figure 3-1. South Africa's provinces.

coastal belt. The central plateau comprises most of inland South Africa, and alternately rises to sharp escarpments that overlook open grassland in the country's heartland, bush to the northwest, and thornscrub to the southwest. The climate of the central plateau of South Africa is mostly semi-arid, with extremely dry portions in the southwest, known as the Karoo, an extension of the Kalahari and Namib deserts.

South Africa's Drakensburg Mountain range forms an eastern spine stretching from Swaziland and extending south to the Eastern Cape Province. South Africa's coastal belt is itself varied. The area around Cape Town has a Mediterranean climate, cooled as it is by the Benguela current. Farther north, the Namib Desert extends to the coastal area of the Northern Cape province on the western end of the country. South Africa also has a temperate south central coast whose shores are cooled where the Atlantic and the Indian Ocean meet, and a tropical coastline along the Indian Ocean on the eastern side of the country.

South Africa has four main rivers, the Orange River and its tributary, the Vaal, that flow through the country's heartland; the Limpopo River in the far north that forms much of the nation's northern border; and the Tugela River that flows east from the Drakensburg Mountains into the Indian Ocean. Despite these natural resources, the South African central plateau often lacks adequate supplies of fresh water. South Africa's new constitution recognizes nine provinces: Gauteng, Northern Province, Mapumalanga, Free State, KwaZulu-Natal, Northwest Province, Northern Cape, Eastern Cape, and Western Cape.

South Africa's population totals some 43.5 million people. Seventy-seven percent of the population is Black African. Ten and one half percent are Caucasian; nine percent are Coloured, or members of a mixed race; two and a half percent are of Indian origin; and less than one percent belong to other races. South Africa recognizes eleven official languages. These include the two Indo-European languages, English and Afrikaans, and nine indigenous South African tongues: Ndebele, Pedi, Sotho, Swati, Tsonga, Tswana, Venda, Xhosa, and Zulu.

South Africa is predominantly a Christian country with 68% of the total population claiming Christianity as their creed. This includes an enormous diversity of sects that split off from mainline protestant groups and around 4,000 African Independent churches. About 28.5% of South Africans practice traditional African or animist religion. Most of the South African Indian population is Hindu, though a small minority does practice Islam. Hinduism accounts for 1.5% of the religious make-up of the country. Islam accounts for 2%, a percentage that includes a small minority of the Indian population combined with some Black African and Coloured Muslims and other persons of Middle Eastern and Far Eastern origin. Most of the European and the Coloured community is Christian, though there is also a sizable Jewish community.

Economy of South Africa

The South African economy presents a paradoxical mixture of first and third world economies, really a first world economy built on the back of a disenfranchised labor class. The contrast is quite glaring. On the one hand there is a modern industrialized urban economy, on the other there is bare subsistence agriculture and petty trading that has changed little since the 19th century. South Africa's organized formal economic sector dwarfs anything else on the African continent. South Africa produces 50% of all electricity consumed on the continent, 40% of Africa's industrial output, and 45% of its mining production. South Africa's agricultural exports also dwarf those of other African countries by a wide margin. The secret of South Africa's success has been its abundant natural wealth and its large pool of underpaid Black labor, both from within South Africa and from the neighboring countries.

South Africa is the world's largest producer of gold and platinum. Mining accounts for 70% of its export revenue and 13% of its Gross Domestic Product (GDP). South Africa's private sector is highly centralized. Rooted in mining, this sector is dominated by the Anglo-American/Anglo-Gold and the De Beers corporations, whose combined capitalization is four times greater than their nearest competitor. South Africa's primary agricultural production accounts for about 4% of its GNP. The country is a net exporter of food and related products including fruit, sugar cane, wheat, dairy products, tobacco, wine, and wool.

Unlike most of the rest of the continent, South Africa has a well-developed system of transportation, one serving local South African and Southern African regional needs. The international airport at Johannesburg also serves as a hub for most international flights serving the Southern African region. As in the rest of the continent, railways were built to carry export commodities from cash crop or mining areas to the coast. The railroads in the Southern Africa region and even some as far north as the Democratic Republic of the Congo and Tanzania eventually link up with South African rail and port systems. Transit charges levied on all these countries is a significant foreign exchange earner for South Africa. Durban harbor in KwaZulu-Natal has the most port traffic in Africa and is the 9th busiest port in the world. And Richard's Bay north of Durban, actually handles more cargo than Durban with less traffic.

Abundant wealth notwithstanding, South Africa is deeply divided along lines of race and class. These persistent divisions threaten to undermine the remarkable political transition that took place in the mid-1990s. South Africa's new government has made a commitment to redress socioeconomic disparities created during South Africa's fractious history of Apartheid while sustaining economic growth. To this end, the government launched an economic program called GEAR, the Growth, Employment, and Redistribution strategy. The program, which features broad market reforms and investment stimulation strategies, has had mixed results.

South Africa's new African National Congress party (ANC) government seems to face almost insurmountable challenges. It must find a way to reassure the business community and the Caucasian minority, while retaining for the Blacks the hope they will see increased prosperity within their lifetimes. With the masses in mind, the government instituted the Reconstruction and Development Program (RDP), an ambitious plan designed to provide new homes, basic services, education, and primary health care for South Africa's majority population.

Economic restructuring has not been easy for South Africa. Per capita income slipped from U.S. $3,545 in 1995 to about U.S. $3,000 in 1999 (U.S. Dept. of State 2001a). The government estimates that the economy must grow at 6% per annum to meet the country's social programs. But growth rates at the end of 1990s, respectable at around 3%, failed to reach set targets.

The value of the South African currency halved during the last 15 years of the 20th century. This was a reflection of conservative world financial markets jittery with regional political transition. And the return of international investment following the transition to Black rule was disappointing. Meanwhile, compounding matters, the prices for gold and other precious metals have fallen at the end of the 1990s. To add to South Africa's woes, the AIDS crisis of the last half of the 1990s has continued unabated into the new millennium. Economists predict the population and the economy will be 25% smaller in 2015 than it would have been without the AIDS pandemic (Smith and Napier, 2001, p.p. 7–8). Indeed by 2005, South Africa will have lost just over 10 % of her workforce to HIV/AIDS. And by 2020, the country 's workforce will have diminished by 25 % (WHO/UNAIDS 2002).

History of South Africa

The fossilized remains of *Homo erectus*, an early hominid, have been unearthed in rock strata in South Africa dating back some three million years. These remains have been found in caves in the Northern Province. It is believed that Stone Age (*Homo sapiens*) people are the descendents of these early tool-using hominids. The fossil record shows evidence 40,000 years old of Stone Age people living in South Africa. Scientists believe these Stone Age humans shared some common traits with the Khoisan, still living today. Scientists attribute an early cave painting dated at 28,000 years to the Khoisan peoples.

The Khoisan are a group of brown-skinned peoples who speak "click" languages. The name comes from Khoikhoi (Hottentot) and San (the Khoikhoi name for Bushmen). In about the 1st century AD Khoisan peoples appear to have migrated down toward the Cape Coast. Archeological evidence shows the KhoiKhoi, who were herders, lived in the well-watered coastal areas near the Cape; and the racially similar San, who were hunters and gatherers, occupied the semi-arid interior directly behind the Cape. Early Nguni-speaking peoples (ancestors of the Xhosa, Mpondo, Thembu, Zulu, Gaza, Ngoni and the Swazi), appear to have left artifacts along the east coast of South Africa as early as 250 to 300 AD. It is speculated that the Khoikhoi originally obtained their cattle from early contact with the more technologically sophisticated (iron smelting) Nguni-speaking groups. These latter peoples, who both herded and farmed, also appear to have traded iron, copper, and tin with the Khoisan.

Relatively little is known about the ensuing 1,000 years though it is speculated that Nguni peoples continued to move into lands occupied by the Khoisan, pushing the latter farther westward and southward. In the late 1400s, Portuguese ships began to stop off at the Cape for food and water, but their movements posed little threat to the indigenous people. But then in 1652, the Domidaris, a Dutch ship bound for India brought the first European settlers to what was to become Cape Town. The aim of this group was to set up a revictualizing station for ships bound for the east. But gradually a colony grew up, taking its toll on the San who either fled, were hunted out, or died of European diseases such as smallpox. In 1657 the Dutch colonists brought slaves from Angola and the East Indies to serve as laborers to help build the colony. Many of these slaves intermarried with Khoikhoi who had become servants and laborers for the Dutch. This group formed the basis of the South African population known during the Apartheid era as the Coloured.[4] The original group of European settlers was joined in 1688 by 150 French Huguenots who fled persecution from Louis the XIV. The colony developed during the 18th century as more European immigrants continued to arrive. As the colony grew, *Trekboers* (pioneers) the most adventurous of the early settlers, moved north and east in search of new grazing lands. In so doing, they came in direct contact first with Khoisan and then with Nguni peoples, all of whom were competing for land. The Xhosa to the west of the Great Fish River encountered the *Trekboers* in 1770. The first of many frontier wars between Nguni peoples and European settlers occurred in 1779.

The Dutch and the French Huguenots were Calvinists who believed in the doctrine of Predestination. The doctrine held that a person's salvation or damnation was pre-ordained. Popular interpretations maintained that a person's social status in the afterlife was manifest in his or her earthly condition.

4. The Coloured also have White Blood, because interracial sexual relations were not forbidden until 1685, see Omond, 1986, p. 13.

Living among the Stone Age Khoikhoi or the Iron Age Nguni, the settlers had no doubt who were the "saved" and who were the "damned." Notions of racial superiority became ingrained in the culture of the early European settlers who referred to themselves as *Boers* or farmers. The Boers, a rugged pioneering lot, developed in South Africa a new Indo-European tongue. Afrikaans developed from a seventeenth century Dutch with a simplified grammar and a vocabulary liberally sprinkled with words and expressions from locally spoken tongues. Cut off from Europe, the Boers emerged as a new white tribe in Africa, a tribe oblivious to intellectual and historical trends brought about by the French and American Revolutions and the Age of Enlightenment.

By the late 1700s, the pastoral life of the Cape Colony began to change as a new European player came on the scene. The British, who were fighting Napoleon on the European continent, seized the Cape in 1795 and ultimately claimed it as a colony in 1806. The British encouraged immigration from Britain in order to assure their control over the land. In 1820 a ship of 5,000 mostly craftsmen and merchants from Britain arrived at Port Elizabeth (then known as Algoa Bay), and eventually settled there and in Grahamstown in the Eastern Cape. The British were arrogant and treated the Boers with disdain and tried to discourage the speaking of the Afrikaans language. In 1834, the British banned slavery, an important cornerstone of the Boer lifestyle. The Boers responded to this perceived threat to their way of life by picking up stakes and leaving the Cape Colony. Their move, known in history as the Great Trek involved 12,000 *Trekboers*. They moved first into Natal on the eastern side of the modern day South Africa where they collided first with the Zulus and then with the British who had established a colony in Natal in 1843. Then the Trek moved inland to the Transvaal and the Orange Free State where these pioneers set up Afrikaner republics in the 1850s.

Afrikaner incursions into the heartland of South Africa were perilous and involved bloody battles with Nguni peoples. The Boers moved forward with ox-drawn wagons. When danger lurked they formed a circle with the wagons known as a *laager*.[5] With their entrenched notions of white racial superiority and their Dutch Reformed Church, the Boer Republics persisted for about thirty years. But the British, who sought to control all of Africa from the Cape to Cairo, were uncomfortable with the two renegade republics at their doorsteps. In 1874 diamonds were discovered at Kimberly (on the edge of the Free State) and in 1886, gold at Witwatersrand (the Ridge of the White Waters) in what was then Transvaal (near Johannesburg). The race to annex the Boers states was on. The Boers and the British fought two Anglo-Boer wars, the first in 1880–81, the second in 1899–1902. The Boers, vastly outnumbered by the British, engaged in guerrilla tactics against the colonial army, tactics they had learned in Africa from their own wars with the native people. The British responded with a scorched earth policy and the imprisonment of Boer wives and children. After more than

5. In later years, as South Africa persisted in its anachronistic racist policies despite world condemnation, it was said the Nationalists were assuming the *laager* mentality.

20,000 Boer deaths, the Afrikaners accepted their fate and signed the Peace of Vereeniging in 1902.

But the British had been so harsh that they were forced to grant concessions to the vanquished. The compromise that ensued paved the way for a self-governing nation. Thus in 1910 the Union of South Africa was born. It comprised the two British colonies, the Cape Province and Natal, plus the two former Boer Republics, the Orange Free State and the Transvaal. Each of the four provinces enjoyed considerable self-government. Ultimately this resulted in severe controls over the movement of Black South Africans in the country, especially in the Free State and Transvaal.

European migration during the eighteenth and nineteenth centuries took its toll on the African populations. From 1779 to 1846, there were six major battles between white settlers moving eastward and northward onto Nguni land into what is now the Eastern Cape and the Orange Free State. This period of time was known as the *Mfecane* ("the crushing"), because it resulted in bitter wars between African groups and the emergence of military states in Black Africa, especially the organization of the powerful Zulus. Three great Zulu leaders, Dingiswayo, Shaka, and Dingaan are remembered for their conquest of neighboring ethnic groups in the formation of a strong Zulu nation. Two other nations grew as they absorbed refugees fleeing from Zulu armies: the Swazis and the Basotho.

The Zulus, under the Great King Shaka (1816–1828), formed a powerful military machine, one that later fought ferociously against the British who would claim the colony of Natal in the 19th century. Despite their legendary bravery and military discipline, the Zulu were outgunned technologically by the British. They surrendered to the British after the battle of Ulundi 1879 and their king Cetshwayo was taken into captivity at Cape Town.

Wars and land claims by European settlers left many of South Africa's Blacks landless. By the late 19th century many Blacks found themselves confined to marginal lands that came to be known first as reserves and later as Homelands. In the different colonies of South Africa laws were passed that restricted the movement of indigenous Africans. As the mines opened, many were forced to look there for work as the only available means of survival.

After 1910, with the creation of the Union of South Africa, racial discrimination, always a fact of life, became more generalized and more institutionalized. A 1913 Native Land Act removed hundreds of thousands of Blacks from land in the Transvaal and the Free State. No Black was allowed to buy, rent, or sharecrop in these areas. Instead, they were "compensated" with land in the aforementioned reserves, reserves whose total area represented a mere 7.5% of the total expanse of South Africa. These reserves would later become the basis for the independent African "Homelands" instituted in 1959. Other repressive legislation also followed. South African Blacks were no longer allowed to strike for better wages or to serve in the military.

If the Boer Wars with the British made the Afrikaner feel insecure, the depression of the 1930s crystallized Boer sentiment into action. Early that decade nearly 20% of the Afrikaners were living in poverty. They launched campaigns for Afrikaner self-help. These formed the basis for Afrikaner nationalism that

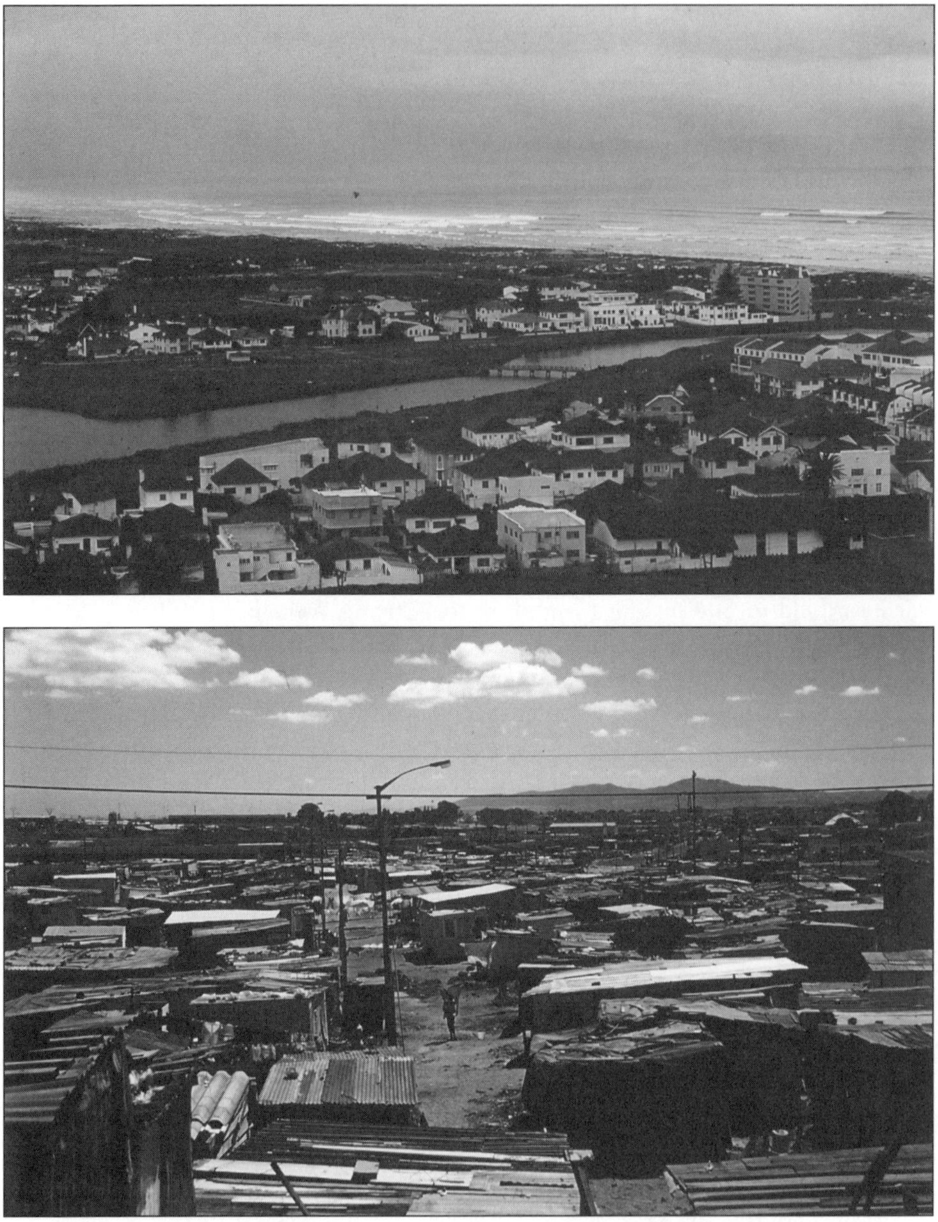

Figure 3-2. The Apartheid systems fostered deep social and economic divisions between the races in South Africa. White (top) and Black (bottom) neighborhoods in Cape Town in 2001. Photos courtesy of Bob Hanson.

would follow. World War II and its heady aftermath of decolonization fever spreading across the African continent did little to steady the nerves of White South Africa, especially the Afrikaners who were in the majority among South Africans with a vote. In 1948 they elected the conservative National Party. The Party's platform included the infamous doctrine of "Apartheid" or "separateness."

After the election in 1948, three legislative pillars were passed. These were the Population Registration Act, the Mixed Marriages Act, and the Group Areas Act. The Population Registration Act of 1950 required all individuals to be entered into a population register and to be classified according to race.[6] The Mixed Marriages Act of 1949 made marriages between Whites and any other racial group illegal. The Group Areas Act of 1950 controlled where each of the racial groups would live. The passage of this act meant that many people were required to move out of their homes and neighborhoods. A patchwork of other pieces of legislation, particularly the Pass Laws and Masters and Servants Laws punished desertion of Black South Africans from their White masters and ensured that the movements of the former were rigidly controlled.

In theory Apartheid meant that each of the four racial groups would be free to develop, each in their separate spheres. In practice Apartheid was a device for ensuring the dominance of the Caucasian race over the other groups in South Africa. Of all of the social services provided by the paternalistic Afrikaner governments over its years in power, Whites consistently received the best, and Blacks the worst. Indian[7] and Coloured services, schools, hospitals, parks, etc. occupied middle positions between the other two races.

Apartheid in South Africa appeared to be based upon four pillars. These included White control of political power; control over space so as to assure racial segregation; the control of Black labor; and the control over people, communities, and social interaction, especially in urban areas. Throughout most of the country's history, White South Africans monopolized political power against the other 85% of the South African Population. From the 1950s onward, after the passage of the Group Areas Act, the government began forced removal of Blacks from their homes to dumping grounds known as "homelands." In theory, these "homelands" represented the places of ethnic origin of distinct Black ethnic groups. In fact, the ethnic basis of many South African groups has long been unclear because of the disruptive events of the 19th century. The *Mfecane* (wars between African ethnic groups), the European incursions, and the industrialization of South Africa, all had led to considerable general mixing of South Africa's Blacks. In fact, the homelands were, in most cases, bits of non-contiguous, inhospitable, unfertile land unwanted by White farmers or industrialists. Some 3.5 million people had been moved to their so-called homelands by the late 1980s, when the program was finally halted.[8] By that time, four homelands, Transkei, Ciskei, Bophuthatswana, and Venda had been declared "independent" by the South African government. It is interesting to note that South Africa's homelands were never recognized by any nation outside of South Africa.

The Group Areas Act was also responsible for the forced movement of Blacks from central urban locations to remote peri-urban ones. With its enforce-

6. Racial classification, always scientifically questionable, was based on such criteria as "appearance, general acceptance, and repute." See Omond, 1986, pp. 24–29.

7. Indians were brought into the colony of Natal in 1860 by the British. As indentured servants, their purpose was to work the newly created sugar cane fields. At the turn of the twentieth century, these Indian workers were joined in South Africa by a second wave of Indians, this new group a merchant class.

8. The movement of Blacks and others peoples in South Africa under Apartheid represented the greatest forced human migration in peacetime history.

ment some Black South Africans with jobs in White areas were forced to endure daily round trip commutes of up to six hours. Over the years, resettlement of Blacks led to high levels of Black unemployment. It also kept Blacks constantly off-balance, making it difficult to create self-sustaining enterprise of any kind—in business, in agriculture, or even in community life. These factors tended to exacerbate social tension, and to foster Black on Black violence, all of which led to emasculation and impoverishment of the Black majority. Geographically displaced Blacks, confined to unproductive homelands or peri-urban ghettos, had few job opportunities other than working in White-owned South Africa in White-owned agriculture or mines. Indeed one of the purposes of the Apartheid system was to prevent Black competition from undermining White privilege.

Temporary housing for Black laborers was sometimes available for rental fees in company-provided hostels. These were single-sex barracks where up to twelve adult men were housed in a single room. Such cramped housing fueled frustration and encouraged violent behavior, all of which was exacerbated by the absence of family life. Unfortunately, because of housing shortages and poverty, same-sex hostel housing for workers continues to this day. Some Blacks, notably domestic workers, were allowed to live in White areas. But such persons were generally forced to live apart from their spouses and families in most cases.

Organized political opposition to White supremacy began in 1912 as a Black leadership coalesced around the imminent passage of the Native Land Act. In the 1920s this group evolved into the African National Congress (ANC). The ANC emerged in a context of growing Afrikaner nationalism. The ANC's support further grew during the 1930s in response to worsening conditions for Blacks during the Depression years. And it was during this decade that those Blacks still on voter rolls in the Cape Province were removed.

In the earlier decades, Black opposition was organized around moderate Black intellectuals. But the legislative agenda of the Nationalists in the 1950s pushed the ANC toward increased militancy. In 1955 the ANC with its allies, the South African Indian Congress and the White Congress of Democrats, drew up its Freedom Charter. This document stood as the basis for the political demands of the African National Congress until 1994.

Protests by racial majorities, particularly the Blacks, continued throughout the 1950s. Particularly hated were the pass laws that required passes[9] of all African adult males and after 1954, all Black females. By the late 1950s it was clear that the South African government was prepared to respond to peaceful protests with violence. Peaceful protests of the 1950s culminated in the massacre at Sharpeville in 1960 when 69 persons were shot dead when White policemen opened fire on a mass demonstration. After the protest, the government declared a State of Emergency. The African National Congress and its offshoot, the Pan African Congress, were banned and security forces detained thousands of people.

9. Passes provided information about the carrier including his/her place of employment. Blacks needed special permission to travel to White areas unless employed there. The passes allowed authorities to control the movements of Black people. Failure to produce a pass on the demand of law enforcement personnel would result in arrest. See Omond, 1985, pp. 122–130.

Top leaders of the African National Congress, including Nelson Mandela were imprisoned in 1963.

From the 1960s onward, Black groups became increasingly militant. Military wings of the ANC, the *Umkhonto we Sizwe*, and *Poqo*, of the Pan African Congress (PAC) purchased arms and worked to overthrow the South African Nationalist government. ANC operatives trained in guerrilla camps in ANC-supporting neighboring countries such as Tanzania and Zambia.

In 1976 school children in Soweto (Southwestern Townships, the teeming collection of Black Townships outside Johannesburg) began to protest against the use of Afrikaans as a medium of instruction in schools. Police responded to the protest with bullets and tear gas, causing some loss of life. The incident set off a chain of revolts that quickly spread across the country. In this context, a new youth movement, the Black Consciousness Movement formed and attracted Black South African youth. The South African group was inspired by Black Power and Black Theology movements active in the United States. One of the South African leaders, Steve Biko, died in detention in 1977, and this sparked off a new wave of protests. The State, under Prime Minister Vorster, used the powers of the Internal Security Act to crush riots and arrest and detain hundreds of people. As resistance to state repression grew, resisters became increasingly more militant. Arms flowed in from shadowy sources in the Eastern Block and were distributed to a smoldering Black population. In the wake of political repression, a culture of violence and lawlessness developed.[10] These habits have proved difficult to curb in the new South Africa.

From the early 1960s, South Africa was considered a pariah by the Western world. South Africa withdrew from the Commonwealth of Nations in anticipation of her expulsion. And in 1974, South Africa saw her seat revoked in the General Assembly of the United Nations. South African sports teams were also banned from the Olympics and from most regional and world competition. And South African Airlines was denied landing rights in most countries. By the 1980s, private corporate disinvestment was putting severe pressure on the South African government. Indeed, in 1986, over the veto of President Ronald Reagan, the US Congress passed the Comprehensive Anti-Apartheid Act which prohibited a range of financial dealing between US companies and South Africa.

In 1978 Vorster resigned his post as Prime Minister. The reins of power passed to Piet Botha. Botha, a reformist within the Nationalist party, instituted a series of cosmetic political changes. Some of these were designed to create a Black lower middle class who would eventually serve as a buffer between the Whites and the Black majority. Black labor was finally allowed to organize for collective representation.

And during the 1980s, symbolic aspects of Apartheid, (so-called "petty apartheid," such as segregated beaches, sports teams, busses, and so on) disappeared. The Mixed Marriages Act (prohibiting marriage across race) and the dreaded Section 16 of the Immorality Act (proscribing interracial sex) were each repealed. During this time Asians and Coloured were also given limited political

---

10. For example, the ANC encouraged Black South Africans not to pay their utility bills. Today, the new government is having a difficult time collecting fees for municipal services rendered.

rights. The response of these groups was lack-luster, the majority preferring to throw in their lot with the Black South African majority.

With the fall of the Soviet Union in 1989, White South Africa lost its claim to protecting the country from a communist threat. As dictatorships fell all over Eastern Europe, the Nationalist government of South Africa began to move toward majority rule. Then President F.W. De Klerk committed the South African government to a negotiated end of Apartheid. Black leaders were released from prison, including Nelson Mandela who had served a 26-year prison sentence. De Klerk began negotiations with Black leaders that ultimately led to a new constitution. The constitution contained a comprehensive Bill of Rights, the naming of 11 official languages, and a restructuring of the armed forces.

In 1994, Mandela stood for president against two rivals, the National party and the *Inkatha* Freedom Party. Mandela won a landslide victory and eventually began a program of Reconstruction and Development. In 1999, Mandela retired, passing on the mantle of party leadership to his ANC deputy Thabo Mbeki. Mbeki won an important victory for the ANC in the country's second post-apartheid election. In mid-2002, Mandela remained a busy octogenarian, an active elder statesman, working tirelessly on a host of important South African issues, including Human Rights promotion and HIV/AIDS care and prevention.

South Africa in 2002 is a society in transition. Its people continue to face the enormous burden of undoing three hundred and fifty years of skewed development. In the last decade of the 1990s every aspect of South African public policy was examined. New laws, particularly those guaranteeing human rights for all people, including women's rights and those of every conceivable minority group, have been passed. It has been a remarkable transition, one far more peaceful than the world could have imagined. But the new South Africa faces enormous challenges. Although there is a growing Black Middle class, there still exist enormous race and class divisions. Unemployment, at 30%, is dangerously high and crime and violence have reached epidemic proportions. The ANC had committed itself to land reform with the aim of providing land/housing to those most severely affected by the excesses of Apartheid. But the mechanisms for reallocating land against competing claims of ownership are proving difficult to resolve and implement.

AIDS Interventions in South Africa

South Africa's rank in the human development index in 1997 was 101. Literacy rates are quite high, 82% of the adult population. South Africa's per capita income was at $3,000 per annum in 1999 according the U.S. State Department figures. There is one physician per 1,529 persons in the population. South Africa's health budget dwarfs any on the African continent. The South African government's budget (national and provincial) for health services in 2000/01 stood at 32.3 billion rand (about $4.5 billion). Per capita spending on health services in 2000/1 equaled 512 rand ($72.58). Expenditures devoted solely to AIDS care and prevention were pegged at 75 million rand for 2000/1 (about $10.6 million). They increased to 125 million rand (about $15.6 million) in 2001/2

(Forgey *et al.*, 2001, p. 228). The nation spent a good deal more on AIDS in 2002/3 with 337.5 million rand (about $33 million) devoted to the AIDS. And AIDS expenditures were expected to increase by 25% for the foreseeable future (Hickey, 2002, p. 1).[11] These increases reflect the growing awareness of the South African government on the worsening HIV/AIDS crisis, an epidemic whose severity continues to grow despite South Africa's considerable efforts.

The first cases of AIDS emerged in South Africa during the late 1980s. AIDS was then regarded as a disease of White homosexual males and of marginalized Black South Africans. At the time the Nationalist government, preoccupied with impending shift to black rule was fairly unresponsive to the impending crisis (Parker, 1994, p. 2). The government did launch an AIDS awareness campaign in 1987 and in the same period it established in Johannesburg the first of several government created AIDS Training, Information & Counselling Centres (ATICC). Meanwhile, a South African Institute of Medical Research (SAMIR) AIDS center was established with private funds.

A model developed in the early 1990s predicted that there would be just under one million cases of HIV/AIDS by 1995. For the year 2000, when presumably AIDS intervention efforts could be expected to render results, it produced an optimistic figure of 3.7 million AIDS cases and a pessimistic one of 4.1 million (Parker, 1994, p. 9). HIV/AIDS growth rates throughout the 1990s, however, have continued to defy even the pessimists. By September 1995, there were already 1.8 million cases of HIV/AIDS in South Africa (Togni, 1997, p. 33). Figures for the year 2000 showed South Africa's caseload at 4.7 million (Whiteside, 2001, p. 3). And the new statistics for 2001 had South Africa's HIV+ rate at five million (UNAIDS, 2002, p. 190, table)! This means that South Africa is the nation that has the highest number of HIV/AIDS cases in the world. The causes for this are complex and can only be broadly touched upon throughout the course of this work.

By 1992, the epidemiological community recognized a growing trend in heterosexual infection rates, particularly in sub-Saharan Africa. At that time, cases of HIV/AIDS in the Southern African region made up 66% of the world's total (Mann, Tarantola, and Netter, 1992, p. 29). It was clear at that time that the majority of Black South Africans exhibited AIDS risk profiles similar to those of their northern neighbors in the region. Meanwhile, a broad array of largely South African based non-governmental organizations began operating their own AIDS interventions.

When the new government took power in 1994, it made sexual health and AIDS a focal point of its health policy, a policy that included the decentralization of health services and the provision of community health clinics (African National Congress 1994). The new ANC government set up the National AIDS Convention of South Africa (NACOSA), a coalition of government offices and of AIDS intervention groups active in health care and HIV prevention. The NACOSA formulated broad policies and channeled increased government funding of AIDS work.

---

11. Historical conversion rates performed on May 16, 2002 through OANDA.COM converter.

One project that has had an important impact on the AIDS struggle in South Africa is a project known as **DramAide**. The project began as a pilot project in a rural part of KwaZulu-Natal Province, in eastern South Africa. Conceived by academics at the University of Zululand, DramAide was launched in 1991. The project used teachers and school nurses to produce a response to the then-emerging epidemic of HIV/AIDS.

DramAide's vehicle for delivering information about HIV and AIDS is "Drama in Action". Funded by the Provincial Department of Health in KwaZulu-Natal, DramAide's approach encourages junior high school pupils to develop skills in drama, and to use these skills to analyze their own social conditions *vis à vis* the risk of AIDS, through the scripting of a play.

The use of Theatre for Social Change has been inspired by the work of Paolo Friere (*Pedagogy of the Oppressed* 1972) and Augusto Boal (*Theatre of the Oppressed* 1979). Both of these Latin American scholars, the first, an educator, the second a dramaturge, stress the importance of conscientization or "consciousness raising" among populations in need of social change. And Boal's work specifically notes the power of theatre in this endeavor. As noted in Chapter 4 (Performance), entire generations of projects in development have adopted the Friere-Boal approach to promoting social change. These two theorists might well be considered the theoretical fathers of Theatre for Development.

Theatre for Development also advocates using members of target groups in the design of their own messages. Development practitioners refer to these techniques as "participatory methodologies." Participatory methodologies, as we shall see, have been the cornerstone of DramAide's approach to the AIDS crisis in South Africa.

DramAide operated in the following way. DramAide teams consisting of trained drama facilitators and nurses/primary health care workers would visit pilot schools and present AIDS information in the form of a play. The children would view the plays and then would be asked to develop over time with teachers their own AIDS dramas. DramAide team leaders would visit the schools on a regular basis to help students with their plays, to give drama lessons, and to explore technical questions about AIDS and social options.

On school "open days," students would present their plays to parents and school officials. Not surprisingly, the students drew on traditional forms of Zulu entertainment including mass choirs and poetry, speeches, sketches, and drama. Schools were encouraged to institutionalize these activities by creating "Health Promoting Clubs." With the assistance of DramAide, Health Promoting Schools organized health festivals for their communities. Again, these festivals are sites for performances including drama, choir, poetry, speeches and sketches, and song, all with deep roots in indigenous South African cultures.

The evolution of the DramAide project in South Africa cannot be divorced from the larger historical context in which it operates. As noted above, the Apartheid government (1948–1994) devoted few resources to the health of the Black communities in the country and fewer still to education and arts promotion. The legal separation of the races into distinct cultural groups ensured a separate development wherein one group had little knowledge/understanding of the lifestyle, cultural and artistic traditions, or problems of another.

Because of the particular nature of South Africa's political situation, the DramAide project used a unique research technique to track its progress and to act as a self-correcting agent. The project chose Action Research to monitor its progress. Traditional research methodologies use the principle of controlled experimentation in which one group or situation receives a treatment and a second receives no treatment or a placebo. Early on DramAide project leaders rejected this approach as inappropriate. In the early 1990s South Africa was in the throes of major political, social, and historical shifts. Such conditions would make it difficult to compare schools across geographical areas, and impossible to cleanly compare cases over time. Besides, as the founder of DramAide noted, it would have been unconscionable to refuse some school children information about AIDS so as to render these groups better experimental controls (Dalrymple, 15 August 1999, interview). Clearly the health of the children took precedence over the needs of a research design. Indeed DramAide felt itself engaged not so much in an academic exercise or experiment but in a mission to save lives in the context of a national emergency. DramAide had opted to use interactive drama in the fight against AIDS. Based on sound theatrical and pedagogical principles, it had launched a social movement. It would now use research not to find out whether its interventions were working, but rather to learn how to better accomplish the project's goals.

The racial mixture of the DramAide facilitator teams helped the project to learn a great deal about the social dynamics of Black South African teens. Most of the nuances of Black social life had been lost to White South Africans. So the early experiences with the school plays were very instructive for project planners, a good many of whom were White South Africans. The plays helped them to understand the depth of the problems surrounding changes in sexual behavior facing the Black majority in impoverished communities. In a sense, the staging of these plays brought DramAide team members closer to one another, to the schools, and to the impoverished communities where they were creating change. The interactive techniques forced all participants to tackle very personal issues they would not normally have discussed with co-workers of a different race. The junior high school students also learned from the plays in ways they would otherwise not have.

Keen to see if their methods were effective, DramAide evaluators measured knowledge levels and action orientation of participant pupils and their parents. It was not altogether surprising that they found the dramas increased knowledge and awareness of the threat of AIDS. They found significant changes in attitudes toward HIV/AIDS in schools with DramAide interventions as opposed to those without them. But the surveys of DramAide projects undertaken in some sites failed to show a difference in students' safe sex practices between those schools with DramAide and those without the project (Harvey, Stewart, and Swan, 1994, pp. 43–44; Hambridge, 1995, p. 87). Researchers and DramAide project organizers explained these results noting that sexual behavior could not change unless both partners in the sex act were equally free to negotiate with one another. Girls, it seemed, could not negotiate. And much of the youth of both genders lacked basic life management skills. They needed to understand their bodies and they needed to learn to organize their lives—to set goals; to prioritize commitments; to make intelligent choices; to resist destructive behaviors; and to negotiate power relations in a confusing and fast changing social landscape. In short, research and practice showed South African youth needed comprehensive sex education and thorough training in "lifeskills." So the DramAide project expanded after 1995 to incorporate lifeskills teaching and sex education initiatives into its project mission. Lifeskills training for youth in South Africa remains a cornerstone of AIDS prevention in South Africa.

AIDS awareness plays had been brought into 772 schools in South Africa by 1995. A further 500,000 persons had been reached through the projects open days and other projects (Dalrymple, 1997, p. 3). This took place in three of South Africa's provinces: KwaZulu-Natal, Gauteng, and Eastern Cape Province. Several other provinces remained under-served.

The DramAide project underwent twists and turns during the second half of the 1990s. In 1996, the project became a national one, and in keeping with its responsiveness to the changing contours of the AIDS epidemic, DramAide instituted two new programs, Act Alive and Go Grow. Act Alive focused on imparting sex education and life skills to high school students by working more closely with both high school teachers and students in health promoting clubs. Go Grow was involved in developing entrepreneurial skills for new groups producing Theatre for Social Change. And in 1997, DramAide began to focus through its Circle Time on Primary School Education. In 1997, Lifeskills delivery was instituted into the National Education Curriculum. This was a testimony to the importance of the link between participatory grassroots methodologies and national policy in South Africa.

In 1997 DramAide joined a consortium of six groups to deliver a national AIDS campaign. The consortium, and indeed the Government Department of Health and the NACOSA, had recognized that the South African public, by and large, was aware of the risks of AIDS and the modes of its transmission. It was agreed that what was needed was a battery of interventions designed to change not just the information environment, but also attitudes and behavior.

So in 1997, after nearly a decade of AIDS news, the HIV/AIDS and STD directorate of the Department of Health of South Africa granted a bid to a media consortium for a Beyond Awareness Campaign. The consortia consisted of CASE, the Community Agency for Social Enquiry, DramAide, The Society for Family Health (SFH), Soul City, (see Chapter 8), the Ulwazi Educational Radio Project, and Syakha Communications. The Society for Family Health was responsible for management of the Beyond Awareness Campaign; CASE was responsible for conducting evaluations on a number of other ongoing national initiatives. Soul City would mount a sophisticated television broadcast series that would treat thematically a number of unhealthy social pathologies that can be conducive to the AIDS epidemic. Ulwazi Educational Radio Project would train Black African radio producers to develop educational material for radio in various South African indigenous languages. Siyakha Communications would provide communication services that were not provided by other communication companies in South Africa. For example it would produce materials for community groups written in simple styles and several languages (Tender Proposal, n.d., pp. 10–11.)

In 1998 the Beyond Awareness Campaign was extended for another two years, with some of the same players plus others who joined the consortium of AIDS media and information professionals (Maart n.d., p. 1.3). The DramAide project remained a key partner in the Beyond Awareness 2 campaign. At this

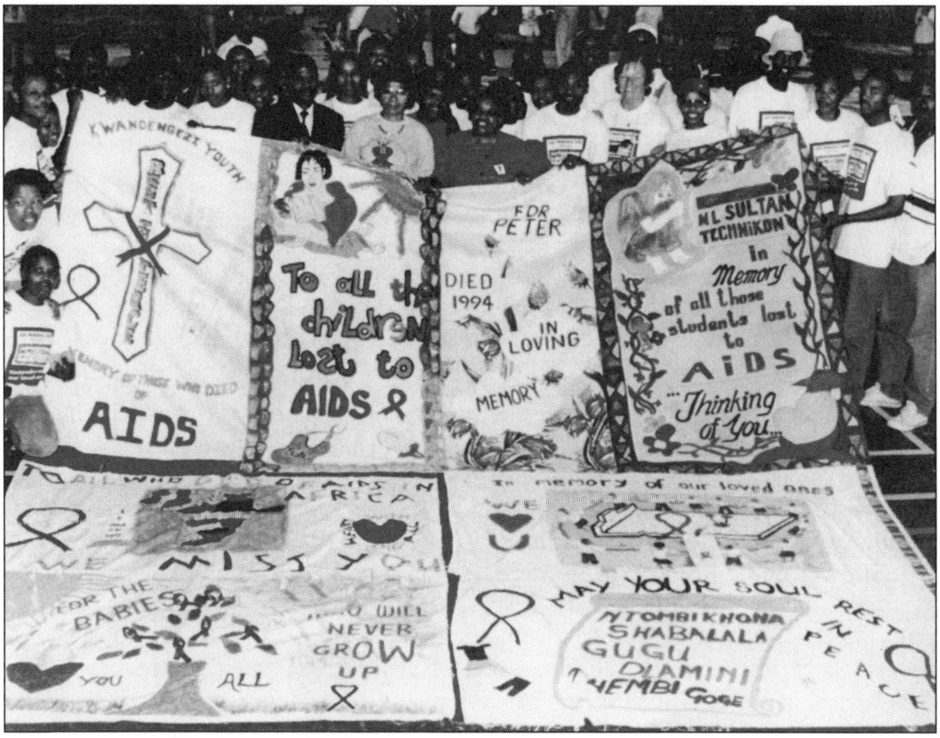

Figure 3-3. South African AIDS memorial quilt. Photo courtesy of the DramAide Project.

juncture in the South African AIDS crisis, DramAide applied some of its revolutionary participatory methodologies to tertiary (university level) institutions. DramAide promoted special AIDS awareness activities at South African technical colleges and university campuses. These include the painting of AIDS awareness murals and the organization of visits to campuses from the NAPWA, the National Association of People Living With AIDS. The DramAide team also launched the South African AIDS Memorial Quilt project early in 1999. In the first decade of the 21st century, DramAide continued its health promotion drama work in schools, training teachers in lifeskills, and helping pupils to create health promotion clubs. It also used its important DramAide methodology in a drama workshop designed to explore issues surrounding masculinity in South Africa. And it continued to work with the NAPWA in a project that positioned NAPWA workers in AIDS information booths established at strategic locations in bus, train, and other public locations. These information workers sensitively answer questions, encourage testing, promote tolerance, and decrease the stigma surrounding HIV/AIDS.

South Africa and its AIDS epidemic is highly visible. It is perhaps more notorious for its errors and controversies than for its innovative approaches to AIDS information and prevention campaigns. Several spectacular blunders are bound up in politics. The first was the commissioning by the ANC of a "Broadway Standard" musical, Sarafina II, by the internationally acclaimed Mbongeni Ngema (see Chapter 8) in the mid-1990s. The Sarafina II project caused a stir in

South Africa because the play was developed with almost no consultation with the NACOSA directorate, a group whose members had long been in the forefront of the AIDS struggle. The play project moreover failed to follow established procedures for message monitoring. It was also an extremely costly venture (10 million rand approximately or about $2.7 million dollars at the mid-1990s exchange rate), "wasting most of the government's 1995 [health] budget" (Tomaselli, 1997a, p. 3). But the worst crime of Sarafina II was that it propagated ambiguous and moralistic messages about HIV and about the AIDS epidemic, thereby undermining much of the more serious work of the NACOSA. The Sarafina II debacle is an example of what happens when politicians or any authorities act, more out of a desire to be ***seen*** to be doing something rather than out of a genuine search to find a solution to the problem at hand.

The second and third causes of South Africa's negative visibility in the AIDS crisis involve the controversial stands President Thabo Mbeki has taken over the cause of AIDS (see Chapter 2) and the refusal of his health minister to fund antiretroviral treatment for pregnant women.[12] In July 2002, a new scandal broke over the alleged funding by the South African government of research on a home grown AIDS remedy. The Mbeki government was reported to have used secret funds to help developers to research a drug known as Virudine. The drug turned out to be medically unsound; and its promoters appeared to be linked to the shady world of arms trade. Once again, the South African government appeared to be desperate to develop alternatives to Western cures about which it is skeptical (Brümmer and Sole, 2002, pp. 2–3). These lapses, notwithstanding, it is worthwhile to scrutinize some of the remarkable work that has been done in South Africa in conjunction with the AIDS crisis.

In many ways, South Africa represents the hope for the AIDS crisis on the African continent. South Africa has a formidable level of academic expertise and sophistication in areas of AIDS epidemiology and AIDS medical research. Academics at the University of Pretoria, at the University of Witwatersrand, and at the University of Natal-Durban (UND) have been particularly active in cutting-edge AIDS social and behavioral research. The Centre for Media and Cultural Studies at UND has a well-established reputation in the field of development communication. It has provided much of the intellectual muscle for the Beyond Awareness Campaigns. It also has a commendable record of scholarship and an enviable list of graduates including experts in the use of media for social change.[13] South Africa has a vast repertoire of intellectual resources, a well trained workforce, and a broad network of long established NGOs. All of

---

12. A course of AZT given to mothers during pregnancy has been shown to result in significant decreases in mother to infant transmission. Following the government's refusal to provide Mother to Child Treatment (MTCT), the Treatment Action Campaign (TAC) of South Africa brought suit against the South African government. In December 2001, the Pretoria High Court ruled in favor of the TAC. Since the ruling, the South African health services are required to administer a course of anti-retrovirals to pregnant women. See Heywood, 2002, p. 13.

13. Warren Parker received his Master of Arts degree from the Center and Lynn Dalrymple received her Ph.D. from the same institution. The Center's Director, Dr. Keyan Tomaselli served as a media expert on the on the South African National Advisory Committee on AIDS and STDs.

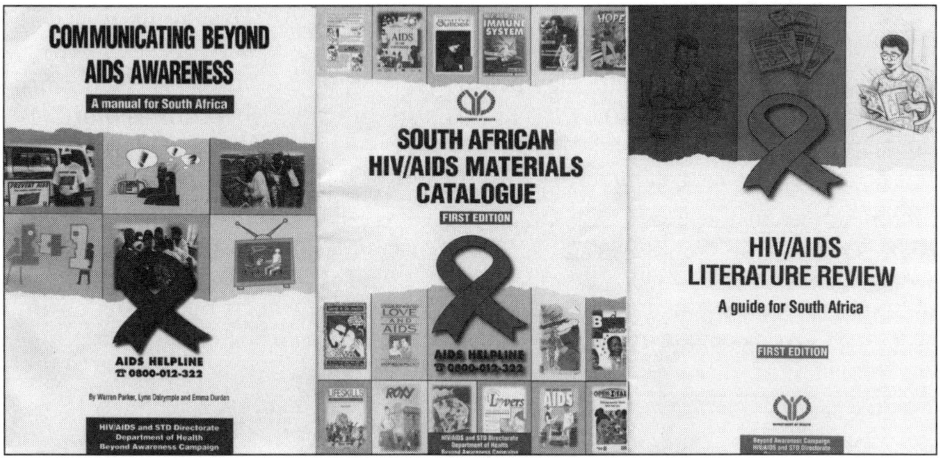

Figure 3-4. South African AIDS activists and scholars have developed comprehensive AIDS information strategies.

these factors help to keep South Africa in the driving seat of its own AIDS intervention campaigns.

What is really remarkable about the South African AIDS media initiative is the sophistication of its strategies. The Beyond Awareness team published *Communicating Beyond AIDS Awareness: A manual for South Africa* written by Warren Parker, Lynn Dalrymple and Emma Durden (1998). The manual is a textbook that combines for the reader both the theory of communication media for social change with a then up-to-date assessment of South Africa's AIDS information needs of the time. The volume presents a discussion of then-existing big and small media; and also discusses dialogue-oriented and participatory media strategies. It illustrates each of its points with examples of on-going projects: the national AIDS taxi campaign in one place (p. 31), the Talking Hands puppetry campaign for children elsewhere (p. 58), and so on. The manual also shows how these different initiatives interact.

What is also exceptional about the South African AIDS awareness initiative is its emphasis on participatory methodologies discussed in Chapter 2. South African communicators recognized, early on, the gulf that lay between various South African target populations. And they understood that all of these groups would have to create their own AIDS messages. Communication experts moreover, understood the importance of giving formerly suppressed peoples the power to address their peers in their own cultural idiom. And it was by using participatory methodologies (namely theatre) in the early 1990s that South African planners learned from their own youth of the need to teach life skills. (See Chapter 8). [14]

14. The plays revealed much about the contexts in which sexuality took place. It revealed sex during "stolen moments" in school playgrounds or on the roadways adjacent to school. It also revealed the performance by pupils of sexual favors for school authorities, such as teachers or headmasters. It uncovered a good deal of non-consensual sex, sex girls felt powerless to refuse. It revealed sex accompanied by violence including violent family members.

It is heartening to see how South Africans toil at the grassroots level with highly democratic methods. It gladdens the observers to watch South Africans refine their methods in response to ongoing processes of Action Research. And it is encouraging to learn that government can be responsive to reports from practitioners and targets in the field.

Indeed, life skill delivery through participatory methodologies has remained a cornerstone of the South African struggle against AIDS. As noted above, the AIDS epidemic in South Africa has been particularly virulent since the mid-1990s. Theater and performance have been involved in the struggle to stem the spread of AIDS. And as we shall see in Chapter 8, the use of theatrical techniques in the struggle against AIDS has also spawned many imitators.

Geography, Climate, and People of Mali

Mali is a landlocked nation in West Africa lying between 10 and 25 degrees north of the equator. Its area is about 1, 240,000 square kilometers (about 480,000 square miles), roughly the size of California and Texas combined. The southern section of the country is dominated by scrubland savanna vegetation, while the north is semi-desert and desert. The River Niger, Africa's third longest river, crosses Mali. The Niger rises in the Futa Jalon mountains in Guinea and flows north to Mali and onward through the nation of Niger before emptying in the Niger delta in southeastern Nigeria. The River Niger waters the nation of Mali, over spilling its banks and creating fertile flood plains along them. The flooding makes this parched Sahelian nation productive. The Niger also forms a rather unique geographical phenomenon, a broad internal delta. The delta is 450 kilometers (280 miles) long in the central portion of the country, and 200 kilometers (132 miles) wide at the city of Mopti.

Mali is surrounded by Senegal to the west, Guinea to the southwest, Cote d'Ivoire to the south, Burkina Faso to the southeast, Niger to the east, Algeria to the north, and Mauritania to the northwest. A single-track railway connects Mali's capital Bamako with Dakar, the capital of Senegal to the west.

Mali has three main seasons that vary according to latitude and decrease in intensity as one travels northward. The rainy season in the south, around Bamako (the capital), begins in June or July and lasts until September or October. The rainy season is relatively cool with temperatures around 30 degrees Celsius (86 degrees Fahrenheit) and somewhat lower temperatures at the height of this season in August. A "cool" dry season begins after the rains in October and lasts to February, where temperatures may also hover in the 30+ degrees (86+ degrees Fahrenheit) Celsius region. From February to June is the extremely hot season with shade temperatures reaching beyond 40+ degrees (104 degrees Fahrenheit) in midday!

Some parts of Mali, the cities of Timbuktu and Gao, and the Bandiagara plateau, home of the Dogon peoples, are among the hottest places on earth. Here, the temperatures can climb up to 48 degrees Celsius (up to 120 degrees Fahrenheit).

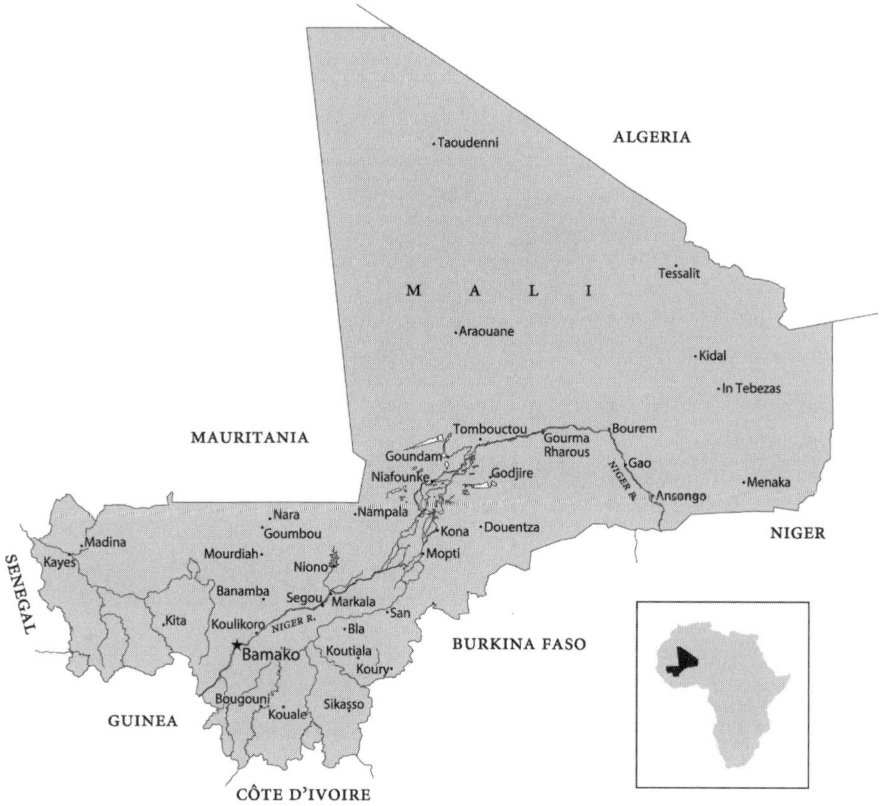

Figure 3-5. Map of Mali, West Africa.

The average annual rainfall in Mali ranges from a low of around 20 centimeters (8 inches) in the extreme northerly regions to as much as 81–145 centimeters (32–56 inches) in the southwestern and southern portions of the country. Like other Sahelian nations, Mali was hit by recurrent droughts in the 1970s and 1980s, prolonged dry spells that have had serious environmental consequences. The effect of these droughts, combined with over-utilization of marginal lands, has led to a steady advance of the Sahara. Most climatologists believe these droughts to be part of a pattern of recent global climate change brought about by human activity, notably greenhouse gas emissions produced by automobiles, industrial activity and the large scale felling and burning of forests. Mali is one of many sub-Saharan countries that will be severely affected by global climate change anticipated over the next 50 or so years it is predicted that arid and semi-arid climates will become even drier and hotter than they are present. Crop failures could become commonplace, and famine will be common (Stock, 1995, p. 33). Vast numbers of persons are expected to move south away from the advancing desert, a pattern that has been occurring in Mali since the droughts of the 1970s.

Mali has a population of 10.686 million people. Like most African countries, Mali's population is ethnically diverse. The largest group are the Mande who represent 50% of the population and whose language, Bambara or Bamanan, is the

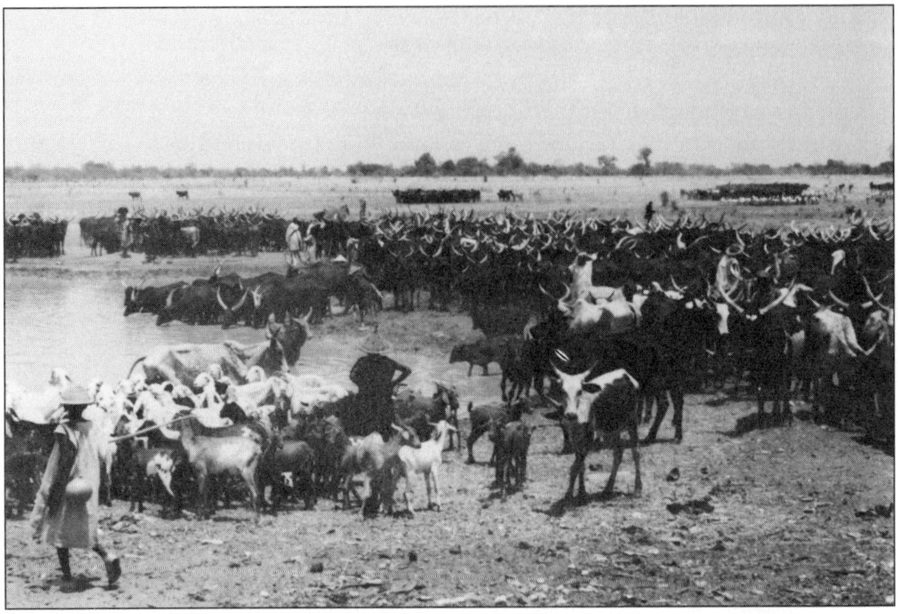

Figure 3-6. The Fulani People of Mali and neighboring countries in West Africa have traditionally been the cattle herders of the region.

lingua franca of the country. Other groups include the Peulh (Fulani), the Voltaic, the Songhai, the Maur (Moor), and the Dogon. French is used as an administrative language and is spoken in the cities. Ninety percent of Mali's people are Muslim; 9% follow indigenous African religious beliefs, and 1% are Christian.

Mali is divided administratively into eight regions plus the district of Bamako, the capital. The regions are subdivided into 55 circles that further subdivide into 702 communes. Once highly centralized in the model of French administration, the government has opted in the 1990s for decentralization and greater local autonomy.

Economy of Mali

Mali is an agricultural nation where four out of five Malians are engaged in cultivation. While rice, millet and sorghum are grown for food, the country's main export crops are cotton and groundnuts (peanuts). Indeed, Mali has become the largest producer of cotton in West Africa in the last ten years. Mali, one of Africa's 34 Highly Indebted Poor Countries or HIPCs, is one of the poorest countries in the world with a per capita income in 2000 of $270 per annum (US Department of State, 2001b). Mali's currency, the CFA franc, was devalued by the French government in 1994 causing widespread misery in an attempt to "adjust" the Malian economy. Like many poor nations, Mali has a rapidly rising population, one that is growing at the rate of 2.98% per annum. Like many poor African countries, the population of Mali is heavily skewed toward youth with almost half of the country's people less than 15 years of age.

The combined youth of the population, its rapid growth per annum, and the country's overall poverty are pushing Malians toward the cities in search of new opportunities. Mali's urban growth continues unabated. The city of Bamako, a quiet sleepy capital in the 1970s, boasted nearly one million people at the dawn of the third millennium. In 1960, only 5% of Malians lived in cities. By 1990 the urban dwelling Malian population was at 23% and was growing at a rate of 3.1% per annum (Drisdelle, 1997, p. 52). Indeed large numbers of young people are leaving their rural areas in search of better opportunities.

Most Malian families also depend upon seasonal migration income. Most have at least one person working outside the country whose remittances help support the family back home. These individuals may work seasonally in Cote d'Ivoire, Senegal, or other nations of the West African region; or they may be employed in another nation of the northern hemisphere, especially France or the United States.

Mali has some of the highest negative indices in the world. It has the highest infant mortality rates, the highest maternal mortality rates, and the highest fertility rates (Drisdelle, 1997, p. 5). A woman has a one in seven chance of dying in pregnancy or childbirth or from an abortion. Life expectancy in Mali is low: 45 for males, and 48 for females. Health services reach a bare 20% of the population; and the adult literacy rate is 31% (UNDP 1999).

History of Mali

Mali has a proud history. Mali stands on the site of the ancient Ghana Empire which was described in the Arabic writings of historian Al Bakri in 773–74 AD. This Ghana Empire was situated on a vast plain stretching between the Senegal and the Niger Rivers. The Ghana Empire peopled by the Soninke or Northern Manding peoples dominated the eastern Sudan region from the 4th through the 13th centuries. The Ghana Empire rose to prominence in part because of its strategic location near to the gold fields at Wangara and to the westernmost trans-Saharan trade route, operated by the Sanhaja Berbers of the Western Sahara. The Ghana empire grew in importance by trading gold and agricultural products gathered on its lands and among neighboring Negro peoples in exchange for salt that was mined in the Sahara (Fage, 1969, pp. 1–17). The earliest origins of the empire are shrouded in mystery.

From the work of Arab historian Al-Bakri, we do know that the empire's capital in 700 A.D., was situated at Kumbi Saleh located about 324 Kms (200 miles) north of modern day Bamako. It was from Kumbi Saleh that the emperors of the Ghana Empire ruled in splendor. Historians G.T. Stride and C. Ifeka draw from Al Bakri's accounts in their description of the empire.

> Both the sanctity and the splendour of the Soninke monarchy were amply demonstrated when the Ghana gave a public audience to settle disputes and hear grievances. On such occasions, the Ghana sat in a pavilion of state wearing gorgeous robes, golden ornaments and a cap of cloth of gold. Around the cap was wound a turban of finest quality cot-

> ton. Tethered outside the pavilion were ten fine horses, each with harness worked in gold; and behind the Ghana himself stood ten pages bearing shields and swords embossed with gold. The entrance to the pavilion was guarded by well-bred dogs wearing collars of gold and silver who were the constant companions of the Ghana. To the Ghana's right were assembled the sons of his tributary rulers expensively clad and with gold plaited into their hair. The royal councillors, with the exception of the governor of Kumbi whose position was in front of this ruler, sat on both sides of the Ghana (1971, p. 34).

It was during the Ghana Empire that Islam began to penetrate into the western sahel region of West Africa. This happened gradually as a result of trade and intermarriage between the Negroid Soninke peoples and their two North African trading partner groups, the Sanhaja, the desert nomads, and the Moroccan Berbers, the ancestors of today's Berbers.

By the turn of the 12th century AD, the Almoravids, members of an Islamic group who lived in Spain and Morocco, were engaged in a Holy War (*jihad*). They attacked Kumbi Saleh and ordered all whose paths they crossed to accept Islam. Many Soninke fled south or west; but many others accepted the Muslim Faith.

Around 1200, Sumanguru, a king of the Susu group of Soninke clans rose up and conquered what remained of the old Ghana Empire. Sumanguru then engaged in a bitter fight with other Mande speaking clans, to control the Upper Niger, so that trade could pass through Timbuktu to North Africa. One of the leaders of the Keita clan, Sundiata rose up and defeated Sumanguru in 1235. With this defeat, the Empire of Mali rose with Sundiata as their king. Much of what we know about Sundiata and the Mali Empire comes from the epic poem the Legend of Sundiata, a portion of which appears in Chapter 5.

The Empire of Mali, a Mandingo empire, united all the clans of the southern Mande (alternatively known as the Mandinka or Manding), and northern Mande alternatively known as the Soninke. It carried on the role of trading both gold and produce with the Arabs in exchange for salt mined in the Sahara.

Some historians have argued that the Ghana and Mali empires were not two separate entities, but rather represented different dynasties of the same peoples. By about 1300, they had extended their power as far as Gao upstream from Timbuktu and down to Kebbi near the border of modern-day Nigeria. Thus the Mali Empire on its southeast flank had access to the peoples and the trade of what is modern day Ghana, Benin, Togo, and Nigeria. On the western front they expanded toward modern day Senegal and the Gambia.

The Mali Empire was at its peak in mid 14th century. At this time, its political power extended east to the borders of Hausaland in modern day northern Nigeria/southern Niger. The empire also stretched northeast and northwest into the Sahara, into what are today parts of Mali and Mauritania. On the west, it extended to the west coast of Africa into what are today Senegal and Gambia. On the southwest the Mali Empire controlled parts of what is modern day Sierra Leone, Liberia, and Guinea. On the southern flank, it controlled parts of modern day Cote d'Ivoire and Burkina Faso.

At the height of its power, the leader of the Empire, Mansa Musa, traveled to Mecca in Saudi Arabia via Cairo. He traveled with 8,000 employees and 60,000 servants and courtiers. Mansa Musa and his retinue spent so much gold from his empire en route in Cairo the price of gold was said to have plummeted 12% (Fage, 1969, p. 22). Historian J.D. Fage quotes medieval historian and traveler Ibn Battuta who journeyed across the Sahara to Mali from his home in Tangiers, Morocco in order to fulfill his mission to visit every country in the Islamic world. Battuta, who dictated his travel memoirs to his secretary in 1353, described the extraordinary kingdom of Mali.

> The Negroes are seldom unjust, and have a greater abhorrence of injustice than any other people. Their ruler shows no mercy to anyone who is guilty of the least act of it. There is complete security in their country. Neither traveller nor inhabitant in it has anything to fear from robbers or men of violence.

Fage continues with his own paraphrase of his ancient Arabic source.

> Not only are the roads safe from travellers and merchants, but it was always easy for them to find good lodgings for the night without prior arrangement, and to buy food, in exchange for salt, spices, or beads, from the many flourishing markets.
>
> The general picture indeed is of a rich, prosperous peaceful, and well-ordered empire, in which effective government and organised communications and trade ran all the way from the Atlantic in the west to the borders of modern Nigeria in the east, and from the fringes of the forests in the south northwards into the desert (Fage, 1969, p. 24).

As successful and prosperous as was the Mali Empire, it encountered internal problems caused by over-expansion. A number of internal weaknesses and succession disputes finally weakened the empire. And by the beginning of the 15th century, the Songhai of the Niger bend (around Mopti) began to assert their power. About 1464 they were united under a Songhai king, Sonni Ali. A ruthless ruler, Sonni Ali defeated the weakened old Mande kings along with those of neighboring West African peoples. Sonni Ali, who died in 1492 (the year Christopher Columbus 'discovered' America), rebuilt a decaying Old Mali Empire before the Songhai Empire dynastic line passed onto the Askias with Askia Mohammed as their first ruler. Fage describes the arrival of the Askias.

> Askia Muhammad was successor not only to the military expansiveness of Sonni Ali, but also to that concept of a universal, peace loving Muslim but Mande-centered empire, able to rank with any other Islamic state, (1969, p. 27).

The Askia's, though nominally Songhai in ethnicity, absorbed Mande values, as they absorbed the old administration of the Mali Empire. The Songhai Empire, however, was fairly short-lived. Succession crises also weakened this empire and it fell to a Moroccan invasion, one that used firearms against Songhai bowmen. This led to the defeat and fall of the Songhai Empire in 1591.

The Moroccan adventure in the Songhai Empire lasted only thirty some-odd years. During that time Moroccan soldiers intermarried with Malian women in the three northern cities of Timbuktu, Djenne, and Gao, while the remnants of the old Songhai empire and the old Mande state regrouped as the Bambara (Bamanan) kingdom of Segou in the late 17th century (Fage, 1969, p. 30).

During the 18th century, rival Bambara (Bamanan) kings were engaged in continual warfare. They managed to wrest power over Timbuktu in the 1780s. *Jihadists* fighting Holy Wars also attacked the Bambara Empire. These disruptions continued almost up to the eve of the French invasion in the late 19th century.

At this time a new Mande empire became important. It was the empire of Samori Touré. Samori Touré was born in a village of what is now Guinea near the Sierra Leone and Liberian border. Samori had been a soldier in a local Mande king's army. By the mid-1860s he was organizing armies and taking slaves and booty. Fage notes that although his birthplace had reverted to animism from Islam, he became more and more Muslim the more he conquered (Fage 1969, p. 157). Samori was building an empire in what is today most of present day Cote d'Ivoire, Mali, and Guinea. Meanwhile, France became a serious contender for territory in Africa after 1879. Samori Touré's empire resisted French encroachment for a time, but it was no match for a 19th century imperial European power. France conquered Segou in 1890, Djenne in 1893, and Timbuktu in 1894. The French finally captured Samori Touré in 1898 and sent him into exile in São Tomé where he died in 1900.

Historians are fond of pointing out and elaborating upon the glories of the Western Sudan from the medieval period to the eve of colonialism. And many enjoy speculating on how these societies would have developed had their progress not been interrupted by colonialism. Alas we will never know what would have happened there without the European colonial adventure. Fage tells us there is no evidence that the Trans-Saharan trade routes were declining before the last quarter of the 19th century. Indeed, it appears that this trade reached its peak by 1875. We do know, however, that after the European conquest of West Africa was complete, the Trans-Saharan trade route shrank dramatically, and maritime trade grew by leaps and bounds (Fage 1969, pp. 157–158).

The French controlled Mali from the 1890s until 1960 in a colony known as the French Sudan. The French were less interested in the landlocked area of French Sudan which would become Mali than they were in some of their other colonies. France established Bamako as the country's new capital. Once a sleepy backwater, Bamako by the year 2000 boasted almost one million people, or one tenth of the population of Mali. And the French built a railroad from that capital to Dakar, the capital of modern day Senegal. The French ambition was to make Mali the breadbasket for French West Africa. They succeeded in this endeavor for a time by overturning the *dina*, a complex set of rules that governed land-use patterns between coexisting groups (nomads, cultivators, and fishermen) along the Niger River. The abolition of the *dina* during colonial times paved the way for the environmental degradation which was to follow and was to wreak havoc on Mali's marginal Sahelian lands (Drisdelle, 1997, p. 19).

The French colonialists left their language, one spoken only by the civil servant and entrepreneurial classes, in the larger Malian cities. Like most of the European colonizers, France left in Mali a somewhat alienated class of administrators sometimes with little patience for the opinions of the common people.

Mali was brought to independence in the years leading up to 1960 by an idealistic pan-Africanist named Modibo Keita (a descendant of Sundiata Keita of epic fame). For a brief period after independence, Mali was federated with its neighbor Senegal. But the West African federation was very short lived, and Mali had become a republic by the end of 1960. Like so many other African states, Mali fell prey to a coup d'état in 1968. Mali was taken over by strongman Moussa Traoré, who maintained power for 23 years. Droughts and corruption marked Moussa's reign. By the early 1980s, severely short of capital, Mali accepted a package of structural adjustment reforms dictated by the International Monetary Fund (IMF). The reform package, which mandated the contraction of the civil service, caused much hardship, especially among urbanites and led to calls for a new government.

In the early 1990s, following the democratic example of Benin, civil associations began to emerge in Mali. Armed with new independent newspapers, groups clamored for political reform. A progressive military officer, Colonel Amadou Toumany Touré toppled President Moussa Traoré. Soon afterwards, elections were held and Alpha Oumar Konaré was elected president of the Republic of Mali in 1992. He was reelected for a second term in 1996. An academic with literary leanings and a former Minister of Culture, Konaré ran a highly civil democracy for a decade. During his two terms in office, Mali former strongman Moussa Traoré was quietly kept under house arrest. In June 2002 Mali again held a presidential election, an election in which Konaré was constitutionally prohibited from running. Amadou Toumani Touré (known affectionately as A.T.T.) ran as an independent candidate and won the election, defeating candidate Soumaila Cisse from Konaré's Adema Party.

Mali in 2002 is at a crossroads. It faces enormous challenges. Gradual encroachment of the Sahara, caused by overgrazing of herd animals, and deforestation for firewood, continues unabated. Ethnic conflict with northern Tuareg, exacerbated by years of drought, is a persistent problem, one that has been with the country since the early 20th century (Drisdelle, 1997, p. 19).

But Mali is an extremely civil society. Mali's ancient history is a history of compromises, of people living together under common Mande culture and values. Mali is blessed with a flourishing free press and a broad array of independent radio stations. At last count, there were over 70 community operated radio stations in the country and an equal number of licenses were held by other groups including private entrepreneurs (Bilodeau, personal communication, July 2001). And Mali is blessed with a wealth of non-governmental organizations (NGOs). Between 1992 and 1996, the number of NGOs in Mali increased from fewer than 100 NGOs to more than 600 (Drisdelle, 1997, p. 29). Surrounded at every turn by calls for decentralization, many young people have rushed to create non-governmental organizations. Eventually, many of these organizations are able to team up with international partners to provide grass roots project implementation.

Mali has a vibrant arts sector that boasts its own special brand of music and dance. It has an abundance of playwrights, puppeteers, acrobats, painters, carvers, and so on. At independence, the socialist leaning government of Modibo Keita created government structures to support these arts. Moussa Traoré's regime followed suit. The nation has four subsidized performing art troupes: *Les Ballets Maliens*, *l'Ensemble Instrumentale du Mali*; l'*Orchestre Moderne: Le Badéma National*; and *le Groupe Dramatique,* the "*Kotèba National.*"

In comparison with many other countries, the AIDS problem in Mali is still relatively small. The country's HIV+ rate is estimated to be between 1.7% and

4% of the adult population.[15] But poverty, migration, and the relative powerlessness of women, key risk profile factors in the worldwide pandemic, are clearly conditions that pertain to Mali. Mali is wise to be vigilant in the face of this epidemic, given that her neighbor, Cote d'Ivoire, a country with which Mali has a great deal of trade, has a soaring epidemic with an HIV+ rate of almost 10%.

AIDS Intervention in Mali

Mali is one of the world's poorest countries, ranking at 165 out of the 174 countries listed in the UNDP's Human Development report of 2000. Mali's per capita income was $270 per annum in 2000. Literacy rates are low (31% overall) with considerable disparity between males and females.[16] Mali has an average of one physician for every 18,376 persons. The government of Mali spends an average $1.50 per person per annum on the delivery of health services to its people. Strapped for cash, Mali must depend upon outside assistance to fund and maintain a viable fight against the AIDS epidemic.

Mali's first case of HIV/AIDS was detected in 1985. In response to the coming epidemic, the government of Mali established the *Programme National de Lutte contre le SIDA* (PNLS), the National Program for the Struggle against AIDS, in 1987. The PNLS carried out a baseline study of HIV rates within the population. These studies showed alarming rates of HIV prevalence among commercial sex workers, rates of up to 40% seropositivity as compared with rates of about 1% of women attending pre-natal clinics. By the end of 1994, the PNLS estimated there were more than 100,000 HIV/AIDS infections in Mali and that there had been 12,000 deaths from AIDS (Amon, 2000, p. 6). By 1995, HIV prevalence rates had risen to 55% among commercial sex workers and 4% of pregnant women at sentinel sites (Family Health International 1998). Clearly Mali had a problem with HIV/AIDS. In 1999 the PNLS estimated that 136,000 people in Mali were HIV + and that there were had already been more than 62,000 deaths (*Plan Stratégique*, 1999, p. 5). Figures published at the end of 2001 showed some improvement. In 2001 UNAIDS reported there were 110,000 cases of HIV/AIDS and that the adult rate of seropositivity had decreased in two years from 2.3% to 1.7 % (UNAIDS, 2002, table). Although these numbers look promising, it is too early to determine if Mali is witnessing a genuine downturn in the epidemic or if these encouraging numbers represent a temporary phenomenon or a counting error. (See note 15).

Unlike South Africa, Mali does not possess an army of trained social scientists and communication specialists on the cutting edge of AIDS research

15. Mali's *Plan Stratégique* of 1999 reported an estimated adult seropositivity rate of 3–4%. The UNAIDS 2000 Report on the Global Epidemic put that rate at 2.3%. The UNAIDS' 2002 reports the Malian adult seropositivity rate to be at a low of 1.7%. Because HIV/AIDS sentinel sites have not been properly established in Mali, HIV/AIDS figures may be woefully underreported. In 2002, as this volume went to press, the USAID was urging Malian health authorities not to become complacent in the light of apparent improvements in the 2002 HIV/AIDS rates.

16. Only 27% of Mali's primary school enrollees are female.

methodologies. There are no academic think tanks comparable to the SAMIR, to the South African National AIDS Research Council, or to the academic departments of the major South African universities studying AIDS. And there exists no blueprint comparable to South Africa's *Communicating Beyond AIDS Awareness* by Parker, Dalrymple, and Durden. Mali's AIDS initiatives do enjoy strong political support from the highest levels. Mali's First Lady, Madame Adame Ba Konaré (1992–2002), created a special foundation in 1995, the *Fondation Partage*, to use Mali's cultural and artistic wealth in the struggle against AIDS (Konaré, 1998, pp. 174–178). Madame Konaré's participation in World AIDS Days and other AIDS awareness events has helped to give a high profile to the pandemic.

Mali's efforts at combating the epidemic are consistent with those noted in Chapter 2 for other countries in Africa. Initiatives support improved health care and case management for those infected; better strategies for handling potentially contaminated instruments and blood products; improved community structures to support the ill and those surrounding them; and Information Education and Communication (IEC) campaigns targeted at the general public and at high risk groups. IEC efforts include social marketing of condoms.

External donors have provided the bulk of the funding for these activities. These include major bilateral sources of aid; a range of agencies of the United Nations; and a plethora of International Non-Governmental Organizations. Bilateral sources of aid include the European Union, the United States, Canada, France, the Netherlands, Switzerland, and The Federal Republic of Germany (GTZ). UN groups include the United Nations Development Fund, UNAIDS Programme, the World Bank, the United Nations Children's Fund (UNICEF) and the United Nations Fund for Population Activities (UNFPA). Major International Non-Governmental Organizations active in AIDS issues in Mali include Plan International, Save the Children UK, Care International, *Enda Tiers Monde,* and Africare, among others. Mali is included in the West African inter-country initiative run by UNAIDS. This is an AIDS prevention project that focuses on axes of migration between and within the countries of Cote d'Ivoire, Niger, Burkina Faso, Mali, and Senegal.

Mali's AIDS interventions tend to be externally driven. INGO based interventions present particular challenges for national campaigns. Each large International NGO has its own particular focus. For PLAN International, for example, that focus is child survival and development; eradication of female genital cutting; family planning; community based health care, and combat of STDs and AIDS. The primary focus of *Enda Tiers Monde* is the environment; while AIDS for *Enda* is a secondary concern. Each INGO also has its geographical territory in which it traditionally operates. Each also operates through a plethora of local NGOs many of which have their own foci and personnel. Interested in fostering grassroots creative products, INGOs in Mali disburse grants to local groups, NGOs that produce AIDS awareness creative products. The result is a smorgasbord of creative, locally relevant, and locally appreciated productions whose technical qualities vary greatly.

Important components in Mali's AIDS sector, the activities of PLAN International are examined here in some depth. PLAN International disburses its own funds, monies derived from donors who sponsor children through Childreach, together with funds matched by grants from USAID.

PLAN International, formerly known in the USA as Foster Parents Plan, had been active in the Malian rural development sector since 1976. In the early 1990s, the organization became concerned about the possibility of an impending AIDS epidemic. In response, it solicited proposals from local (Malian) non-governmental organizations. Ultimately it selected eleven local organizations (NGOs) and gave them grants to produce creative informational projects within PLAN's zones of operation.[17] These activities included people's theatre, music, video announcements at sporting events and the like. PLAN considered these early interventions as pilot projects in the areas of AIDS intervention.

Between 1995 and 2000 PLAN operated several programs for HIV/STD prevention and control. PLAN's informational approach involved both edutainment strategies and participatory strategies. For the latter, the organization also recruited and trained village heath workers from local NGOs to give talks on HIV/AIDS *(causeries)* and to sell condoms. This activity was consistent with both Malian national health policy aimed at decentralization and PLAN International's goal to promote community based health initiatives. Research moreover has shown the important contribution of interpersonal communication as an antecedent to behavior change (Singhal & Rogers, 1999, pp. 151–152). And research conducted by PLAN International shows that individuals in rural communities, particularly women, rely on community health workers for important information on STDs and AIDS (Diarra and Diarra, 1996, p. 52).

IEC activities at the community level comprised the great bulk of PLAN's activities and input during the early life of the project (Amon, 2000, p. 18).[18] PLAN International has produced a great wealth of materials including seven video taped plays, a twelve part audio soap series, a children's quiz book, documentary video, games, and miscellaneous printed materials. (See Amon, 2000, p. 29). This material is circulated through PLAN's local NGO based network of community health workers who organize viewer sessions and discussions with the materials. Much of this material was produced by local NGOs, some of them partners of PLAN.

PLAN International's year 2000 report lists an impressive array of information activities conducted over a five-year period.

> During the lifespan of the project, PLAN has reached more than two million people in over 2,000 communities with information concerning HIV/AIDS and the prevention and treatment of sexually transmitted dis-

17. Typically, INGOs operate by gentlemen's agreements within certain parts of a country in which they have projects. PLAN will take over one region while CARE will take another, and Save the Children will take a third. The division of territory makes it possible to INGOs to develop close links with local partners. It also avoids costly duplication of services.

18. Between 1995 and 1997, 80% of the PLAN projects were devoted to IEC activities. In 1998, PLAN International responded to high rates of knowledge about AIDS in the general population and began to broaden their IEC to include general health information.

> eases (STDs). Working through more than fifty local NGOs, the project covered PLAN program zones in the regions of Koulikoro and Kayes and non-PLAN zones in the regions of Sikasso, Segou, and Mopti. More than 73,000 group discussions, 56,000 household visits, 20,000 video presentations, 4,000 theatre performances, 1500 radio emissions, 250 school presentations, and 350 presentations to women's and youth groups took place. In total, nearly 175,000 IEC sessions were held (Amon, 2000, p. 4).[19]

PLAN is conscious of philosophies of edutainment and participatory methodology when it commissions media products. Many of PLAN's productions are done by CESPA, the *Centre de Services de production audiovisuells*, a center established by the UN, and one that specializes in participatory methodologies. CESPA producers and videographers were trained in formative research techniques (Dagron, 2001, pp. 115–120). In cases where there is no formal pre-testing, the development of information materials is carefully supervised by PLAN staff, all Malian nationals. After production, materials are circulated through the networks of community health workers. These individuals provide feedback as to what works and what does not. This information is recycled into the next creative project.

PLAN International, like so many INGOs, has built up a formidable record of accomplishments in the area of AIDS awareness in Mali. They have worked to destigmatize HIV/AIDS and in so doing have promoted care and support for the ill. And they have begun to tackle questions related to particular cultural aspects of Malian society and the danger of AIDS, namely levirate and sororate marriages and the risks that female genital cutting poses for the transmission of AIDS.

Mali has a wealth of dedicated operatives working to stem the tide of a growing epidemic. Mali benefits from the talent of clever artisans and gifted musicians, trained playwrights, and skilled audio-visual producers. Theoretically, these and other media are coordinated at CNIECS, the *Centre Nationale d'Information, Education, et de Communication pour La Santé*. A few times a year, CNIECS sets aside time on the calendar devoted to AIDS information. During these focal points, all the media are enjoined to participate in AIDS awareness activities. Unfortunately, there appear to be months of "dry spells" where there is relatively little attention placed on the AIDS issue. This is caused partly by a lack of funding and partly by the absence of an overall AIDS media plan.

The CNIECS seems to act more like a clearinghouse than like a campaign organizer, more like a cheer-leader than a master-helmsman. What Mali lacks is a master campaign strategist overseeing Mali's national Information AIDS campaign.[20] Those responsible for the coordinating the AIDS awareness campaigns in Mali have medical rather than media backgrounds. More effort must be made to coordinate the efforts of sizable networks of rural NGO, national radio and television, and 148-odd community, private, religious, and party owned radio sta-

---

19. PLAN International administered a project worth $7 million over a five-year period. One half of the funds came from USAID and one half was raised from PLAN's donors.

20. Evaluation reports bemoan the lack of coordination of the AIDS awareness campaigns in Mali at the government level (See *Plan Stratégique* 1999, p. 13; see also Amon 2000, p. 44).

tions. This is paramount if Mali is to retain her relatively low infection rate and avert the heartbreaking epidemic of some of her neighbors.

Review Questions

1. How have aspects of South Africa's history, its economy, and its social and political life combined to foster in 2002, the world's highest number of cases of HIV/AIDS?
2. How does the DramAide methodology help to diagnose social problems surrounding HIV/AIDS in South Africa and how does it help to change the social conditions it addresses?
3. What aspects of Mali's social and economic profile make it vulnerable to the HIV/AIDS epidemic? Are there aspects of Mali's country profile that you think may help to protect that country from the kind of devastating HIV/AIDS epidemic plaguing South Africa?

Chapter 4

Performance

This chapter provides an overview of performance, and is designed to introduce the four substantive performance chapters that appear in Part II of the book. The chapter is divided into several parts. Part 1 defines performance and then looks at the nature of performance in Africa. Part 2 considers how African performance traditions differ from those of the West. By way of contrast, it also briefly surveys the role of literacy and other forces of modernity in the evolution of Western historical and spiritual traditions. Part 3 considers the historical neglect of popular cultural studies by academics and relates this to the study of performance. Part 4 presents a range of communication theories that incorporate notions of drama and performance. And part 5 reviews theories of theatre and performance in development. In so doing, it raises the question that asks what gives performance its special power in Africa. This question informs all of the substantive performance chapters that are to follow. The theoretical discussion concerning the power of performance in Africa is again be taken up in Chapter 9.

Nature of Performance in Africa

Performance involves the intentional use of the human body (or parts thereof) by human actors in a series of structured or patterned actions designed to create meaning for a community of participants or spectators. Performance in Africa involves such obvious genres as singing, recitation, and storytelling; dance, drumming, and puppetry; and various forms of mime, masking, and theatre. Performance is also contained in the more "mediated" arts such as radio, TV, film or video production, and some of their "streamed" multi-media and interactive variants. Finally, performance in Africa also includes religious worship, religious and secular rituals, festivals, and parades.

Anyone who has attended a genuine African performance, one performed in its natural context, has been struck by the dynamism of African performance, by the power it holds over both performers and audiences. One may wish to know why this is so. This chapter explores these issues and is inspired by the power African performance has had on me.

The Oral Tradition

As noted in Chapter 1, Africa is a continent that lived, until quite recently, predominantly in the oral tradition. This means that entire traditions have grown up without the aid of texts as storage devices for information. Elsewhere I have argued that the oral tradition has made interpersonal communication in Africa somewhat different from that of the West.[1] I have shown that where there are no libraries, no places where people are able to look up stored facts, people's knowledge about the environment, their history, their genealogy, their means of survival, their religious beliefs, their moral codes, and so on, are all stored in non-text form. Some of this knowledge is entrusted to specialists who guard the information jealously and in secret, passing it down by word of mouth to their successors. Religious rites, healing lore, and rituals of divination are traditionally handled in this way. Other knowledge is more openly shared with the general public. Local history, environmental information, or moral teaching, for example, might be manifest in the form of stories, songs, or proverbs recited by elders or by historical specialists known as bards or griots. (See Chapters 5 and 6). Still other knowledge might remain the purview of distinct groups segregated by age or occupation who would each possess a body of lore encoded in such oral forms as songs, stories, or proverbs.

What must be understood about all this cultural material in oral societies, all of these genres is, once again, that they have no prior existence somewhere else as texts. Rather they exist in the individual and collective memories of the people and that these memories are stirred up or recalled through performance. Indeed in such oral societies people call up knowledge through the use of rhyming proverbs, rhythmic refrains, assonanced couplets and other pneumonic devices. Performers also remember stories through the use of cliched characters and archetypal tales. And they call up this knowledge, (i.e. they draw it out of storage) by reciting it, by telling it aloud, and by performing it with their bodies. *It is through externalization, through performance, that knowledge in these societies is made present.* The creation of knowledge through performance is then, in most senses, artistic.

It is equally important to note that the creation of knowledge in oral societies is a social preoccupation as well as an artistic one. A performance requires the participation of at least two persons. One performer and one audience member at the very least are needed, though bigger groups are better. This means that knowledge or reality in traditional societies is essentially dialogic. It is not recognized as fact unless at least two people share or confirm it. Africans regard knowledge as well as artistic production as something "which is called to be" i.e., something that is generated from the sociality of the community (Ojaide, 1996, p. 20). The private aesthetic vision of the artist, so typical of Western artistic forms, is alien to the traditional African mindset.[2] Indeed the notion of community suffuses all African art and performance. For art and performance must always have a social purpose, at the very least to pay tribute to the community and its values, the values which have nurtured its citizens. Indeed, Africans expect functionality in their art and in their performance. And that functionality should be a moral one.

---

1. See Bourgault, 1995, Chapter 1.

2. Persons who spend too much time alone, and/or persons with highly idiosyncratic worldviews are considered powerful and sometimes dangerous. Such is the behavior of the diviner who consorts with positive life forces and of witches or wizards who consort with evil.

The oral tradition that helps to foster communal values is also useful in explaining how knowledge operates in oral societies. With its dialogic discourse, the oral tradition insures that tales are told in "story like" ways for easy recall, and that these "story like" ways, having a narrative rhetorical style, govern thought. Stories told aloud structure information in such a way that the listener knows who the "good guys" are, and who the "bad guys" are. And their performance ensures that the audience knows for whom to root. Stories feature characters that are larger than life and therefore whose motivations are fairly unambiguous. Sensitive to group dynamics, storytellers are careful to make their audience feel they are part of the "in crowd." They do this by attributing evil, bad weather, poor farming to the out-group, to "those people over there," to the alien neighbors. Orally held information is sometimes seen as being aggressive. Agonistic is a word that is used to describe it (Ong, 1982, pp. 43–45).

Non-Discursive Symbol Systems

The oral tradition, as I have just described, accounts for or provides for verbal knowledge in traditional societies, including African ones. But the question of how non-verbal or non-discursive knowledge is stored is even more intriguing and complex. How is knowledge stored kinesthetically? What are the meanings of the complex rhythmic steps and slaps that make up the South African gumboot dance? What does the audience of a South African male gumboot dance understand when male dancers lift their legs and stomp their boots. And what does it mean to post-Apartheid audiences when they see females performing the gumboot? How does a troupe of Dan dancers of Cote d'Ivoire, West Africa, know which movements to use in order to call given spirits in a stilt dance? And what happens to the meaning of this dance when steps are altered? What is the significance of mythical animals depicted in a masquerade? In which ways is the significance of such a performance diminished when a masquerade is performed in a non-sacred context? The interpretation of these intricate patterned non-verbal symbol systems involves complex semiotic questions that can only be answered through painstaking historical and contemporary analyses of each genre. But a primary step along this path involves an appreciation of the overall spirituality that is the foundation of performance in Africa.

Africans are generally spiritually minded people, and the life of the spirits is generally ever present in their consciousness. While this is especially true of African villages, it can also be true in Africa cities.

African traditional life is focused around family and kin groups who are intimately tied to the cosmos through departed relatives or ancestors. Africans are expected to honor their ancestors, and by extension, the gods through the frequent observance of a number of rituals, both large and small. The relationship is one of reciprocity and the ancestors are expected to respond to their commemoration by showering blessings on the living. The ancestors are considered to be ever present and rather deeply involved in the affairs of the living. Those ignored are expected to wreak havoc on hapless living kin, sending them job loss, debilitating pestilence, freak accidents, ill health, foul weather, or a host of other calamities.

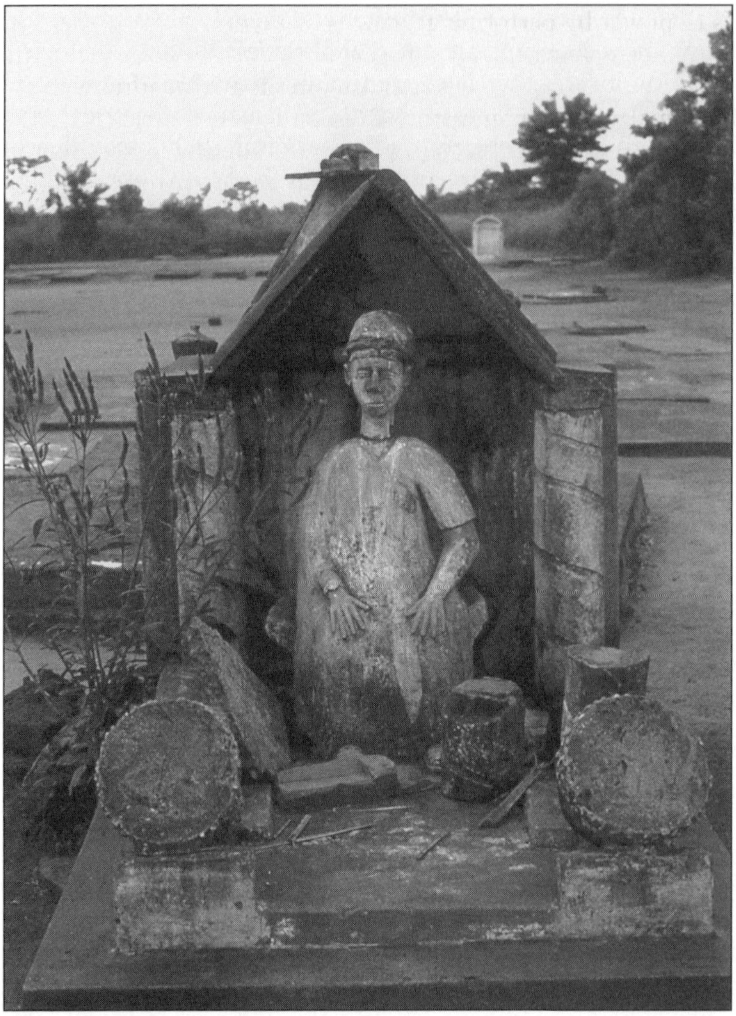

Figure 4-1. Family graves in coastal Togo are built to show respect for deceased elders. This grave-shrine bears evidence that appropriate rituals to this ancestor have been performed.

Besides having contact with departed kin or lineage members, many Africans, especially artists and performers, enjoy a special bond with deceased patrons. These might be unrelated persons, master drummers, dancers, diviners, drama instructors or even academic teachers or other persons who played an important role in imparting artistry to a pupil. Living protegees of these masters are expected to publicly acknowledge their deceased patrons within the course of any live performance.

In many traditional African societies power was maintained through secret societies. Secret societies were the place where human power and spiritual power met in order to govern the affairs of the community. Human members of these societies, through the collective power vested in the group, would tap into spiritual power in order to govern effectively. These society members would often gain access to power by performing secret trance or masquerade performances in hidden places outside normal social boundaries. Such performances often helped members of the secret society to assume an alternative identity, such as the identity of an animal spirit or ancestor (Bellman 1984; Bourgault 1989; Schwab 1947). Even in societies not steeped in secrecy, political power in Africa is regarded as intimately connected with spiritual forces (Arens and Karp, 1989, xvii). Performance, always done for a social purpose, should therefore underscore the moral order. Performance in Africa is on some level, then necessarily didactic. It is intended to convey information and instruction.

Nature of Performance in the West

It may be difficult for Westerners to grasp some of the concepts described herein. This is because our consciousness has been deeply affected by historical processes that began in the 1400s, trends that led to secularism and materialism. These historical shifts were related to the development of Protestantism, the invention and spread of printing, and the birth of industrial capitalism.

Westerners with any religious training or background are most likely to have experienced the religious traditions of Reformation Protestantism.[3] Most of these Protestant churches have historically featured denuded and ascetic worship styles, an emphasis on literacy and rationally-based approaches to religious knowledge, and a reliance on a distant male God and his local (and largely male representatives), the clergy.

Those schooled in the Roman Catholic/Eastern Orthodox faith may find some of the African concepts of spirituality somewhat easier to grasp or appreciate. This is because many medieval traditions, or remnants of them, persist to this day in Catholicism. The relationship of the African ancestors might be similar to the relationship held between a medieval Catholic settlement and the patron saint of that community who may have founded a monastery at that site. The relationship between an individual Catholic and his/her private patron saint (or his/her guardian angel) in the Middle Ages would be akin to that of say an African drummer to his deceased teacher.

The special power of the Catholic priest to transform the bread into the body of Christ is akin to the ability of a diviner to transform a set of ritual objects into an arrangement with predictive power. It is fitting to use the Catholic example because the Roman Catholic or Orthodox mass incorporates an ancient ritual of transformation in which the sacrifice of the crucifixion is believed, not merely to be symbolized, but indeed to be reenacted through the mystery of the transubstantiation.[4] Christians, whose religious background is Reformation Protes-

---

3. Reformation Protestant groups are thought commonly to include Lutheranism and its various branches; Calvinism in its various manifestations, i.e., Presbyterian, Baptist, and Dutch Reformed Conventions; Anglican or Episcopalian Conventions, and certain branches of Methodism, among others.

4. Webster defines the transubstantiation as the miraculous change by which according to Roman Catholic and Eastern Orthodox dogma, the eucharistic elements at their

tantism, are accustomed to worship services that merely recall through symbolism the sacrifice of the Redemption. Only the Catholic and Orthodox rites claim to recreate it.

The Reformation is an important watershed in this discussion because it signaled the end of the Middle Ages and ushered in the era known as "modernity." The movement towards Protestantism began in 1517 with the posting of Martin Luther's 95 complaints against Roman Catholic Church practices. In issuing his complaints Luther hoped to bring about reforms that would purify the Catholic Church and cleanse the Church of its artistic, performative, and ritual excess. Luther started a firestorm in the church that eventually led to his excommunication. This was not a consequence he anticipated. Meanwhile Luther's Protestant Reformation did lead to new trends in art, fashion, and religious worship. And religious movements and sects inspired by Luther are indicative of the rather modest and unceremonious religious tastes of 16th century Europe that he brought into fashion. Puritan churches, puritan fashions, and puritan values as depicted in early American colonial history and literature are also reflective of these trends.

Spirituality in these Protestant contexts was decidedly stark. Worship involved somber singing in stripped-down, undecorated churches; sermons from dour male authority figures, working as stand-ins for a distant male God; complete with private contemplation of Christian mysteries and individualized prayer.

The Protestant Reformation is noteworthy in this context for another reason. The Reformation of the 16th century gave rise to the so-called "Protestant ethic" that was so supportive of the nascent mercantile capitalism. The Protestant ethic endorsed hard work, eschewed excesses of celebration and pageantry, and generally launched the Western world on a trajectory that separated work from play (Weber 1958).

Historians also closely relate the Protestant Reformation to the development of printing. Printing, it should be recalled, was developed in 1455 and it had spread throughout Europe by the early 1500s. It was because of printing that Martin Luther's 95 complaints about the Catholic Church came to be disseminated so widely throughout Europe. And it was because of the availability of new Bibles, printed in vernaculars, that people were in a position to read for themselves. The development of printing led to the end of the Middle Ages, an age in which knowledge had been rhymed, the accounts had been read aloud, and the law had been what local custom said it was.

Meanwhile printing made information a commodity and began a revolution in knowledge that paved the way for several other historical processes. Besides the Reformation of the 16th century, these included the Age of Enlightenment of the 17th and 18th centuries, the Industrial Revolutions of the 19th century, and the Scientific Revolution of the 19th and 20th centuries (Burke, 1991, pp. 67–77; Crowley and Heyer, 1991, pp. 79–123). By the 18th century knowledge had become text based. Unwritten knowledge, the knowledge of the unschooled (that of women and peasants) was less and less respected.

---

consecration become the body and blood of Christ while keeping only the appearance of bread and wine.

Printing, the literacy it fostered, and the historical developments that came in its wake served to distance the world of spirits, the non-material world from the world of Western humankind. And over the centuries the Western world came more and more to rely on texts, i.e., written documentation as the basis of knowledge. As the Western world grounded itself in texts and text-based knowledge, the value of folk art and folk wisdom attenuated. Indeed, the history of the modern Western period (roughly 1500–2000 AD) is a history of the decline of belief in non-codified systems of human knowledge and interaction: common law, folk medicine, midwifery, and women's intuition (Thompson, 1989, pp. 3–42). Meanwhile, over the course of 500 or so years, performance became a specialized form of expression associated chiefly with entertainment and leisure.

Popular Culture in the "Academy"

If concern for the arts has seemed frivolous during much of the modern period, the study of folk and popular art has appeared even more so. This is because these forms were associated with common unlettered folk. And performance art, including improvisational music, street theatre, folk and popular dance, mime, and storytelling have suffered the most because these forms were not scored and therefore lacked the respectability of the "high arts." [5]

The academic study of popular performance genres is a phenomenon that dates only from the twentieth century. And serious attention to African performance on its own terms dates only from the last half of the last century. The study of popular performance or rather its neglect can be understood by taking a look at the attitude of the West regarding performance art forms. For the popular performing arts have suffered from a number of biases in Western scholarship. These include an inherent secularism in the Western social sciences, a preference for the study of texts, and a class and gender bias.

African performance has also been a field vastly understudied in the humanities and social sciences. Apart from the sheer logistical difficulty of studying African performance, the area has also been neglected for the same reasons that account for its neglect in the West. Many African performance genres have long been perceived and classified as popular art or popular culture, and hence have been deemed unworthy of study until the late 1960s. And African performance genres, moreover, bereft of scripts or scores, lack a textual basis for study.

---

5. High arts are art forms that are thematically complex and often require special training or knowledge in order to be appreciated. Displaying the virtuosity of an individual genius, high art forms depict a rather singular view of the world through the lens of the artist. Bearing the hallmarks of a literate world, high performance art was typically scored. Some examples include opera, ballet, symphonic and liturgical music. These were performance genres that got the attention of scholars, though until quite recently, such scholars concentrated more on the texts of performances than the actual performances themselves.

Popular Art in Africa

Popular art is a type of art that emerged in the Western world in conjunction with urbanization and industrialization. Sometimes called kitsch, popular art lacks the thematic complexity of high arts and the cultural authenticity of folk art. Popular art emerged in the 19th century as an art form designed to serve the leisure needs of the newly industrialized masses. Mass produced popular art is sold for profit.

Although Africa never witnessed an industrial revolution similar to that of Europe in the 19th century, it has seen enormous movement to the cities in the 20th century. Art that has emerged after colonial contact, especially in urban multi-ethnic contexts is called African "popular art." Such genres include, for example, the visual arts of painting and photography; the performing arts of popular street theatre, concert parties, and electrified musical concerts; and the processional genres of parades, fairs, and rallies. It also includes such hybrid genres such as photo-novels, radio narratives, television serials, feature-length "video-films,"[6] and cinema. Although this art in Africa is commonly referred to as popular art, it tends to be more quirky, less manufactured, and less standardized than its Western counterpart. This is because its production is still executed at the hands of individual artists rather than by a manufacturing process. Moreover, as noted above, the product or artifact of African popular art is likely to contain a moral lesson intended by the creator and expected by the consumer. Indeed even modern popular African art anticipates group, rather than private, enjoyment in building the moral sensibility of a community. For these reasons, the profit motive of this African popular art may be less evident than in its Western counterpart. At best it is the product of a cottage industry (rather than a multinational corporation) which still retains it craft-approach to its product.

Ethnic Art in Africa

African popular art exists in contrast to what has been called in the context of African studies, "Ethnic Art." This is the art that existed on the African continent prior to the colonial period. This is the art that comes to mind in the West when the subject of African art is raised. This art includes masks and carving and the performances they suggest; bronze and clay statuary and pottery; ornamental decoration for the body and for the dwelling; weaving and textiles; music and dance; storytelling and song; and poetry and recitation. This art was initially included in studies of different "tribes" by colonial officers who used ethnographies to classify the peoples whom they governed.[7] The officers were often helped by anthropologists who produced surveys of geographically contiguous peoples.

6. The term "video film" refers to a genre of locally produced feature-length fictional format productions made with analog or digital video equipment, distributed on VHS format for private use and also shown in renovated cinema halls to paying customers. The "video film" industry is a cottage industry in West Africa, notably in Ghana and Nigeria.

7. The field of anthropology was founded during the imperial period of Western history and is tainted with its participation in the colonial past. The term "tribe" was used extensively during the colonial period and has been criticized for its imprecision and its

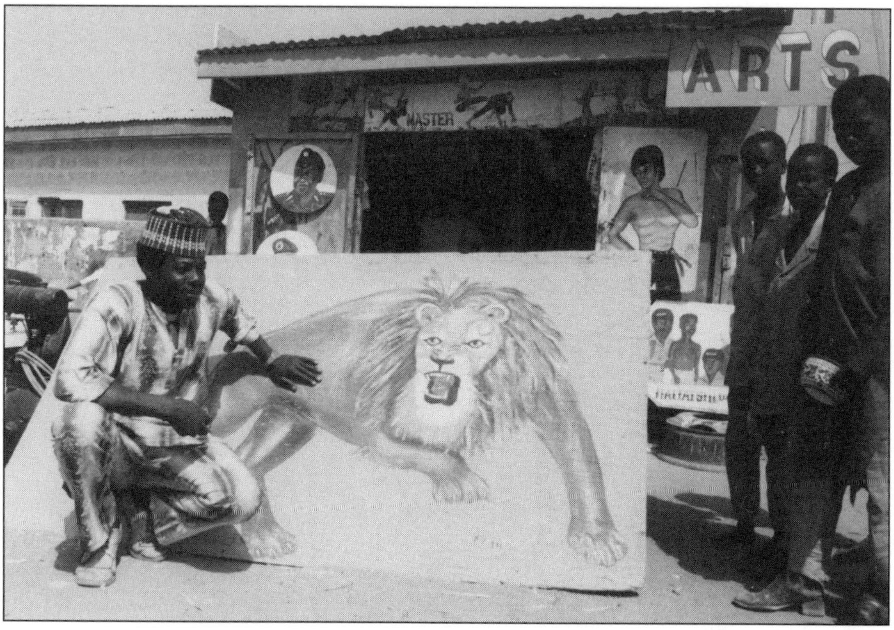

Figure 4-2. Sign painting is a form of popular art commonly found in African cities.

This volume will concern itself with performance genres, genres that clearly span the divide between African popular art and so-called African ethnic art. This is because village performance traditions still thrive in their own right and because they continue to underpin and to inspire performance in Africa's cities. Indeed the study of the way these traditions have adapted to new urban conditions falls well within the realm of performance studies and is touched upon in several of the genre chapters.

Although popular urban African art has suffered from scholarly neglect, (for reasons already mentioned), village based performance in Africa has fared somewhat better. The field of anthropology has been described somewhat derisively as the study of people and societies most unlike ourselves (Worth 1972, p. 351). Long preoccupied with studies of kinship (who has blood ties to whom, and how they are related to those in power), it did give some attention to performance, particularly as it related to religious ritual and to the maintenance of power.

Indeed, like any discipline, anthropology has enjoyed its share of fads and fashions over the years. For many years anthropology's primary interest in performance lay in explaining how ritual and other symbolic behavior was functional to the maintenance of individual psychological balance[8] or to the mainte-

over-determination of differences between peoples. Because of its association with imperialism and its implied notions of inferiority and "governablity," when applied to a group of people, the term "tribe" is considered politically incorrect. The term ethnic group is today the preferred term used today to refer to people who ascribe their descent to a common ancestor.

8. See Malinowski, 1948, pp. 1–67.

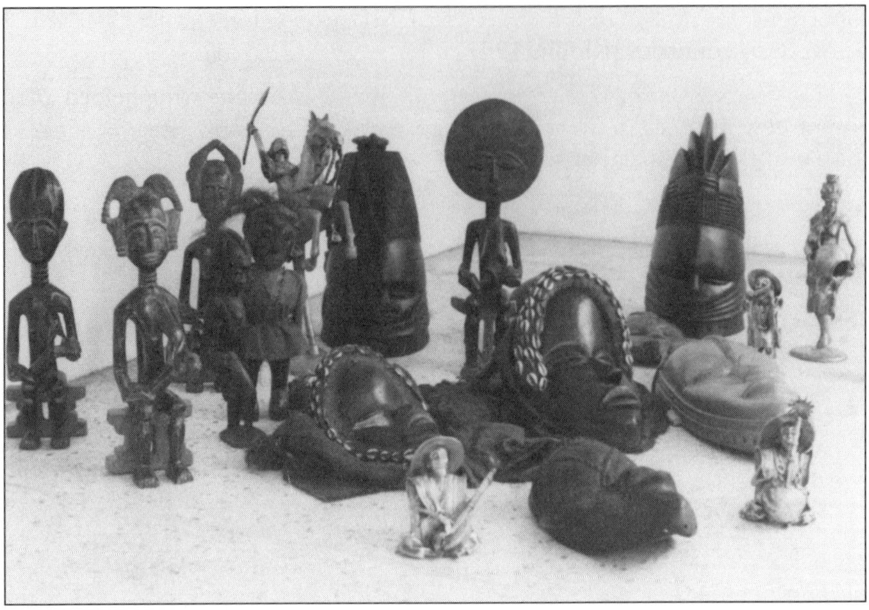

Figure 4-3. Most African art that is referred to as "ethnic art" was intimately connected to the maintenance of continuity between African life and the world of the ancestors.

nance of social ties in the existing social order of a given ethnic group.[9] The problem with both of the paradigms of functionalism and structuralism in anthropology is that each failed to account for social change that was clearly happening all of the time. Indeed these anthropological studies, failed to look at how "ethnic arts" and performance mediate experience for people. Moreover, they eschewed the study of African performance in urban contexts presumably because urban Africans were somehow too much like Westerners.

The 1960s appear to have been a great watershed in many scholarly fields including performance studies and anthropology. For one thing, social criticism took a decidedly demonstrative twist, as people marched in rallies, sat in "sit-ins," loved in "love-ins," and generally communicated their thoughts and feelings about social phenomena in communal, public, and performative ways. The 1960s was also a time in the United States of growing consciousness of diversity within American society. Again, our diversity became apparent through a series of *Movements* (emphasis to be noted) which drew strength from marches and other performances. The first of these, the Civil Rights Movement eventually gave rise to numerous movements of the 1960s/1970s: the Black Pride, Black Consciousness, and Black Power Movements; the Indian Rights Movement; the Feminist Movement; the Gay Rights Movement, and so on. All of these groups had long celebrated and maintained their identity at least in part through the use of non-lexical (non text-based) codes. The sixties, incidentally was also a time when U.S. immigration proportions shifted for the first time, away from high

9. See Durkheim 1961.

proportions of Europeans, to include higher proportions of new arrivals from non-Western countries (Kloph, 1991, p. 6).

This chapter will now review a number of scholars who helped to bring about a new appreciation for performance and its role first in human communication and then in social change.

Theories of Ritual, Communication, and Performance

Origins of Ritual

One scholar whose work on ritual is seminal to this discussion is Harvard philosopher Suzanne Langer whose *Philosophy in a New Key* (1976) laid out her theory of symbolism. Langer argued that there are two important types of symbolism. Language, or discursive symbolism, which communicates rational propositions, and ritual, or presentational (non-discursive) symbolism which transmits emotions or feeling. Langer noted that discursive symbolism was made up of individual units that could be combined and recombined in order to create meaning. Presentational symbolism, she argued, could not be divided into distinct units or bits. One had to experience the entire ritual to derive its meaning. Langer's work was important because it focused academic thought in the area of emotion in human experience. Moreover, it attributed rationality to feeling (generated by ritual) (Langer, 1976, pp. 79–143).

Langer's groundbreaking work was a study in the symbolism of reason, rite, and art. Langer was concerned among other things with the origin of ritual. She argued that rituals originated in ancient times in self-expression. Primitive humans looked around, contemplated the universe, and became excited by the power of some aspect of the cosmos: the brightness of the stars; the power of ocean currents; and the fierce cunning of hunted animals. Their first utterance was an affective gesture or cry: a shout, a prancing, or a rolling on the earth, i.e., demonstrations of feeling. Langer argued that these expressions were contagious and were soon taken up by the individual's neighbors, who wished to fall into step with the expression. Such expressions soon became routinized, (i.e. *they turned into ritual*). The gestures, no longer expressions of sentiment, came to symbolize the referents (the great powers) which first inspired them (Langer, 1976, p. 152). Drawing from Langer then, *ritual is be defined herein as a patterned enactment of symbolic behavior performed by a group.*

Two scholars of non-verbal communication, Paul Ekman and Wallace Friesen are important in this context for the work they have done on non-linguistic-based communication. Ekman and Friesen's (1975) work shows there is remarkable consistency across cultures in the ways humans facially display six basic emotions of fear, anger, sadness, disgust, happiness, and surprise. And these sentiments are readily recognizable across cultures and appear to be universal. Even more compelling is the research conducted by these same scholars among primates, particularly chimpanzees. These studies demonstrate a remarkable likeness between chimpanzees and humans in the way both groups facially express the basic six emotions. Ekman and Friesen conclude from the above studies that these emotional displays are biologically based (i.e., "hard wired") into the human limbic system. As we shall see further along in this discussion, these hard-wired expressions (innate responses) appear to have been ritualized into important public performances of myth and religious belief. This fact alone suggests that the raw material of ritual display is of very ancient origin, and may even pre-date modern human consciousness.[10]

Interpersonal Communication as Performance

The field of interpersonal communication has contributed handsomely to performance theory. This is particularly true of those scholars known for theories of symbolic interaction and theories of drama. Broadly, these authors argue that meaning is created through, and sustained by, interaction in the social group. Interaction establishes, maintains, and alters certain conventions—roles, norms, rules, and meanings—within a social group or culture. Those conventions constitute the reality of a given culture.

One communication scholar whose work laid the foundation for the dramatistic school was George Herbert Mead. Mead argued that people are actors, not reactors. And he defined a communication act as involving two persons and three movements: one person/movement to initiate the act, one person/movement to respond to the act, and two persons/movements to perceive the meaning. Human beings use symbols in their communication, the meaning of which is negotiated in the process of interacting with others (Mead 1934). Symbolic interactionism, like many theories of the first half of the 20th century,[11] stressed the importance of ***conscious*** interpretation of symbols and behaviors. As we shall see below, many ritual theories taken from the anthropologists allow for the transmission of ideas *not* consciously processed. It should be noted that the ritual view of communication grew out of many sources including the symbolic interactionist perspective.

Symbolic Interactionist theories came to influence a set of communication theories known as dramatistic theories or theories of dramatism. Dramatists see people as actors on a metaphorical stage interacting with others, all playing out roles. Two important dramatistic communication theorists were Kenneth Burke and Erving Goffman.

Kenneth Burke put forward the theory of social drama. Burke recognized that humankind's ability to manipulate sophisticated symbols helped people to rise beyond their pure animal nature. He recognized two levels of activity in humans, motion: which humans and animals have in common, and action: the pur-

10. The search for evidence of symbolic behavior, especially ritual behavior in the immediate ancestors of modern humans continues. At this point it is unclear to what extent *Homo erectus* manipulated symbols. And less is known about whether this species buried their dead.

11. George Herbert Mead's *Mind, Self*, and *Society* was published posthumously.

poseful and voluntary behaviors of individual humans only. The second makes use of symbol systems through which humans create societies that are inherently hierarchical or otherwise unequal. Individuals must find ways of coping with their neighbors who occupy different positions in the pecking order and from whom they are inherently divided. People's social interactions are dramatic enactments of their positions in society. Social interaction is infused with four conditions listed by Burke: ***guilt, mystification, victimage,*** and ***redemption.*** An individual feels guilt, (alternatively shame, embarrassment, anger, self-loathing, disgust) because he or she is less powerful, less good, or less accomplished than someone else with whom he or she interacts. Individuals communicate to purge their guilt, i.e., they devise explanations for their failings. These explanations are proffered to others. Individuals feel a sense of mystery when interacting with others who occupy different positions in the social hierarchy. The differences fascinate both parties. This is mystification. But hierarchies, (i.e., social systems with built-in inequality) must supply mechanisms to purge individuals and the group of their collective guilt. Hierarchies find scapegoats that they punish for the collective guilt felt by everyone. This is victimage and it leads to group redemption wherein the group is collectively purged of guilt.

Another dramaturgical communication theorist is Erving Goffman. Goffman argued that people structure every day events as performances designed to make an impression on others (their audiences). When people approach a communication situation, they first ask themselves what sort of a performance is going on. They define a situation in terms of the way they are able to organize in their own minds what they see happening on a kind of social stage. Events, according to Goffman, are made up of strips of arbitrary activities. Several strips make up a frame. A man reading on a sofa get up, picks up a leash, calls his dog, attaches the leash to the dog's collar, and leads him outside. The last five strips make up a frame Goffman would call "walking the dog."

Goffman pioneered the technique of Frame Analysis that is a technique for examining the way an individual organizes experience (Goffman 1974). Frame analysis is a very useful tool for communicators because it sensitizes them to the need to know where others are "coming from." It has excellent application to the developing world where persons may be assigned to fairly fixed social roles,—mother, wife, village blacksmith, chief, for example. Clearly each of these individuals would frame experience differently from one another and would communicate accordingly. And all of their public behavior would be judged in terms of whether each fulfills the expectations of his/her roles.

Goffman argued that those engaged in conversations were not so much exchanging information as telling a story starring themselves. He allowed that we all have many "selves." To be effective, he observed, communicators need to make both judgments about the nature of the frame at hand; and selections of the appropriate "self" to frame. In other words they need to respond effectively to two questions: "what is going on here?" and "which self will I present in this story?" Goffman stressed the importance of self-presentation in the management of a person's image. Goffman's discussions stress the *cognitive* capacity of the self to organize mini-dramas of self-presentation. And he assumes that those perceiving information about the presented self are also making a *cognitive* assessment of the performance (Geertz, 1983, pp. 23–26).

A Ritual View of Communication

The field of communication is concerned with how human beings use codes to inform one another of their needs and desires, to create a community, and to ensure the survival of the group. For a long time, the field of communication looked mainly at the way messages were created and extended through geographical space from one individual to another or to the group. This view of communication placed great emphasis on the content of the messages, particularly their ability to inform or to influence. This approach to communication has been called the "transportation view of communication." More recently, communication scholars have focused their study on the way communication supports society in time. This view is less concerned with the content of these messages than with "the creation, representation, and celebration of shared beliefs" (Carey, 1975, p. 177). It is a ritual view of communication.

A ritual view of communication is especially concerned with the human tendency to wrap oneself in symbols, or as anthropologist Clifford Geertz has called them, "webs of significance" (1973, p. 5). A ritual view of communication is fully conscious of the fact that people use symbolic codes both to make meaning, and to find meaning in their lives. Humans do not just eat their fill, as do animals, humans surround the act of eating with symbols. They dine. Humans do not simply satisfy sexual urges through mating, they surround biological sexuality with courtship rituals or dating games. Sometimes, they even "fall in love!" Humans don't just walk away from a deceased member of their community, they organize a funeral to send the deceased off to the afterlife. And they construct a belief system to make that afterlife plausible. The ritual view of communication studies how communication is used to sustain these "webs of significance."

The ritual view of communication is useful because it describes both how rituals communicate and why communication is so ritualistic. Briefly, rituals operate by muting individuality so as to bind people together with a common set of beliefs, values and practices, into a cohesive group. Communication is ritualistic because its power lies less in the content of its messages, than in the comfortingly familiar form it takes among people who share common social bonds.

The ritual view of communication is also useful because it can account for social change. The view argues that all communication occurs through an exchange of symbols. Some of these symbols are denotative, i.e., they are signs which stand for discrete things. The sign appearing in a parking lot and showing a wheelchair, for example, stands for, or denotes, the idea of parking for the disabled. Other symbols are connotative, that is, they contain meanings which are both concrete and meanings which are emotionally charged. The American flag, for example, denotes or stands for the country of the United States of America. The flag conjures up many different feelings in the hearts of beholders. The same flag may create feelings of pride and loyalty among Gulf War Veterans, but sentiments of ambivalence and shame among some Vietnam Vets. Because communication occurs between at least two persons, each can and does use symbols to which they attach slightly different connotative meanings. This is because (as observed by Burke) meanings are "negotiated" between speaker and listener. In the "negotiation" there is great flexibility. What a symbol means one day can easily change by the next day, depending on what the two speakers bring to the joint experience at any given moment. In effect, the meaning of symbols is shifting all the time without the speakers giving much thought to a given interchange.

It is within this shifting definitional ground that professional communicators—advertising professionals, press attaches or public relations practitioners, and the like, operate to engender subtle shifts in meaning for use by their clients. These meanings are unleashed into the public record and then become part of the national discourse.

Consider the national debate over the inclusion of coverage in many health insurance plans of reproductive services for women. Some insurance companies refuse, arguing that the use of birth control devices is as elective as piercing one's ears. These same companies also argue that to cover birth control is to imply that pregnancy is a disease. With opposing views, proponents of this same coverage argue that birth control is an essential component of women's total health care needs. They add further that to refuse birth control coverage is to discriminate against women, the only group whose bodies are affected by pregnancy. This debate, really a debate about money, is being fought over alternative sets of definitional symbols.

Rituals, which are patterned symbolic enactments, combine whole sets of symbols whose meaning may shift over time. The Oval Office was once a symbol of respectful, sober power in American society. The meaning of this symbol has been over time "negotiated" between the American presidents and the American people. The Clinton affair with Monica Lewinsky is said to have tarnished the image of the Oval Office. If one would believe the pronouncements of pundits early in the new century, the Oval Office connotes ideas of illicit sex, marital infidelity, and public prevarication. These new shades of meaning henceforth will be factored into the meaning of the Oval Office symbol by the public for some time to come.

The President's signing of bills into law in the Oval Office is a civic ritual. It combines several symbolic elements. These include: the presidency itself, the Oval Office, the ceremonious presentation of the bill; the dramatic handing over of the pen; the theatrical flourish of the presidential hand signing the bill; and the ever-present flash of photographers' cameras documenting the historical event. All these elements are arranged in a certain processual order. If the meaning of any of the symbols has shifted or if the order of the symbols is switched, the meaning of the ritual will be altered. To proceed with our analogy, the fact that the image of the Oval Office was tarnished by Clinton's activities therein will alter the meaning of the signing of a bill. So would an extreme flourish of the presidential pen before signing. And if the cameras were to snap before the bill was signed, this would also involve a meaning shift.

The ritual theory of social change says that communicative/ritual events can shift slightly the meaning of symbols and or recombine them in new ways. Through these processes people can accommodate change in society or even usher it in. The rituals allow people to process symbolically their changing world. Ritual is seen then as a meta-communicative genre. In other words, it is a grander form of communication than that which occurs in a simple two person interchange. But it operates in the same way and has the same properties.

Ritual seems to be one of the oldest forms of communication, a form that calls us back to our early days at the dawn of civilization. It is a powerful tool for imparting group norms and imparting group solidarity. The subject of ritual will be taken up in the final chapter of the work.

Theatre and Performance in Development

Related to ritual, performative genres appear to possess some of the transformative power of ritual for those who take part. The idea that performance can promote positive development in individuals as well as groups is ancient in origin. Plato believed that education should be based upon play. And education from the 5th century BC in Greece included reading, writing, and recitations of the Greek dramatists. Greek theatre was considered an important educational instrument for the people.

During the Middle Ages, the Catholic Church used mystery and morality plays to educate the people about their faith and its core values. The plays were resurrected during the Counter-Reformation as a means to mystify the faithful, to dazzle them with drama, and to lure back Protestants possibly starved for pomp and pageantry in worship.

Performance was incorporated in formal education as a result of a number of movements. Early in the 20th century, C. Cook devised a pedagogical methodology called "the play way." This theory argued that youth should be encouraged to be active in the educational process, to experiment, and to play with ideas and lessons (Mlama, 1991, p. 26). Proponents of the American Creative Dramatics Movements and the British Theatre-in-Education Movement have worked to make performance part of the curricula in American and British schools throughout much of the 20th century.

In Africa during the pre-colonial period, as noted in Chapter 8, various forms of performance were used to socialize the young (Mlama, 1991, p. 27). During colonial times missionaries ignored or suppressed these performative genres because of their connection with traditional African religion. But when it suited the colonial masters, they promoted African performance, albeit in secularized and generally urban entertainment contexts (Mlama, 1991, p. 58).

For the last 20 years or so, the body of literature promoting the use of performative genres (particularly theatre) in development projects has been growing. Some of the impetus for using Theatre for Development has been inspired by the work of Augusto Boal. Boal's work, *Theatre of the Oppressed* (1979) advocates the use of theatrical techniques known as Forum Theatre. The Forum Theatre workshops were designed as consciousness raising exercises among the participants (poor Latin American peasants). According to Boal's theory, peasants would first be 'conscientized' through the theatrical process. With their consciousness raised, they would begin to see the source of their problems, chiefly the inequitable distribution of wealth. This would constitute the first step in their empowerment and encourage them to begin to work out solutions to their problems. In subsequent workshops, they would start to devise new plays in which

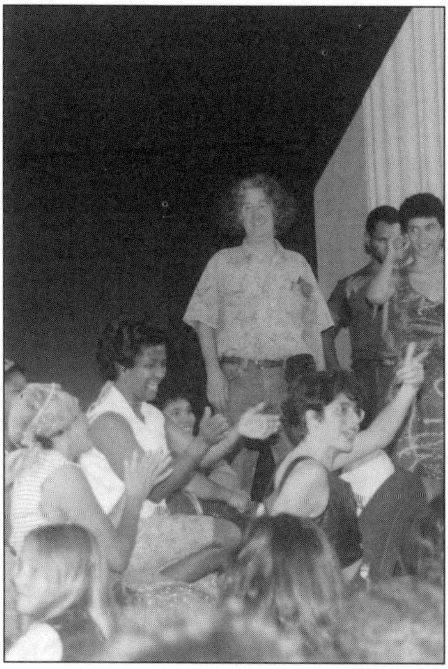

Figure 4-4. Augosto Boal conducts a Forum Theatre workshop. Photo courtesy of Doug Paterson.

the oppressed would play new and stronger roles, confronting in some fashion the oppressive individuals or the social situations the latter had created. Plays would be constructed around local problems and incidents. Plays, for example, could be crafted around issues of housing or other resource acquisition. Some examples of such problems could be, for example: the need to convince a landlord or a local official to repair leaking sewage pipes or the need to enjoin a husband to accept his wife's use of family planning techniques. Another issue might be the need to secure local entitlements such as pipe-born water or a local maternity clinic from politicians or local government representatives, for example.

According to Boal's theory, merely devising the plays was empowering to individuals. This is because it permitted the poor to imagine a world in which they exerted a bit more control over their environment. Boal saw these performances as rehearsals wherein peasants would also practice taking control over their lives. This rehearsal process can be compared to that of an employee in the corporate world who practices in private in front of a mirror the act of approaching his or her supervisor to request a pay raise.

Beyond the level of individual effectiveness, Boal argued that performing these plays was socially empowering ("conscientizing"), because plays often galvanized an entire community to address long-standing problems. And sometimes the plays could also be immediately effective in redressing long-standing grievances, as when landlords or other officials caved in to performers' demands under the pressure of public theatrical exposure. Boal's techniques, if properly implemented, are extremely powerful, even revolutionary. They should ultimately lead the oppressed to question the power structure that sustains their suppressors.

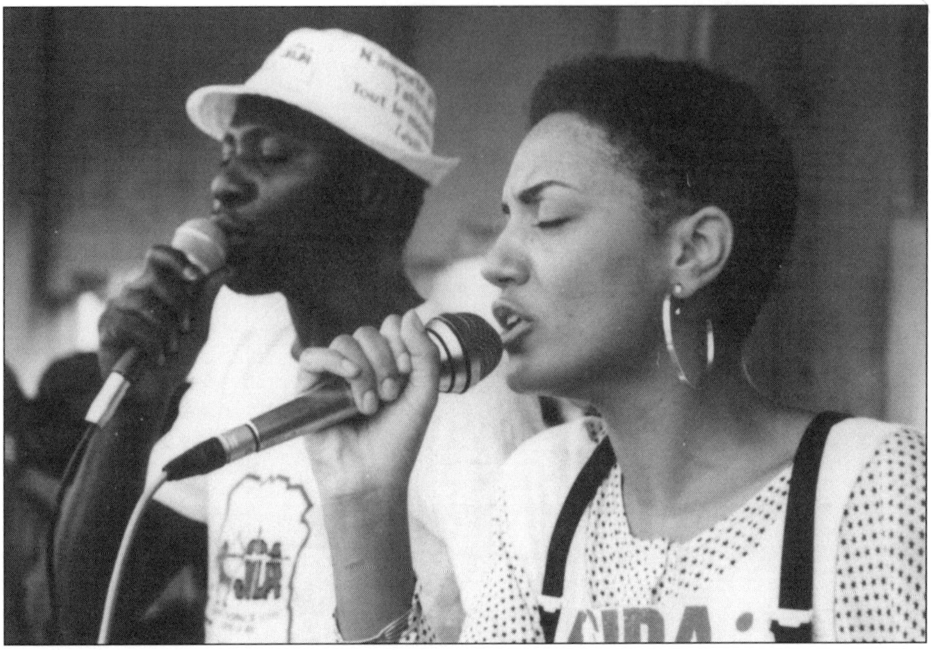

Figure 4-5. AIDS Awareness concert, Democratic Republic of the Congo. Photo courtesy of Population Services International.

Less overtly politicized, many scholars and development practitioners have advocated the use of local performance in development projects without the critical theatrical underpinnings advocated by Boal and his colleague, radical pedagogue, Paulo Freire. Such theorists and practitioners promote popular Theatre for Development not because they hope to promote radical structural changes, but because they see drama as an educational tool that seems to be both effective and practical. Locally based performance, moreover, seems inherently democratic. It avoids the pitfalls that have arisen in other development projects where communication materials produced by outsiders (both foreigners and local urban élites) have been ill suited to the needs and interests of audience members. Indeed the literature of development projects in Africa is riddled with programs gone awry partly because they were badly communicated.[12] Theater for development is seen as offering hope for better outcomes in development projects. Conceived by the people and for the people, it is inherently popular in the sense of being pleasing to audiences.[13] David Kerr's excellent volume entitled *African Popular Theatre* (1995) contains a chapter on Theatre for Development. The Kerr work details a vast number of applications of theatre to the problems of socio-economic advancement in southern Africa. And Penina Mlama's *Culture and Development* (1991) recounts her experiences "workshopping" Theatre for Development projects in Tanzania, Cameroon, and Zimbabwe (1991). Indeed theatre has emerged as a well-respected tool for development and adult education on the

12. See for example, Hornik, 1988, pp. 14–26; see also Stevenson, 1988, pp. 1–33.
13. See for example Wilson 1987; see Pratt 1989.

African continent. Gurav Desai has described a number of theatre projects used in the service of development, even though he faults these projects for falling short of their revolutionary potential as described by Augusto Boal and Paolo Freire (1990, pp. 65–92).

Today many international non-governmental organizations (INGOs) and bilateral aid agencies are actively promoting the use of theatre in their African development projects. Oxfam supports the Association for the Promotion of Senegalese Women (APROFES) that produces grassroots theatre designed to empower women (OXFAM n.d.). Plan International, ENDA Tiers Monde, and other INGOs use Theatre for Development to warn people against the spread of AIDS. So do a host of other projects supported by the bilateral aid wings of the U.S., the Canadian, and the European Union. Indeed, performance of all types is being used in conjunction with AIDS communication campaigns. The subsequent chapters will attempt to detail some of the major performance genres that are to be found on the African continent. These chapters will also examine how performance is being used to stem the spread of AIDS on the African continent.

It is unfortunate that most of the literature promoting the Theatre for Development movement fails to focus much attention on the association between ritual and performance and the profoundly transformative power of the two genres. The literature is indeed lacking in this way. Elsewhere I have argued that performances produced in Theatre for Development projects in Africa can sometimes approximate the feel, power, and transformative capacity of ritual (Bourgault 1991). Indeed as Wole Soyinka has noted, “The question of the supposed dividing line between ritual and theatre should not concern us much in Africa, the line being one that was largely drawn by the European analyst” (Soyinka, 1976, p. 5).

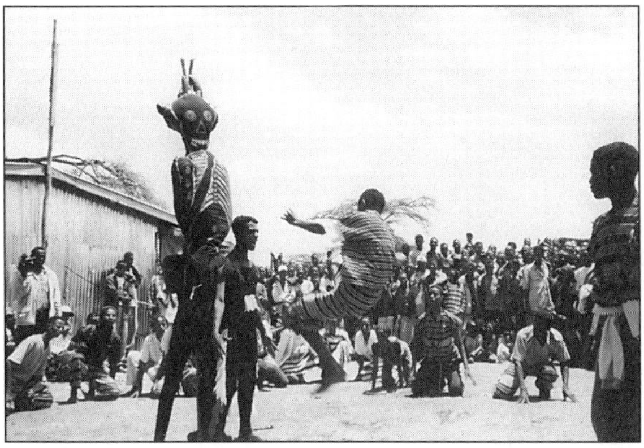

Figure 4-6. *Debub Nigat* AIDS Education Circus, Awassa, Southern Ethiopia. Awassa is supported by German and French INGOs. Photo courtesy of David Schein, Awassa Children’s Project.

Review Questions

1. In which ways is performance especially important in societies with low levels of literacy? How do these considerations impinge on the importance of ritual in such societies?

2. How did the development of literacy and texts alter the use of performance in the Western world, especially during the “modern period”?
3. How, according to Boal, does Forum Theatre work to empower people?

Part II

Performance in Africa

Chapter 5

Oral Narratives

Chapters 5 and 6 of this volume treat a subject known in literary circles as "orature," or "aurature." It refers to the vast body of African cultural forms, that existed in African societies before contact with the West and which still persist today. By and large, these forms are not housed in libraries, for they are not written down. They are stored in the memory of human beings who pass down the history, the stories, the religious knowledge, the prayers, the rituals, and the moral values of society without recourse to written records. As we shall see, they are easily applicable for use in the AIDS crisis. They can easily serve as edutainment when featured, for example, on radio. And the facility and familiarity of oral narratives renders them prime candidates for participatory methodology.

In explaining oral cultures, such as those of rural African societies, Professor Walter Ong invites us to consider a world in which "no one is ever able to look anything up" (1982, p. 31). Here knowledge must be stored in easy-to-recall formulary expressions, expressions with rhythmic patterns whose utterance triggers the recall of additional bits of information. This chapter will treat oral narratives, recitations that tell a story, often with music, sometimes without. Chapter 6 will investigate some of the stylistics of oral performance to which Ong is referring. Then it will briefly review the vast territory of chants and songs.

Social World of Oral Artists

The first point a reader should appreciate is the social nature of oral narratives. Almost without exception African performance in the form of tales, chants, or songs are meant for public consumption. If some of the renditions supplied in this text seem somewhat colorless, it may be that folktales supplied in this volume came from anthologies that eliminated the lively oral elements of the tales. This is because early scholars of folklore in the 19th and early 20th century tended to privilege the written word and considered orality a sub-standard version of the more "civilized" literary text. But we shall see that these oral tales are anything but substandard and have a particular artistic essence all their own.

Before examining the forms themselves, it is useful to look at the storytellers or oral bards. Although traditionally most persons had some ability to tell a story, genuine oral artists had considerable skill and underwent a good deal of training. The training consisted of observation and practice. A would-be bard would try to spend as much time with the story-telling elders and the village musicians as possible, listening to their tales and their music and practicing whenever he/she could. More formal training would involve a trainee moving into the home of a gifted bard and learning at his or her feet in exchange for performing domestic chores.

In many African societies, oral bards enjoy an ambivalent position. They are revered for their talent but they may be kept at a distance because of their power to use words, to speak or to sing what others by convention are not allowed to utter. And like performers in Western societies, oral bards are known to prefer their art to more conventional work, be it farming in Africa or computer programming in Western countries. So the larger public often looks upon performance artists with a dose of admiration, a hint of jealousy, and a touch of derision.

There are, of course, a wide range of social arrangements that are possible for traditional performance artists in Africa. Many societies once had court poets, whose job it was to raise up the king or the ruler. Court poets were often rewarded for their lofty words by being given a place in the chief's house, land to farm, or other valuable benefits. Some of the societies who enjoyed court poets include the Hausa of northern Nigeria, the Ashanti of Ghana, and the Zulu and Xhosa of South Africa.

In the Mande speaking areas of Guinea, Mali, Senegal, and the Gambia, court poets belonged to a hereditary caste. The court poet caste members of the Mande are called griots or *djelia* (singular *djeli*). During the time of the great empires of the West African savannas, these griots sang the praises of the kings, serving as forerunners of today's press attaches and public relations operatives. They also played a lesser role of advising the king and could even be known to provide subtle criticism of him. Today, in the absence of kings, many griots serve a range of patrons especially politicians. Indeed just as griots and other court poets used to prepare rulers psychologically for war,[1] bards of today incite politicians to campaign.

Politicians notwithstanding, many artists today simply perform for whomever will pay. Such artists are called upon to perform for religious rituals or secular ceremonies, and generally to entertain at festivals and social gatherings. One of the important roles of the griots is to maintain family histories. They do so by remembering histories of families for whom they sing. In keeping with tradition, noble families in Mande speaking and neighboring areas of West Africa,[2] may well retain a long standing relationship with a griot family who serves the family's official singing and speaking needs. The nouveau riches may seek to establish such a relationship among itinerant griots whose services are available.

Dr. Thomas Hale's volume, *Griots and Griottes* (1998), contains a job description for the modern griot. Some of the modern occupations he lists include

1. The Epic of Sundiata contains vast sections about the role of Sundiata's griot. See Okpewho, 1992, p. 26.

2. Some of the West African groups with griots include the Wolof of Senegal, the Fulani of several West African countries, the Senufo of Cote d'Ivoire, the Sonike of western Mali and southern Mauritania, the Khassonké of western Mali, the Songhai of western Niger and eastern Mali, the Moor of Mauritania, the Mossi of Burkina Faso, the Bariba of northern Benin, the Dogon of eastern Mali, the Hausa of Nigeria and Niger, the Dagbamba of northern Ghana, and the Tuareg of northern Mali, Niger, and southern Algeria.

genealogist, historian, adviser, spokesperson, mediator, interpreter and translator, musician, composer, teacher, witness, praise-singer, and ritual participant. To these might be added marriage broker, journalist, anchorperson/announcer, tourist guide/entertainer, and change agent/development communicator for government or non-governmental organizations.

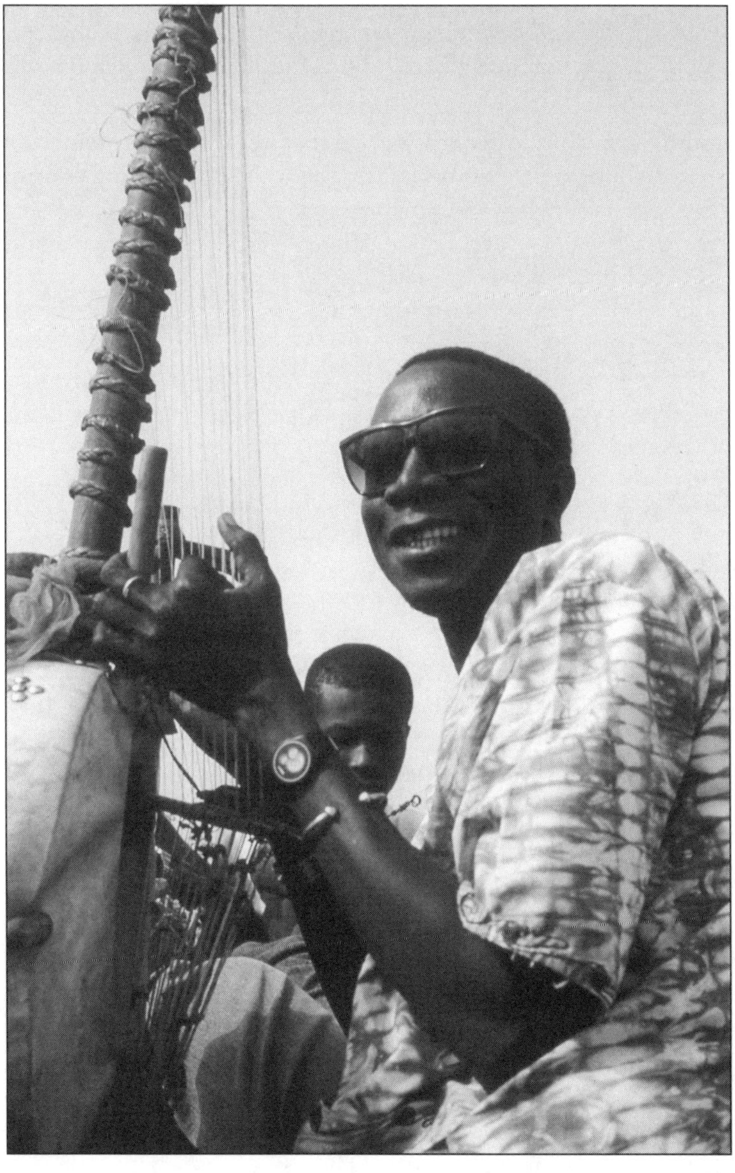

Figure 5-1. Gambian griot with 21 string kora. The Legend of Sundiata is told with accompaniment on this instrument.

Griots are part of a major social grouping in Mande society that work with well defined spiritually charged materials. This grouping, the *nyamakala*, according to Charry, include artisans who work with metal, wood, clay, leather, words and certain types of music. The second group, the nobles or *horon,* by tradition, do not engage in these craft occupations but rather practice farming, governance, and military activities. The two social groups, *horon* and *nyamakala* enjoy a complex relationship with one another that allows for checks and balances within the social system of Mande society. The *horon* class may well govern, but their behavior is controlled with great subtlety by the powers of the *nymamkala* class, particularly the griots whose power with words is both respected and feared by Mande nobles (Charry, 2000, pp. 29–62).

This author was able to record a griot that uses his art to entertain tourists who dine at Bamako, Mali's Grand Hotel. Refer to Oral Narratives.

Video 1. Griot Songs with Kora
Djeli Mory dit "Fa" at the Grand Hotel

This chapter is concerned with stories told in Africa. It will explore the nature of some of these stories together with their themes and social purposes. The chapter will conclude with two examples of the application of storytelling techniques to the struggle against AIDS.

As with any and all of the performance forms covered in this text, the classification of oral tales into types can be a problem. Some analysts, for example, have classified stories based on the protagonists, the main character, of the tale. Such a view has led to a four-part division that includes 1) animal tales, 2) human tales, 3) fairy tales, and 4) myths. But there are difficulties with this system because the categories often overlap. Animals often behave like people; people can act like animals; and spirits [fairies] can turn into people or animals during the course of the tale. Myths are stories about the gods and are thought to inspire in people awe and reverence for their origins. But the problem of classification persists with myth. Some of the gods may begin as animals or as humans or may transform into them in the course of the telling!

A second way to classify tales is to consider them according to purpose. Here it is the social function of a tale that is important. Is the story a lesson in history, in power, or in morality? Does the tale seek to help a certain group cope with their lot in life or better understand their role? Does the story play a part in a ritual of diagnosis or cure? The difficulty with using social purpose for classifying tales is that the tool is not very precise. This is because many tales give several lessons simultaneously.

A third method of organizing tales is by way of their outstanding characteristics. Here the folklorist might ask whether the tale deals with trickery, for example, or whether it presents a dilemma or riddle to solve. Often a tale's most outstanding characteristic is the morality or immorality it showcases. Alternatively, it is the history of a village, a town, or of a profession (potter, blacksmith) which it highlights. But this method of sorting tales is also problematic because of the problem of overlap. And the reader should note that dilemma tales are open-ended and may not have a solution. They are designed to foster discussion.

Other scholars have classified tales based on the context of their delivery. Thus hunting tales are told when hunters stop to rest. Divination tales are told when a diviner seeks to diagnose an illness for an individual or a group of people. Women's laments are told when women gather for communal cooking or washing. Moonlight tales are told in the evenings when families or age-graders[3] gather after evening meals. Praise stories are told when a great man is honored in a title taking ceremony or when he is sent off to the land of the ancestors at his death. This way of sorting tales equally lacks precision and fails to deal adequately with overlapping categories.

Aurature scholar Isidore Okpewho has devised a scheme that he believes eliminates most of the problems already mentioned, and simplifies the classification process. He has arranged narratives into three large groups: 1) Legends, 2) Explanatory Tales, and 3) Fables (Okpewho, 1992, pp. 183–22).

Legends

Legends refer to stories about people or events that are so fantastic they must be memorialized. Some of these legends, according to Okpewho, are historic, i.e., they happened more or less within the span of people's memory, and they adhere more or less to fact. Analysis shows how a skilled bard recounts a recent story using stylistic devices similar to those used in the telling of a mythological tale.

Professor Okpewho also speaks of romantic or mythic legends. The events in these tales happened long ago, in an ageless era when things were then not what they are today. So it is possible to include in these mythic legends incredible flights of fantasy, where heroes perform seemingly magical feats and have superhuman powers. The Mande[4] story of Sundiata, the founder of the ancient Mali Empire of the 13th century, is a mythic legend.

3. The term "age-graders" refers to age and gender-based social groupings who have undergone initiation rituals at the same time.

4. A number of related West African groups trace their descent from the ancient Mali empire, united by Sundiata. Folklorist Charles Bird gives us an excellent account of the Mande region. There is the core of the ancient Mande kingdom that extends from Segou (Mali) in the north down to Boundali in Cote d'Ivoire and from Segou (Mali) in the east to the River Falémé in the west. The core area has western extensions which run into Senegal, Gambia, and Guinea, northern extensions running into Mopti in Mali, eastern extensions spreading to central Burkina Faso and the north of Ghana, and southern extensions as far as Abidjan in the Ivory Coast (1972, p. 275).

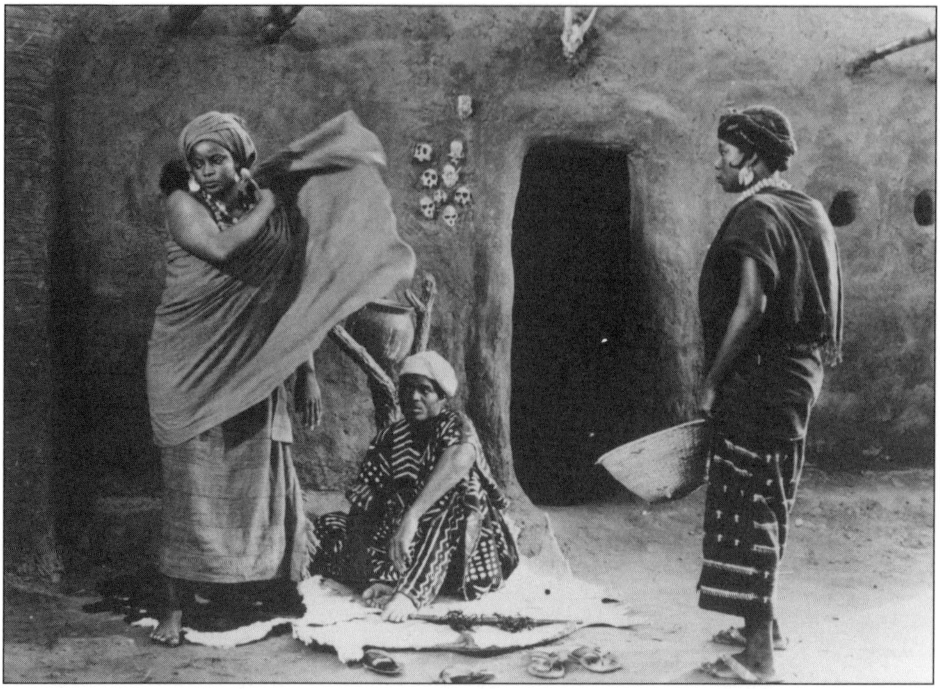

Figure 5-2. Scene from "Keita: The Heritage of the Griot," produced by Dani Kouyaté. "Keita" recounts the Legend of Sundiata. Characters from the video are (left to right): the Queen Mother, Dankaran Touman (Sundiata's half-brother), and Sologon (Sundiata's mother). Photo courtesy of California Newsreel.

The story takes place in the mid-thirteenth century AD after the fall of the ancient Ghana Empire in the eleven hundreds. At the time, the Mandingo were governed by individual princes each of whom ruled a given village state. Meanwhile, the neighboring Susu clan had their dreams set on ruling the entire Mande territory.

The Legend of Sundiata

> There was once a Mande boy named Sundiata who lived in the village-state of Kangaba. Sundiata was the son of Nare Magham, the ruler of Kangaba. Sundiata's mother was Sologon, Nare Magham's second wife. Sologon was said to have married Nare Magham in mysterious circumstances. When Sundiata was a boy, it was prophesied that he would be a great leader. But as a child, he seemed to offer little hope for his parents. A cripple, he learned to speak only at a late age. Sundiata's father Nare Magham died, and Dankaran Touman, Sundiata's half brother was given the rule of the village-state. But Dankaran was weak and ineffectual so Dankaran's mother, Nare Magham's first wife, (the Queen Mother), ruled the kingdom.

> Magically, Sundiata's legs healed during this time and he grew very strong. Threatened by Sundiata's newfound power, his stepmother, the Queen Mother, planned to kill him, his mother Sologon, and his sisters. Sologon learned of the plot and fled with her children. The Queen Mother sent envoys to pursue and kill the family but the envoys always failed in their missions.
>
> Sumanguru, ruler of the neighboring Susu, began to conquer Mandingo village states. He laid waste to the Mandingo capital Jeriba. A cruel ruler, he was said to sit on the skins of the chiefs he had defeated.
>
> Sundiata meanwhile began to unite Mandingo warriors. He also plotted in other ways against the Susu. He sent his sister to Sumanguru's bed to seduce the Susu ruler and to learn the secrets of his magical power. Sumanguru continued his conquest of the Mandingo village states and invaded Kangaba, Sundiata's birthplace. Sundiata's weak half brother Dankaran Touman fled and the cruel Sumanguru assumed direct rule over the people of Kangaba.
>
> Sundiata's sister, Sungulan Kulankan returned to her brother successful in her mission to seduce Sumanguru and to learn the secrets of his magical power. The people of Kangaba send messengers to Sundiata to ask him to be their leader. Armed with the knowledge of magic and the hope of his people, Sundiata led his cavalry and his bowmen across the plains. Finally in 1235 he met the Susu army commanded by Sumanguru in person. Although outnumbered, Sundiata and his men razed the well-garrisoned city of Susu. Defeated, Sumanguru disappeared and was never seen again. Sundiata went on over the next five years to crush resistance from the Susu and to build a great Mali empire, which remained the dominant power in the Western Sudan for the next 150 years.[5]

The Legend of Sundiata, a lengthy tale that can be told or sung, is the most important piece in the repertoire of a griot from the Mande region of West Africa. Romantic or mythic legends that cover a great deal of time, a broad geographical or political area, and describe super-human feats, usually helped through magic, are also called epics. Several African ethnic groups tell epic tales about the exploits of their leaders. These include among others: the Mande peoples of Mali and some neighboring states (see endnote 4), who tell of Sundiata; the Zulu of South Africa who recount tales of Shaka; the Banyanga of the Congo who sing their Mwindo epic tale; and the Ijo of Nigeria who recite their story of the Ozidi. Legends, romantic myths, and epics are important to societies because they tell people about their rulers and help to reinforce social pride and group identity.

---

5. Derived from Stride and Ifika, 1971, pp. 47–51. See also D. T. Niane. 1965. *Sundiata: An Epic of Old Mali,* trans. G.D. Pickett. London: Longman.

Explanatory Tales

Okpewho's second category includes explanatory tales. An explanatory tale is a tale that tries to explain the origin of a whole range of elements in a culture. Foundation myths, for example, represent an important category of explanatory tales. Foundation myths tell about the origins of a people and they consider larger philosophical questions about the meaning of existence as a given people see it. The tale below comes from the Fulani, the main herding people of West Africa. The reader should note the importance of milk in this cattle-loving group.

Fulani Foundation Myth

At the beginning there was a huge drop of milk.
Then Doondari came and he created the stone.
Then the stone created iron;
And iron created fire;
And fire created water;
And water created air.
Then Doondari descended the second time. And he took the five elements
And he shaped them into man.
But man was proud.
Then Doondari created blindness and blindness defeated man.
But when blindness became too proud,
Doondari created worry, and worry defeated sleep;
But when worry became too proud, Doondari created death, and death defeated worry.
But when death became too proud,
Doondari descended for the third time,
And he came as Gueno, the eternal one,
And Gueno defeated death (Beier cited in Okpewho, 1992, pp. 203–204).

The Zulu foundation myth tells of the creation. Like all creation stories, it reflects the reality of contemporary society in which it finds itself. This one was recorded by Dr. Wilhelm Bleek, a Cape Town librarian. It clearly reflects a South African world well after the Zulu had encountered Europeans.

Zulu Foundation Myth

I
The Great One came out of the Earth beneath.
He came out with the sun and he came out with the moon.
He placed them in the sky saying: Let the sun travel by day...
Saying: Let the moon appear after sunset.
II

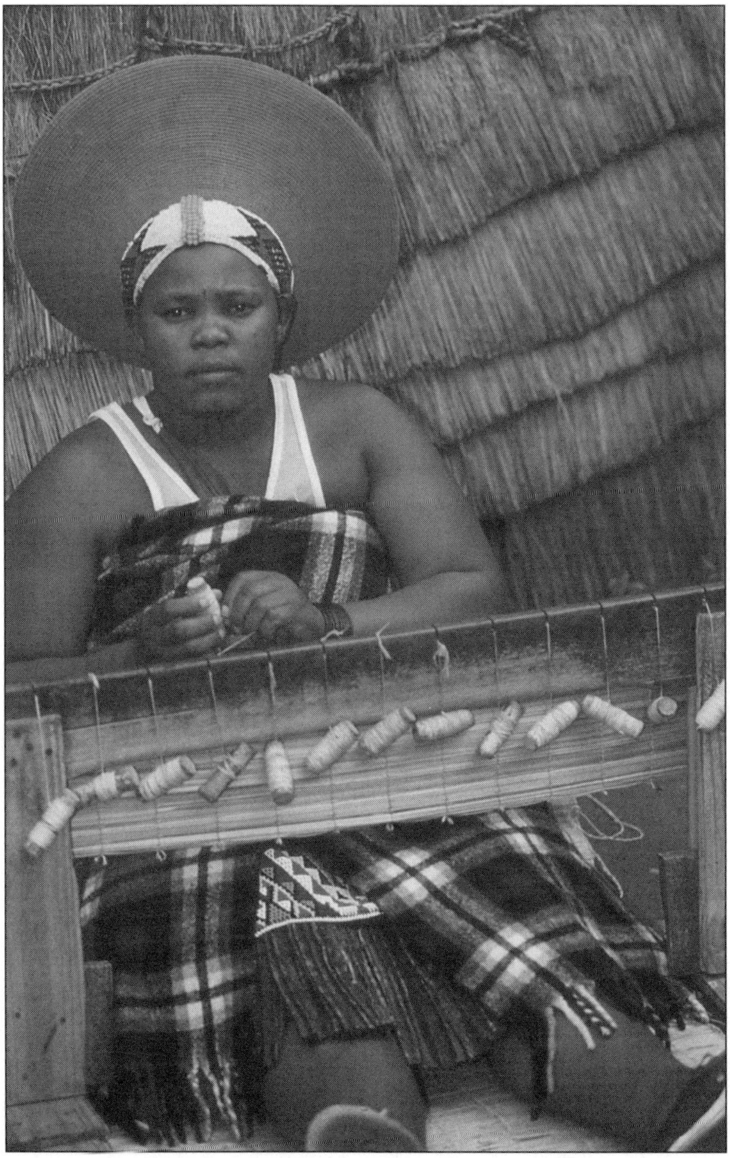

Figure 5-3. When a Zulu woman married, her hair was plaited with clay, rendering her headpiece irremovable. Today, married Zulu women cover their heads instead with a red woolen beret. Photo Courtesy of Bob Hanson.

The Great One rose out of the Earth underneath.
He brought forth people (Bantu) and white people;
He brought forth cattle, goats, sheep, dogs.
He brought forth the animals of the wilderness and many other things.
    The Great One called Unwaba the Chameleon.
Saying: 'Go to Bopapa on Earth and tell him: People shall not die.'
The Chameleon went on its way downward, treading careful.
    The Great One called Intulo the Lizard.

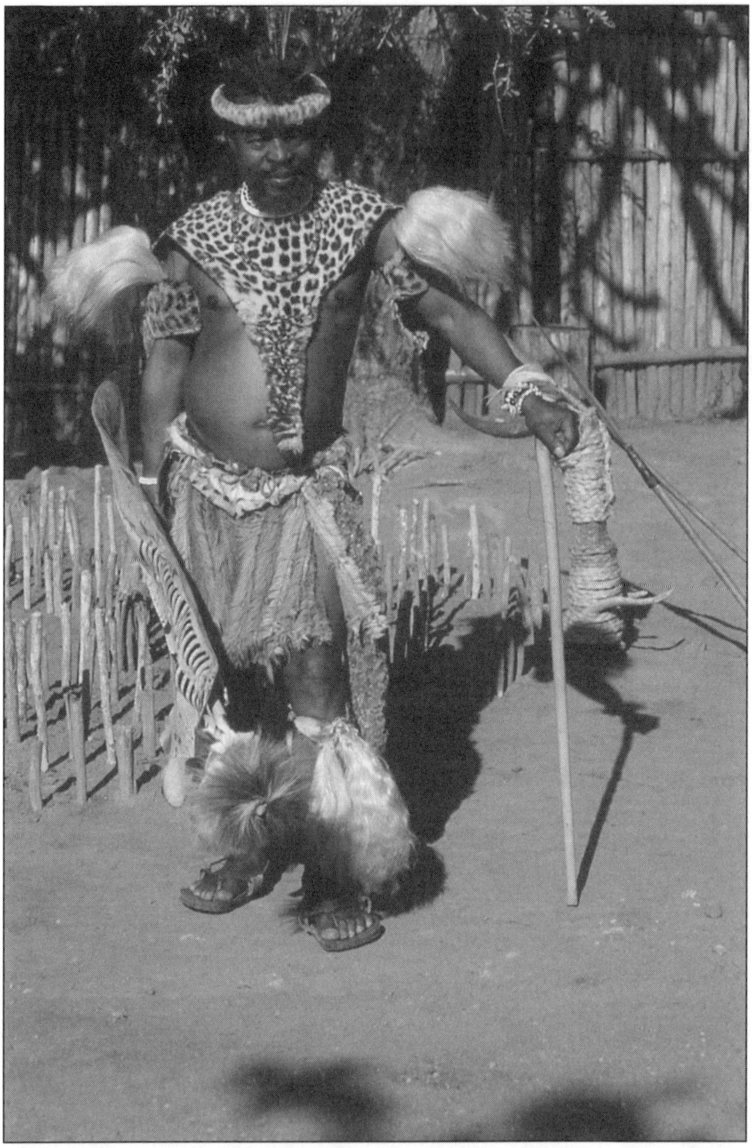

Figure 5-4. A Zulu elder. Photo courtesy of Neil Cumberlidge.

Saying: 'Go and speak; The people (Bantu) shall die.
The white people shall die as well as the black people.
The cattle, the sheep, the dogs will all die. Nothing will remain.'
Intulo the Lizard set off running rapidly down to Earth.
There it spoke: All the people must die, all who inhabit the Earth,
And all the animals upon the Earth.
Meanwhile Unwaba the Chameleon trod carefully.
Then it stopped and nibbled the leaves of the shrub Bukwebezane.
III
Meanwhile the Lizard Intulo ran in great haste, because

The Great One had spoken: 'Intula, arrive on Earth
And say unto the people that they must all die.'
The Lizard Intula arrived on Earth, obeying the Great Lord.
It spoke there: 'All the people shall die, white and black.
All the animals will die, tame and wild. Nothing will remain.'
The word of the Great One cannot be taken back. It stays.
People and animals die, leaving behind their little ones.
IV
The Great One created: a white man and woman
Saying: The white man shall marry the white woman
And they will beget more white people.
And He created the Bantu-people, man and woman,
And they begat the Bantu, the black people.
The Great One spoke: the White people shall live near the Ocean
And the Black people shall live in the middle of the land,
They shall build kraals to keep cattle, goats and sheep;
They shall breed dogs and go hunting.
V
The Great One spoke: The White people shall own clothes and guns.
The Black people shall wear skins and the men will carry spears.
The married women shall wear a red headdress.
The married men shall wear a headring.
VI
The Great One broke out of the Earth, out from beneath.
He rose up from the reeds, from the water's edge,
He created many nations: the Sun people, the Elephant people,
The Bushmen, the white men and the Black people, the Bantu,
In many tribes did he create them: the Zulu, the Swazi, the Ba-suto, the Xosa, the Sembu, Tembu and Pondo and twenty-four other tribes.
VII
The Great One spoke: Let water come forth that the people
May drink from it and the animals as well
Let fire come forth so that people can cook their food.
There is the Earth, let the women dig it.
Let the men cut trees and build houses.
The men shall make hoes and give them to the women
So that they can plant seeds, so that the millet may grow.
The women must fetch firewood, grind the corn and cook food.
VIII
A woman shall be obtained from her father in exchange for cattle.
If a man dies, his younger brother shall marry his wives
Lest they be married by men from other tribes.
If a man knows how to keep his people
He will how to keep his cattle
So that his sons may inherit the shining beasts after he dies old (Knappert, 1995, pp. 267–269).

Reprinted by permission of Harper Collins Publishers, Ltd. ©Jan Knappert, 1995

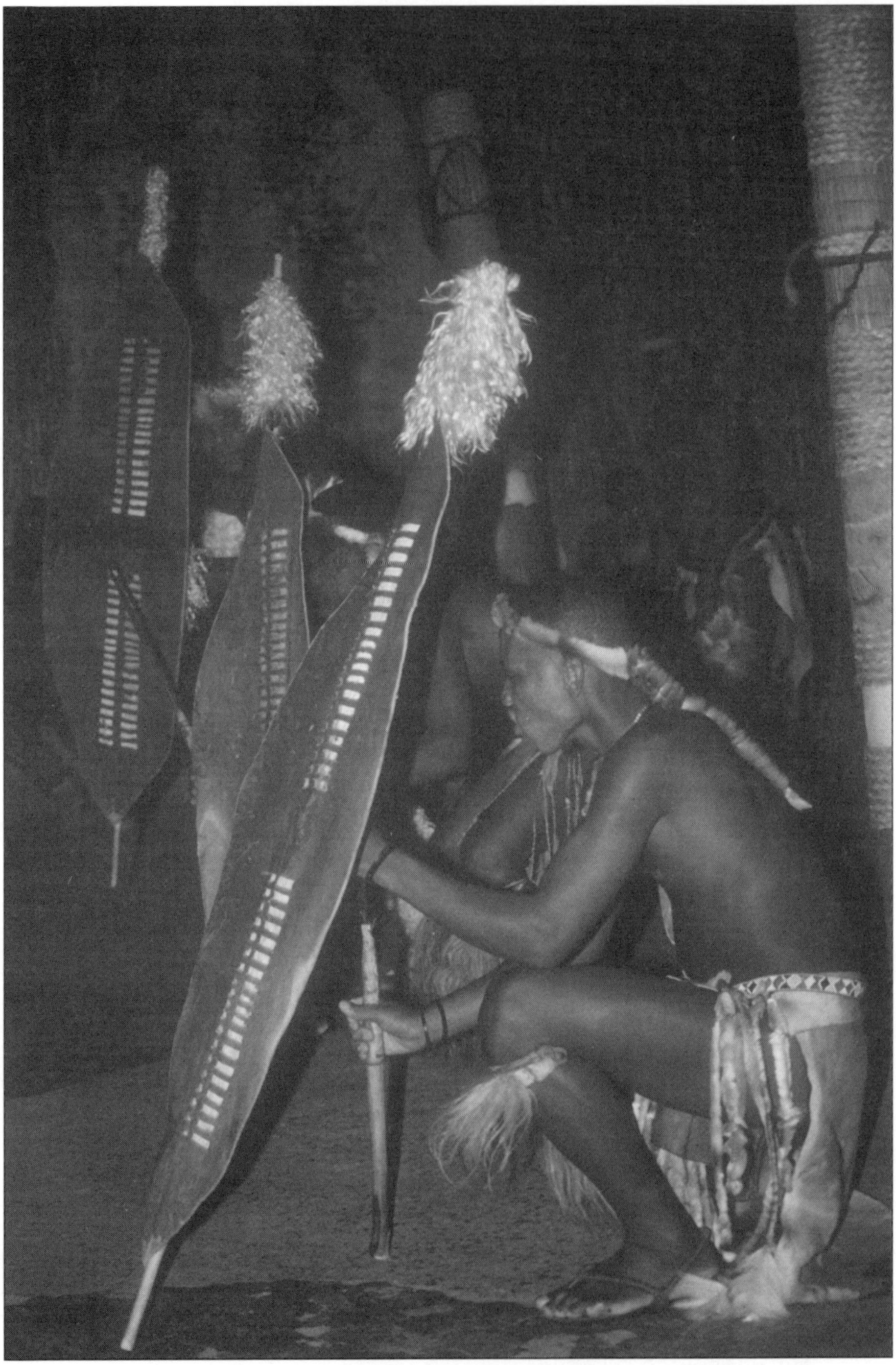

Figure 5-5. The Zulu Foundation myth recounts the creation of a great warrior nation. Photo courtesy of Neil Cumberlidge.

The reader should note the power of the foundation myth to impute divine intention to arbitrary social practices. Today, most married Zulu women sport red wool berets rather than the red clay headdress (plaited into the hair) to which the myth refers. And few Zulu married men wear the head ring (leopard) as this is reserved for special ceremonies.

The Mande creation myth is particularly interesting in that it makes mention, among other things, of the first bard, Soukoura, playing the first drum. This fact goes a long way to underscore the importance of oral performers in Mande society.

Mande Creation Myth

God first created the seed of the Balanza tree (*Acacia albida*). Then he created eleusine seed in twin varieties, as they say, 'He made the egg of the world into a pair so they would multiply.' Next, God made three more pairs of seeds, and placed each pair in one of the four corners of the earth. He enclosed them in a flower in one of the egg-seeds where there were two boys and two girls. The eldest boy wanted to rule the world, so he came out prematurely and descended to earth. Earth was his own placenta from which God quickly made the earth. Pemba, that was his name, sowed the seeds, but only the red eleusine germinated because the earth was stained with placenta blood. Pemba's twin Faro became a twin fish, a pair of *mannogo*. One fish was cut into pieces and scattered on earth where they became trees. From the other fish God made a man, a new Faro who atoned from his brother's sins. God sent him down in a ship from heaven. It came to rest near the mountain Kouroula, where there was a cave, Ka, and near it the first pool was formed. Faro, the first of eight people, four men and four women, disembarked. The eldest was called Kanisimbo, 'from the womb of Ka.' They saw the first sunrise. God had made the sun out of the other half of Pemba's placenta. Down from heaven also came the first bard, Sourakata, playing the first drum. Then the first blacksmith came down, and seeing the drought he raised his hammer and struck a rock, and rain poured down from Heaven filling the pool Kokoro with fresh, fertilizing water. Simboumba, brother of Kanisimbo, began to speak, saying *nko*, 'I speak,' while he was sowing the seeds after the first rain. He took the clay from the pool and built the first sanctuary on the hill, The Egg of the World. Its roof was made of bamboo, Faro's hair. Kanisimbo sowed the first rice, *malo*. They built their first village called Kaba 'maize'. By causing the floods of his body, Faro created the Niger, so that river is his body, both male and female. In it he left his seed for the future generation, which will be like fishes at first (Knappert, 1995, pp. 150–1).

Reprinted by permission of Harper Collins Ltd. © Jan Knappert, 1995

Apart from foundation myths, there are explanatory stories that are used to account for the surrounding environment, including plants, animals, or even neighboring groups. The following narrative, "Why Birds Have Different Colors," is a story published by the People's Educational Association of Sierra Leone.

Why Birds Have Different Colours

Once upon a time, all the birds of the world competed for a chieftancy. The requirement was to fly from Bafodea to the end of the world and back before all the other competitors. Bafodea was struck by famine. So when they set out most of the birds were distracted by the different kinds of food they came across in their flight.

No sooner did they take off than the vultures came across a carcass. They crowded around it and started to eat while the other birds continued on their journey. Some miles away, the hens too came across some rice. Like the vultures, they came together and started to peck the rice and forgot all about the competition.

The others continued with the flight and soon came across some wild fruits which attracted the "Kodo-Kodos." They stayed behind eating the fruits while the others continued the flight. The Koma bird which is normally very slow, slower than all the other birds, was the first to reach the end of the world. At the end of the competition, the 'Koma" won the first prize, that is, a gift of many beautiful clothes. On his return journey he gave out some of the clothes to the other birds leaving the best ones for himself.

That is why all birds have beautiful feathers but the "koma" is the most beautiful and the king of birds (Hinzen, James, Sorie, and Tamu, 1987, p. 156).

One of my students provided the next story that she heard as a child in South Africa. It is an explanatory tale as to why there are differences between black people and white people.

Why There Are Differences between Black People and White People

Everyone in the world started out black, and then one day they happened upon a flowing stream. Some people were so excited they immediately jumped into the water. When they came out, their hair was straightened, and their skin had turned white. Others were afraid and decided only to put their palms and the bottoms of their feet into the water, which is why black people are lighter on their palms and the bottom of their feet (Mashinini 2000).

A third type of explanatory tale looks at the behaviors, beliefs, and values of a given society. Like many such stories, the one below is a moral tale, taken from the Abron peoples of Cote d'Ivoire and collected by Alexander Alland, Jr.

There was once a woman who had no children. For ten years she had none. And then, one after another, she had three sons. She loved her sons very much, but after several years they died. After this, the woman could do nothing but cry.

One night a dog came to her and said, "God calls you; follow me." She followed the dog, and when she came before God, he said to her, "Woman, why do you cry so much?" "It is because I lost my three sons," she replied. God then asked her if she would recognize her three sons if she saw them again. She answered that she would of course know her sons. Then God said, "Go with the dog and find them in my village." The woman was led by the dog to God's village. Soon they came before a leper who had no hands and feet. "Is this one of your sons?" asked the dog. "No," replied the woman. They went farther. The dog took her before another man, who was destitute, a man who was despised because he did not pay his debts. "Is this one of your sons?" asked the dog. "No," replied the woman. They went farther into the village. The dog took her before a third man, who was mad. "Is this one of your sons?" he asked. "Surely not," replied the woman. The dog then took her back to God, who said to her "You have seen your three sons and you may take them home with you if you wish." "No," replied the woman. "I prefer to have no sons." She returned home to her village and recounted all that had passed to the villagers. After this she had many daughters, all of whom were beautiful (Alland, Jr., 1990, p. 144)

The story shows the importance of accepting life as it comes. The woman chooses not to disturb the dead, and is rewarded with many daughters. The story also shows the attitude of the Abron toward leprosy, madness, and debtors.

Another of my students, from Kenya, supplied the following explanatory tale.

The Maiden

The sun blazed upon the earth; there was no rain. The crops died and hunger was manifest among the people. This happened one year, again the next, and then for a third year. So people gathered at the praying place and asked of each the reason for their plight; then the question was posed to the Medicine Man. He spilled his gourd of its contents, upon the ground again and again. Then he declared that the rains would come only when the maiden Wanjiru was bought. He told them that each, from the youngest lad to the oldest man, must bring, on the appointed day, a goat to purchase Wanjiru from her family. The day arrived, and all the people were present, with each man leading a goat. The people gathered in a circle, and the relations of Wanjiru stood together, and she herself stood in the middle. As they stood there Wanjiru began to sink to into the ground. Soon she was in to her knees. She cried, "I am lost!" The people pressed close and placed goats in the keeping of Wanjiru's parents. She sank lower to her waist. Again she cried out, "I am lost but much rain will fall!" More goats were thrust upon her family. She sank to her breast, and still no rain came. Wanjiru cried out another time, "A great rain will come!" Now she sank to her neck, and then the rain poured down. The people should have come forward to save her, but instead they placed more goats upon the family. Then Wanjiru said, "My people have undone me," and she sank down to her eyes. As one or another of her family moved toward her to save her, another of the people would present him or her with a goat and that family member would step back. Wanjiru cried out for the last time, "My own family has undone me!" Then she sank from sight. The rain poured down in a great deluge and the people hurried for shelter in their homes. There was a young warrior who lamented the loss of Wanjiru. He swore to find her and bring her back. He wandered for a long time, and eventually returned to the spot where Wanjiru had disappeared. Here as he stood where she had stood, he slowly began to sink into the ground; and he sank lower and lower until the ground closed over him. He found himself on a road beneath the ground, and as he trod down the road he came upon Wanjiru, all muddy and disheveled, and without her clothing which had disintegrated. He picked her up and carried her upon his back to where they had sunk beneath the ground. Here they rose up together into the open air. He took her into his mother's house where she was fed the fat from slaughtered goats and clothed with their skins, until she, again, was beautiful and well dressed. It came to pass that the village was having a dance, and she and her warrior attended. When her family saw her they attempted to approach her, but her lover beat them off. When her family made repeated attempts to see her over the course of the next few days, the warrior repented. He paid the family the purchase price and allowed them to reconcile (Kimama 2001).

The Maiden, according to Kimama, shows the importance of deference to the gods, even at the cost of sacrificing a family member. The story also highlights the values of respect for tradition, authority, and kinship obligations (Kimama 2001).

A great many of the moral tales are out and out didactic. A good example is the tale of the dog and His Shadow from the Sierra Leone collection.

The Dog and His Shadow

Once upon a time there lived a very gluttonous dog. He would never go satisfied however much he ate. He would eat for years, continuously without going satisfied. One day, his owner brought plenty of beef. The wife was told to cook all of it with plenty of rice. This was the time of harvest when there was enough food in the land. This greedy dog's owner was a hunter, and was a well-known hunter. He would bring home game every day. This dog would eat and eat and eat. There were times when he could not even breathe because there was no space left for breathing. He would not allow any other dog to even come around. If any dog or cat, or even a hen came near where he ate, he would tear them to pieces.

One day his owner got a very big game, the biggest he ever got since his career as a hunter. As usual, all of it was cooked with plenty of rice. When the hunter sat down eating, the biggest lump of meat in the soup dropped from his hand on to the ground. Before the hunter could wink his eyes, the dog had grabbed the meat and run with it. He ran and ran until he came to a bridge in the outskirts of the town. When he came to the bridge, he looked in the water, and he saw a reflection of himself. The greedy dog thought this was another dog with a big lump of meat in his mouth. He looked, and looked and looked; he wanted that meat too. But this was only his own shadow. He convinced himself that the lump of meat he was seeing in the water, in the mouth of his fellow dog, was bigger than his. So he must have it as well.

He barked at the reflection in order that the dog he was seeing in the water would drop his meat and he would take it. When he barked, his own meat dropped from his mouth and went deep down the river. He looked down again in the river and saw that the dog in the water too did not have meat any more. He barked and barked and barked until he was tired. He then returned home. When he got home his owner flogged him mercilessly. So the greedy dog lost on both sides—he could not eat the meat and he was beaten for taking it away. This is why you end up missing all if you want all at the same time (Hinzen, James, Sorie, and Tamu, 1987, p. 195).

Fables

Okpewho identifies a category of stories he calls fables. Here, the interest of the bard is in presenting an imaginative drama or story, or in simply delighting the audience. Dilemma tales are among those that can be described as Fables. Dilemma tales present listeners with a problem for which there is no single correct answer. The purpose of the tale is to invite reflection and discussion.

The following is a dilemma tale from the Grushi of Togo, told to folklorist A.W. Cardinall and summarized by William Bascom.

A chief's daughter fell in love with a python that appeared in the form of a handsome man. During the night it resumed the form of a python, swallowed the girl, and carried her off to its home in a large lake. In the morning the chief ordered his people to follow, but they found no tracks. A man who could smell everywhere followed their trail to the lake. A man famous for his thirst drank the lake dry. A famous worker dug out all the mud, revealing a hole so deep that its bottom could not be reached. A man whose arm could reach all over the country pulled out the python; it was killed, but when they cut open its stomach, the girl was dead. A man who had medicine to raise the dead restored her to life. Now, which of these five men did the best? (Answer: They were all equally good, and the girl never married again). (Adapted from Cardinall, as cited in Bascom, 1972, pp. 203–204).

Another tale, The Three Fast Brothers delights the audience, shares the values of the community, and generates lively discussion. The Three Fastest Brothers comes from a collection of tales from Sierra Leone.

The Three Fast Brothers

Once there lived a woman and her husband. The woman was very fast and agile and her husband admired her very much for her agility. They lived happily together for a very long time, without having any children.

Some time later the husband died. Bur before he died, he called his wife and said "My dear, we have been married for quite a long time now but we have not been blessed with any children. Now, I am praying that when I die the Lord will give you a child who will be more agile than you."

Three months after her husband's death, she married another man. She was lucky to have three children for this man, all boys. The first was named Birma, the second Abdulai and the youngest Amadu.

When they had grown up their mother would always call them together and ask them who was the fastest and most agile among them. Each one wanted to prove to their mother that he was the fastest.

The eldest was the first to try. There was an apple tree behind their house so he decided to pick some ripe apples from it. He climbed the tree. Instead of picking them one by one, he just shook the branches and the apples fell down. Many apples fell, but before they fell on the ground, he had climbed down, removed his clothes and spread them out so that all the apples fell right onto his clothes. None fell on the ground.

The younger one said he was faster. So the eldest challenged him. While they were arguing an eagle was hovering over their hen which had just hatched its chickens who were out finding something to eat. Before the eagle came down to snatch one of the chickens away, he had run into the house, collected a basket, and within a second had collected all the chickens, put them into the basket and closed it.

The youngest one said: "I am sure I am faster than you two." So they challenged him. One day he went hunting with his father. While they were going, the weather suddenly changed. It was going to rain. They were in an open field and there was nowhere they could take shelter. He said to his father: "Wait a minute, let me try and do something." He hurriedly went into a nearby bush, took out his cutlass and cut some wood. He came back, cleared an area, and in no time had built a hut for them before it began to rain. Among these three boys, who do you think was the fastest and most agile? (Hinzen, James, Sorie, and Tamu, 1987, p. 251).

After hearing this story, listeners will spend a good deal of time enjoying a friendly debate as to which of these brothers is the most agile. The discussion will be open-ended, expanding according to the time available for it.

Trickster tales are also included among fables. These tales typically pit a small clever animal against a larger or more ferocious one. Audiences delight in seeing the powerless win against the odds in a competition of wits. Favorite African tricksters include tortoise, spider, hare, and cat. Lee Haring collected this tale from a Kamba informant in Kenya in 1968.

Trickster Tale 1

The crocodile asked the monkey to visit him. The monkey asked the crocodile, "How shall I reach your home when I don't know how to swim?" The crocodile told the monkey to jump on his back.

On the way, the crocodile felt hungry and asked the monkey, "Can you give me your heart? Because I am feeling hungry." The monkey told the crocodile, "this is what we are going to do: We are going to go back. Because when we become friendly to somebody we leave our hearts at home." Now the monkey told the crocodile, "You see, I am very weak. I cannot be eaten. So we have to go back and I'll get you my heart."

The crocodile agreed that they should turn back. When they reached the shore, the monkey climbed into a mango tree and picked a mango. He threw it and said to the crocodile, "there is the heart;" but the mango got into the water. He picked another one, but when the monkey threw this one the crocodile dived into the water. That is the end of our story (Haring, 1972, pp. 166–7).

According to folklorists, trickster tales follow a certain pattern involving a series of predictable events or conditions. Some folklorists have listed these as 1) false friendship; 2) contract or pact between protagonists; 3) violation of the friendship, usually by the trickster; 4) trickery or deceit of the story characters by one another; 5) escape of the trickster; 6) reward of the trickster (Haring, 1972, p. 166).

A second example of a trickster tale comes from Clement M. Doke's 1927 collection of Lamba folklore.

Trickster Tale 2

They made friends, Mr. Little-Hare and the Guinea-Fowl. Then one day Mr. Little-Hare made a crate and got in, and Mr. Little-Hare said to the Guinea-Fowl, "My friends, won't you pick me up?" Then all the Guinea-Fowl came and couldn't pick him up. Then Little-Hare came out and said, "Now all of you get in!" Then indeed the Guinea-Fowl all got in. When they had finished getting in, the Little-Hare tied it up where they had got in and carried it.

Then the Guinea-Fowl said, "Mate, put us down!" And Little-Hare answered, "No, because a certain person wants you!" Then the Guinea-Fowl, when they heard that, cried out bitterly. Then Mr. Little-Hare went in search of Mr. Leopard. When he reached the outskirts of the village, he hung up (the crate), and came to Mr. Leopard, and said, 'I want to become your friend." And he agreed saying, "All right!" Then Little-Hare said, "Let us go, you shall receive some relish." Then indeed they went and found a number of guinea-fowls in the crate and took them, and ate them as relish (Haring, 1972, p. 167).

According to Okpewho, a final category of fables includes tales of ogres and monsters. Members of the underworld, they inspire terror, awe, or simple curiosity in humans. People believe these creatures emerge in dark forests, the bush, or in unsettled spots. The following is an ogre tale of the Masai of Kenya supplied by N.L Kipury in 1983.

Ogre Tale

Once upon a time, there lived a young woman who eloped to meet her warrior lover out in the wilderness. The warrior directed the young woman to a place in the forest where he would meet her. He said to her: "If you get to a fork along the path take the right path." Then the warrior went ahead to await her arrival in the forest.

The young woman took off, and when she got to the fork that the warrior had mentioned, she followed the left path, forgetting which path the warrior had instructed her to follow.

As the girl walked on, she came upon an ogre who said to her: Hey young woman, where are you going; do you have anything to say, now that I'm going to eat you? The girl answered in song:

(Song)
Not here my bead
Let us go to the water hole
Where you can eat me
And have a drink
O my dear warrior, where was it?[6]

And so it happened that this was very bushy country. The ogre led the young woman on, and when they got to another spot, he said to her:

6. The ogre does not realize that she is calling out to her lover, rather he must assume she is calling *him* warrior.

"I am now going to eat you here." The lady again broke into song, urging him not to eat her yet.

They went farther on, and the young woman kept hoping that the warrior would hear her voice. As they walked on, the ogre asked the young lady: Shall I eat you here?" The girl sang again:

(Song)
Not here my bead
Let us go to the water hole
Where you can eat me
And have a drink
Oh my dear warrior, where was it?

But the warrior still had not heard her. When they got to a cave by the river, the ogre collected branches and leaves on which to place the young woman's flesh after he had slaughtered her. When he brought one type of leaf, the girl objected to having flesh laid on ordinary leaves, preferring the sweet-scented leaves of the *matasia* plant. The ogre brought another type of leaf, but the girl rejected them until eventually the sweet smelling leaves of the *matasia* plant were brought. When the ogre asked the girl whether those were the right type of leaves she said: "Yes, these are the ones." The ogre then laid the leaves down on the ground and lit a big fire. All this while, the girl was continuously singing the same song.

Just when the ogre was about to jump on the young woman, the warrior suddenly emerged from the bush. The young woman said to the ogre: "It is now your skinny flesh that will be laid on those leaves." The warrior killed the ogre and placed him on the bed of leaves and took the lady away. And that is the end (Kipury cited in Okpewho, 1993, pp. 219–220).

This story is like the trickster tales in that it stars a non-human character that takes on human characteristics. It functions mainly to amuse the audience, all the while elevating the role of male, especially warrior, in relation to female protagonist. The reader should note the use of song in conjunction with the recitation of this tale. The song is used as a stylistic device to mark the progression of the story, and to heighten the drama of the woman's predicament. But it also serves to break up the spoken narrative with a refreshing tune, thereby holding audience interest. The combination of narrative and song is very common in the performance of African tales.

It is worth noting that scholars who have collected these tales have not always been sensitive to the performance dimensions of these oral arts. Many of the narratives provided above might seem quite different in a performance context than how they appear on the printed page. This is a discussion that will be taken up in the next chapter where the presentation of tales and other forms of orature is treated.

Traditional Oral Artists and the Struggle against HIV/AIDS

It is clear that the African oral tradition is a vast cultural repository suitable for the transmission of messages of great importance. Not surprisingly, the oral tale is being used in the fight against AIDS. Malian radio has long transmitted the tales told to a musical accompaniment told by griots, so it seems quite natural to adapt this genre to an AIDS message. The following story emerged in a radio workshop conducted by the author for Malian Radio broadcasters in 1998.[7]

The story was written in French which I have translated.

Herebougou

The story took place in a village called Herebougou. It is a prosperous village where it rains abundantly. In this locality nothing happens by chance. All events can be explained.

One day Konyini, a young man of the village decided to go and discover the world and seek his fortune. Everyone in the village was happy for Konyini and they gave him a big send-off party. After all, Konyini was going off for a great adventure.

Konyini settled in a city named Kunbengougou. Here, he worked. He was astonished by the attractions of the city. Unfortunately the company he kept led him to contract a terrible disease. Konyini got thinner. He weakened. He decided to return home.

When he arrived in the village of his birth, the people no longer recognized him because he had so withered away. Everyone shied away from him because of his health. He was abandoned, marginalized, and excluded from society. In the meantime, misfortune fell upon the village. There was famine and misery. Desolation and despair could be read on the faces of the people of Herebougou.

The population decided to consult the oracles to learn the source of the evil that was ravaging the people. And doing this, the people learned that misfortune was befalling them because they had abandoned a son of the village. The inhabitants of Herebougou decided to aid the sick one, to assist him and to support him in every way. And this was how good fortune returned to the village. The village became normal again. Everything returns to order.

Moral: We must never abandon the sick, even if that person has AIDS.

---

7. I conducted a one-week workshop on development broadcasting for broadcasters from independent radio stations and for selected Peace Corps volunteers. The idea of the joint workshop was to hone the skills of broadcasters in the techniques of development communication, to introduce the Peace Corps volunteers to development and independent radio in Mali, and to promote collaboration between these two groups.

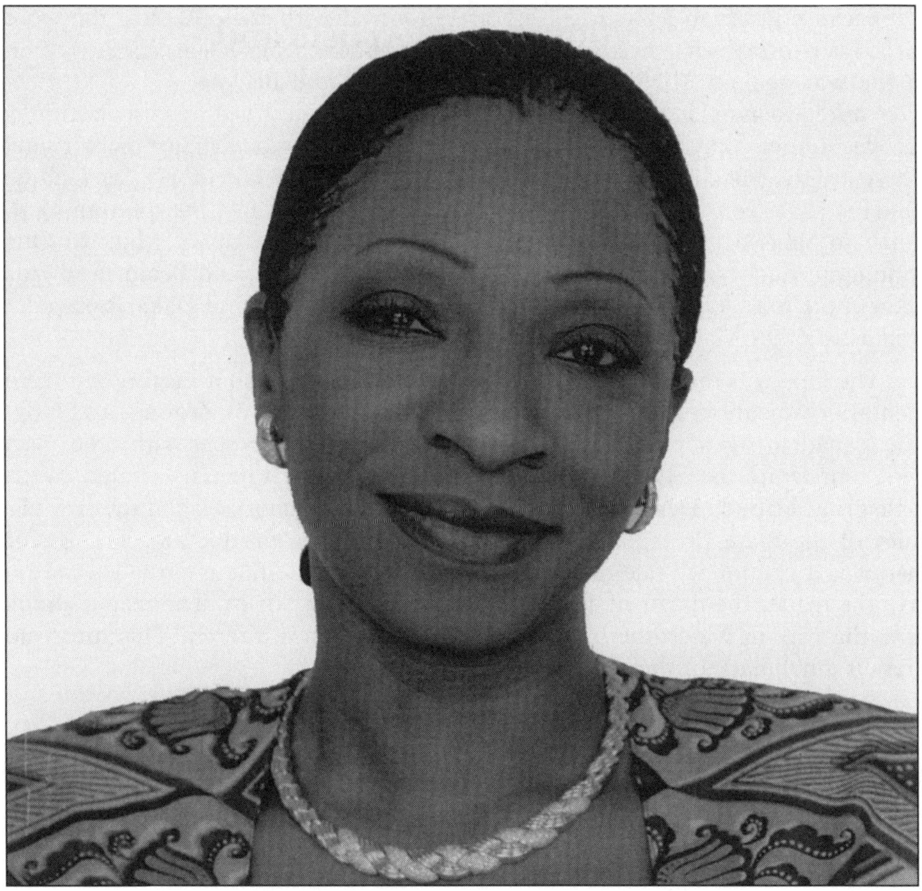

Figure 5-6. Madame Adame Ba Konaré, Mali's former first lady (1992–2002) and founder of the Partage Foundation. Photo courtesy of Editions Jamana.

Slogan: Always help a sick person consumed by AIDS (collected by Bourgault, "*Manuel de Radio Rurale*, 1998, p. 28).

This story, with its strongly moralizing approach is fairly typical of tales as we have seen. Like "The Dog and His Shadow," it shows how a violation of social/moral norms has negative social consequences while the pursuit of righteousness leads to a just reward. Elegant in its simplicity, it reinforces the importance of kin and village solidarity, something that the fear of AIDS has helped to undermine. Herebougou, a mythological village of good fortune, appears in a number of tales, many about AIDS. Typically, a young person, usually a male, leaves Herebougou to seek his fortune (often the funds for a bride-price). These young men are seduced by the city and the attractive females who live in it. Eventually, they fall ill and die of AIDS.

Mali's Partage Foundation, which actively promotes the use of the arts against AIDS, holds competitions for the best AIDS tales. This helps to preserve the genre while engaging people competitively in storytelling about AIDS.

Because griots in Malian society are endowed with the power of the word, the power to say what needs to be said, they emerge as excellent spokespersons in the war against AIDS. Djeli Daouda Dembélé and his wife Hawa Dembélé were asked to assist in preparing and recording a tale destined for distribution on cassette among long distance truck drivers along the region's major truck routes. These are the truck routes along the West African "AIDS corridor." (See Chapter 2). This route consists of the road from coastal Abidjan in Cote d'Ivoire to the north to Sikasso in Mali. The route extends east from Sikasso, Mali, to Ouagadougou, Burkina Faso, and onto northern Ghana, Togo, and Benin. And from Sikasso the road leads the truckers west to Bamako, Mali, and Dakar, Senegal as well as to other Malian and Senegalese cities.

The tape was distributed through a partnership between a local non-governmental organization, the Association for the Development of Zégoua, and CIDA (the Canadian Agency for International Development), together with other partners supporting the SIDA2 project.[8] The thirty-minute tape is narrated by the male griot, Daouda Dembélé. His wife Hawa sings the choruses and the two play roles of the main protagonists at intervals during the production. The performance is a cautionary tale to truckers. A portion of the tale is provided here to give the reader the flavor of such tales as told in West Africa. The reader should note the way in which the bard addresses his audience directly. This direct address is a hallmark of the oral tradition.

Yiriba

(*NGONI*, FOUR STRINGED HARP, MUSIC UNDER THROUGHOUT)

Daouda: I, Djeli Daouda Dembélé and my wife Hawa Dembélé have produced this cassette to give useful information to all drivers of long distance vehicles. I am the great bard of truck drivers. The drivers who promote the intermingling of people, give us your hand. It is together that we can do something good. With my wife, we are with you night and day for all your problems. The work of a driver is very hard, and this is information that is useful for your health.

The Whites who have come from Canada to help us have called this project AIDS 2 [SIDA2]. This project has not overlooked drivers. We thank this party for their assistance in seven African countries: Guinea, Senegal, Mali, Cote d'Ivoire, Burkina Faso, Ghana, and Benin.

Hawa's Refrain: I have traveled to the East, to the West, to the North, and to the South. I have never encountered a similar fever, Father of the griots.

Narrator (Daouda): Project AIDS 2 has worked with the big doctors in our seven great West African countries. I greet the doctors of Mali, of

---

8. SIDA2 is a seven-country AIDS prevention project supported by Canadian government Aid (CIDA the Canadian International Development Agency or ACDI *Agence Canadienne pour le Developpement International)*. By 2002, the project had entered into a new cycle and was known as SIDA3.

Commune VI and Commune V. There are sexually transmitted diseases and we must not hide them. The dispensaries are at our disposition. If we are feverish and have a sexually transmitted disease, let us go to the Health Center in Koutiala. They are there, these doctors to help us. The same applies to Sikasso, Bougouni, Zégoua, and Kadiolo. The story I will tell you, information disguised is called the Story of Yiriba. He is not just anyone—for there where he is people follow his story, be they women or men. I thank him before the customs office in Bamako, in Bougouni, and in Koutiala. During his voyage from Yopougon via Koutiala and Segou to the Port of Abidjan he felt a fever overtake him, so he went to Abobogare. There the doctors prescribed him medicine and he went on his way.

Hawa's Refrain: I have plowed all the big cities from the west to the east, from north to south, and I have never encountered such a great fever.

Narrator (Daouda): Cured, Yiriba attacks Zankologodenni and stops at Toumodi, then Yamoussoukro, Bouaké, and Zégoua. All the drivers meet at Zégoua, all the truck drivers possible. We observe Ivorians, Guineans, Malians. And we see the apprentices putting water in radiators. As they were seated, Korotouma, plump like a Mecca salad, with a firm, high butt and pointed breasts passed in front of them. Exclamations were proclaimed and each one (drivers) looked at one another. Yiriba followed the girl, greeted her, and inquired as to her plans.

Korotouma (Hawa): I have gone to Abidjan via Burkina [Faso], and today I'm at Zégoua looking for a lift to Bamako.

Yiriba (Daouda): No Problem. I've got my rig here ready to leave for Mali. But there won't be a convoy today.

Korotouma (Hawa): Big Brother. I can wait until tomorrow.

Narrator (Daouda): Sexually transmitted diseases are diseases that harm a person. Korotouma had some of these diseases: white discharges and gonococcus. Apparently her conditions went unnoticed because she had a good figure [was plump and healthy looking].

My objective is the health of drivers. A sick driver means that ten families are in trouble. The driver's family, the apprentice driver's family, the family of the merchant who sells the diesel, the family of the policeman, etc. If twenty drivers stop driving, the road will feel the effects. Money for food will be lacking. Even the washer-women will be affected. We are with you brave drivers, and your health is on our minds.

After he had completed customs formalities—vaccination proof, *laissez passer*, transit visa,—Yiriba took a date with Korotouma in the Babemba Hotel of Zégoua. When night fell, they came to the room. Wanting to wash, Korotouma was given money by Yiriba to pay for a second towel rather than let her use his. This is because he said two persons should not use a single towel. Once in bed, Korotouma caressed Yiriba from his neck to his thigh. The man jumped from bed, grabbed his travelling bag, and handed Korotouma a condom that she did not appreciate.

Korotouma (Hawa): What is that? It's because you do not love me.

Yiriba (Daouda): Far from that.

Korotouma (Hawa): Imagine presenting a condom to a grand lady such as myself!

Yiriba (Daouda): Prudence is the queen of mothers. I did not say that you are sick. But I, what do you know of me? Both of us travel a lot, and we meet many people every day. This condom will protect you and me. I must say we hardly know one another.

Korotouma (Hawa): You believe that I have AIDS?

Yiriba (Daouda): Are we even afraid of AIDS? It is other STDs we should fear. There are medicines for these in the health centers along the way. But my faithful companion is the condom.

Daouda: Upset, Korotouma abandons the room, leaving Yiriba by himself.

Hawa's Song: I greet all the drivers of Mali, of Cote d'Ivoire, of Guinea, of Burkina Faso. From Conakry to Senegal. Those of Tambacounda and the capital. Everyone should listen and adhere to the advice of one another.

Narrator (Daouda): The next morning, the boys who did not know where she had slept, followed her when she walked around the yard of the customs office. Seydou, debauched and stubborn, spoke to her.

Seydou (Daouda): Hey little sister. Yesterday you passed by us in the yard here. I looked in vain for you.

Korotouma (Hawa): I went to sleep near the hill.

Seydou (Daouda): You did not find a ride?

Korotouma (Hawa): There is a driver named Yiriba whom I lost. He had promised me.

Seydou (Daouda): I am going this afternoon. It's no problem.

Narrator (Daouda): He was not leaving that day, but he did not want to say so. The girl followed him to the hotel and after some caresses the two entwined themselves and remained so until the next morning. Many drivers were saying morning prayers at 7:30 AM. In performing his ablutions[9] Seydou noticed that his urine was burning him. He asked himself what could be wrong. He had not thought about a condom. Korotouma's STDs had infected Seydou. Gonococcus. This disease can stay a long time [be asymptomatic] in a woman but rapidly infects and is symptomatic in a man. From [contamination] one morning the harmful infection was detected that same afternoon. The man left for Bamako, and Korotouma went on her way. Seydou changed the tires for Ghana. After Bako (Here I greet these doctors, those of Burkina Faso, of Bobo Diolasso and Nyangoloko, I greet driver Salvador of Nyangoloko, the drivers of Pountin, of

9. Muslims pray at fixed intervals throughout the day. Ablutions (washings) involve the washing of all orifices. To be ritually and actually clean, Seydou would have passed urine before washing for prayer.

Ouaga[dougou], and Koka[10]) Seydou arrived in Benin where he lives. He bedded down with his wife whom he infected and who detected nothing.

On the other side, Yiriba, always with his condom traveled here there and everywhere.

Hawa's Refrain: I have traveled from east to west, from north to south and I have never seen a fever like this one, Father of the Griots.

Narrator (Daouda): It is rare to see men like Yiriba, but of the likes of Seydou, the world is full. Seydou remained ill in Benin. He resorted to self-medication which some call the "Walking Pharmacy," "Dust Pharmacy," or "Anything Goes [Pharmacy]."[11] Does not "Anything Goes" mean "Go Everywhere?" He puts them in tonic: 20 tetracyclines, 10 to 14 [*sic.*], five "blue-blues"[12] hoping to augment your speed, certainly, but there when your speed is finished, you will no longer move. After this treatment, he stayed put.

Yiriba, after Ghana, proceeded to Benin where he looked up his buddy Seydou whom he found ailing in Porto Novo [Benin]. Seydou had entrusted his rig to his apprentice driver for a trip to Ghana, then Abidjan [Cote d'Ivoire], and Bamako [Mali]. Seydou tells Yiriba "I am sick and I don't know how I got this because I have a girlfriend at Vridi [Cote d'Ivoire], another at Abobogare [Cote d'Ivoire] and another at Zégoua [Mali]. Really I do not understand," said Seydou.

But Yiriba said, "Big brother, I had told you. Every time you are with a woman, you must always be wearing a condom. It will protect you. There are contagious diseases, gonorrhea, etc., diseases, which will make you impotent and sterile. These diseases make you susceptible to AIDS.

I, griot say that these diseases create a path for AIDS. If you are infected by any STD, it weakens you and causes you to lose weight. Death can follow. Thus, lets join hands to combat this mortal disease.

Hawa's Refrain: I have searched all the big cities from east to west from north to south, and I have never seen any disease like it.

Narrator (Daouda): The driver's apprentice who had been entrusted the vehicle never even returned to Benin to visit his supervisor. Seydou's wife, who fell ill, never gave birth again. She could not get surgery because she had had the disease for such a long time. Let's join hands. Because listen. If your vehicle leaves with another because you are ill, you will never get the rig back. Beware. It's generally Toumani Kone of Sikasso of Somatrie; Toegoue of Kenedougou Voyages, Bamadou Simaga of Segou. These people [rig owners] do take care of the drivers [they employ] and give

10. Towns and cities on the long distance routes in Burkina Faso.

11. Pharmaceuticals, often expired, are readily available in the markets, taxi stands, and long distance truck and bus stations in many parts of Africa. Sometimes medication is sold from a tray that is carried on the head of the vendor who ambles about the stations, hence the name Foot Pharmacy. Because markets and stations are dusty places, these "pharmacies" can also be called "dust pharmacies."

12. Stimulants.

> him back his keys. Also Batio of Mopti.[13] Rig owners. Take care of your drivers.
>
> The story of Yiriba is about seeing and meeting women and men every day. Prudence must reign supreme. Always have a condom whether you are a woman or a man. This will avoid many disagreements. (Daouda Dembélé and Hawa Dembélé, 1999 translated from Bambara to French by Moutaga Ly and from French to English by Louise Bourgault).

Selections from Yiriba can be heard on the compact disk that accompanies this text. Refer to Oral Narratives.

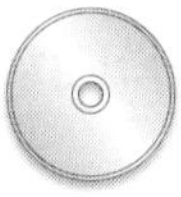

Audio 1. "Yiriba" AIDS Awareness for Truck Drivers
Griots Dauda Dembélé and Hawa Dembélé, Mali

The story of Yiriba raises in an entertaining way, many of the social, interactional, and health factors that contribute to the spread of AIDS. Sexually transmitted diseases, rampant on the African continent, are discussed. Their symptoms, or the lack thereof, are noted. Their relationship to the spread of AIDS is discussed, their proper treatment and cure encouraged. Self-medication is roundly discouraged.

The story also treats the issue of the all too common denial, usually by women, of a sexual past. Korotouma regards herself as a "*grande dame*" apparently excluding "sex for a lift" as a form of prostitution. Whatever her self-identified occupation, her behavior in refusing the use of the condom is all too common. It represents one of the serious impediments working against the containment of the AIDS epidemic. Korotouma's sexual aggressiveness is noted though not overtly condemned while Seydou is said to be both stubborn (for refusing to use a condom) and depraved. He is depicted as morally reprehensible because he puts his family at risk.

The consequences of falling ill with any STD are shown to be both financial and social. Seydou loses his rig and hence his livelihood. He also loses a comrade, his apprentice who obviously graduates to driver as a result of Seydou's misfortune. This is a disappointment for folks living in the "people-oriented" societies of West Africa. More importantly, Seydou's wife becomes barren, a great tragedy in societies where the birth of a baby, even to a poor unmarried woman, is usually considered a joyous event. The threat of infertility is a powerful motivator for condom use.

Griots use techniques of oral presentation that make their tales and songs particularly appealing and particularly memorable. Daouda Dembélé and his wife Hawa address the audience directly. They honor their listeners, long distance truck drivers with praise and flattery. They list the cities, towns, and coun-

13. In praising the owners of rigs who do assist in the health care expenses of their drivers, Djeli Dauda is putting subtle social pressure on other owners who are less socially responsible.

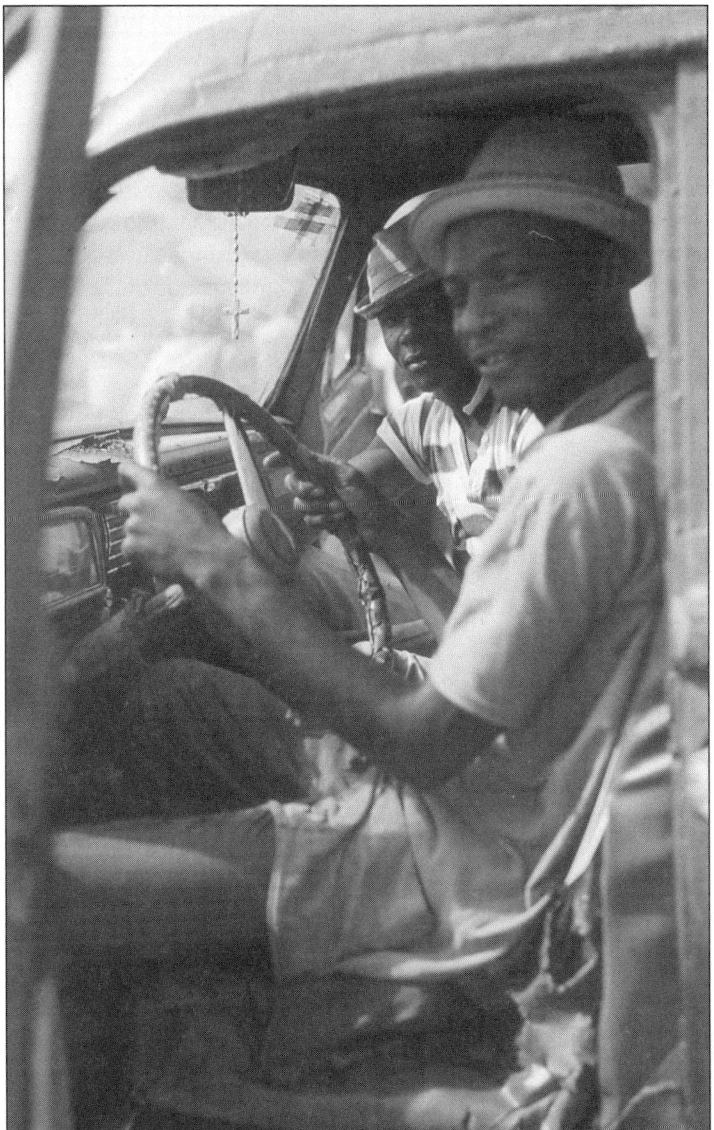

Figure 5-7. Migration and mobility are important factors in the spread of HIV/AIDS. Truck drivers are considered a high risk group.

tries whence the drivers originate or through which the drivers pass. They thank their sponsors. They praise the rig owners for caring for their drivers. They certify the value of the doctors and clinicians that will treat the truckers for STDs. They commend the rig owners who help their drivers when these latter fall ill. Daouda and Hawa's presentation is careful to affirm the importance of all members of society. It promotes the communal values of harmony and plurality.

The griots use a number of stylistic devices to attract and retain interest while getting the message across. They accompany the tale on the *ngoni*, a five stringed lute. They use musical interludes, sung by Hawa to break up the narrative and to reinforce the main message about the severity of the epidemic. There is a cyclicity to this musical arrangement which is built up through repetition. This is characteristic of the oral tradition, one that both restates African notions of cosmology and reinforces group sentiment (Brown, 1998, pp. 66; 107–8; 135; 150–1,184).

The Dembélés also vary their styles of presentation. Although Daouda serves as narrator, the two performers also act out the character roles of Yiriba and Korotouma; and Seydou and Korotouma. The listener must be attentive to these shifts in point of view which are typical of the oral tradition, and which help to give the presentation a kind of "you are there" feel. These and other stylistic issues will be discussed in Chapter 6. Clearly the *djeli* (or griot), the socially sanctioned advice-giver, tale-teller, news-carrier, with his magical gift for words and music, is an excellent medium to use in Africa's cultural arsenal against AIDS. And clearly the griot's musical story recitation resonates well within the community.

The idea for the development of Yiriba originated from a local NGO, the Zégoua Development Association. The folks at Zégoua, a border town, proposed the idea of using Daouda Dembélé because he is himself both a griot and a former truck driver. The staff in the NGO knew a work of his would be a hit among his peers! Daouda Dembélé and his wife Hawa spent some time at the SIDA2 headquarters training in HIV prevention strategies. This production approach appears to have insured the authenticity of this folk genre while assuring a clear high quality message. Using a familiar and popular genre and a locally originated product is key to producing effective edutainment.

SIDA2 produced 4,000 copies of the cassette to be distributed at cost (500 CFA francs or about $.80 US) to truck drivers, and to be supplied to NGOs throughout the region. The NGOs were free to make and sell official copies in order to raise funds for other projects. But the response to Yiriba has been excellent. Radio stations throughout the West African region are playing Yiriba, and bootlegged copies regularly appear in the Zégoua and other markets. SIDA2 staff estimate that probably up to 4,000 additional bootlegged copies had already been made, less than a year after the official copies were released (Sylla, June 2000, interview). Truck drivers from all ends of the ancient Mali Empire, from Côte d'Ivoire, Guinea, Burkina Faso, Senegal and the Gambia) were reportedly clamoring for the Yiriba cassette ("AIDS Control/AIDS in Mali" 2000).

Review Questions

1. What is the purpose of the Legend of Sundiata? How does this legend instill pride in the Malian people, and by extension, the people of the Mande diaspora?
2. What are the multiple roles for the griot in Mande society? What oral stylistics do griots employ in their oral art forms?
3. What subjects are tackled in the cassette recording Yiriba? How does this production use time-tested storytelling methods from the Mande culture to warn truck drivers about the dangers of HIV/AIDS and other health risks?

Chapter 6

Chants and Songs

Stylistics of Oral Performance in Africa

The previous chapter treated the subject of oral bards on the African continent and surveyed the kinds of tales they may tell. This chapter examines the stylistics of oral performance and reviews two additional oral performance genres: chants and songs. It should be noted that all three genres, that is, stories, chants, and songs benefit from similar techniques of construction and presentation. In the struggle against AIDS, artists are adapting chants and songs just as they are adapting oral narratives. This chapter will demonstrate why these oral genres lend themselves so easily and so well to social comment, edutainment, and social participation.

Role of the Audience

The first item of note in the study of African oral performance is the social nature of performance, the fact that performance in Africa reflects the communality of life. Almost without exception, the works presented in Chapters 5 and 6 and indeed in all of the genre chapters, are designed to foster ***group*** enjoyment through communal action. An oral bard expects his audience to participate in a narrative or a song. And audiences usually oblige a performer in various ways. They shout cries of encouragement to the narrator; they cheer the hero; they boo and hiss at the villain. They gasp in fear during a frightening interlude. They laugh with relish during an amusing scene. They call out warnings when a character is menaced. Audience members may well join in the delivery of recurring lines or refrains, and they will clap and stomp rhythmically or dance during musical interludes.

Audience members may assist in delivering a performance. They may pose questions to a narrator to encourage him to begin, or to extend the tale. They may help him with a forgotten line or word. A performer who fails to generate obvious audience response may be unable to continue, attuned as he is to the social dynamics of presentation. Ever sensitive to audience tastes and sensibilities, performers shift the content of the tale to suit the tastes of the audience. This is why there are so many different versions of oral tales.

Music

The reader should also note that many of the oral narratives provided may be accompanied by music. The music will vary according to the ethnic group, the availability of musicians, and the suitability of the pieces. Music often provides a context within which to situate the tales. Sometimes the narratives are highlighted by a group chorus, or punctuated alternatively, as we have seen in last chapter's "Yiriba," by a lone voice. The narrator himself or herself may sing a tale as well as narrate it in prose. And at intervals between movements of a tale, a good storyteller may even mime or dance what is about to come. It should be noted that performers, particularly those who also dance, might use costumes or props associated with the story.

Innovation versus Fixed Text

The content of certain types of oral narratives is highly prescribed. This includes some royal poetry and some divination ritual for example. But generally speaking, the performance of oral tales, chants, and songs involves a great deal of improvisation. The storyteller, for example, has the bare outlines of a story around which he fashions his art. The performer uses his skill with the language, and its delivery to render the tale. He also uses his voice, his face, his gestures, his whole body, or even a few props to heighten the impact of the recitation he is giving. He may demonstrate an action in his story by miming the action of stabbing, of beating, for example, with his head, with his hands, or with his whole body. He may break into song or dance if the mood of the piece or the audience calls for it. Closely connected with the storyline, these musical interludes would advance the narrative.

A good African bard can approximate the sounds of his world. He can hear the sound of the pounding of the pestle against the mortar in the kitchen. He can render the slashing of the cutlass against the brush in the forest. He can recreate the thumping of the fish nets against the rim of the canoe in the sea. His presentation will celebrate the trumpeting of the elephant; it will recall the laughing of the hyena; it will call to mind the rumbling of the hornbill. For indeed, the performer fashions the narrative not for the eye but for the ear. Griots and other bards use certain identifiable styles and techniques to appeal directly to the sense of hearing. In the audio clip provided in the accompanying compact disk, Liberian village actors orally produced the sounds of a machete hacking through the rainforest in a village-based drama produced for radio.[1] Refer to Chants and Songs.

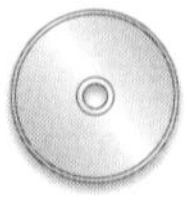

Audio 1. Ideophones of Machete from "Mother Swamp" Village Theatre of Gwemble, Liberia

1. For a detailed account, see Bourgault 1991. See also Brooke 1989.

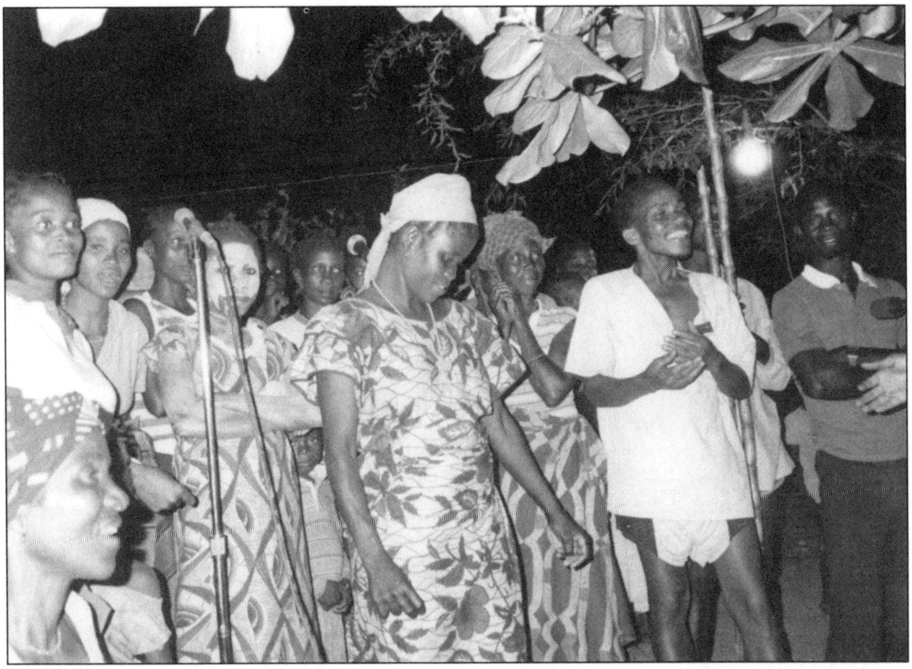

Figure 6-1. Liberian women singing for the village-based drama, "Mother Swamp," produced by the Liberian Rural Communications Network (LRCN).

Repetition

Repetition is one of the important stylistic devices exploited by the oral performer. It is used for several reasons. First, it helps the bard to build and maintain a rhythmic delivery. Second, repetition adds emphasis and creates drama. And third, it promotes audience comprehension and encourages their participation. A repeated chorus or refrain, moreover, can be used to separate different messages of a narrative or separate episodes in a folk tale.

Okpewho explains the use of repetition in the oral tale as compared to its use in writing.

> Whereas the writer generally makes every effort to avoid repetition (whether in phrase or in logic) and carefully eliminates any noticeable instances of repetition in the fear they might cause the composition to drag and so to bore its readers, the oral performer cultivates repetition both as a means of achieving auditory delight in listeners and as a convenient framework for holding the distinct elements of the composition together (Okpewho, 1992, p. 78).

And as noted in the last chapter, repetition creates a sense of circularity, one that replicates the African world view.

Agonistic Toning

Bards make use of high contrast (sometimes called agonistic styling) in drawing their characters. Pitted against one another, these personalities are larger than life. Their memorability provides for easy recall for the bard and rapt identification for the audience. Thus bold heroes defeat sniveling cowards; fast and clever animals compete with slow and dim ones. Young and beautiful maidens suffer at the hands ugly old crones.

Parallelism

Bards make liberal use of a technique called parallelism. Parallelism or parallel form refers to the balancing of images and ideas. This balancing is clearly evident in poetry, chants, songs and even prose narratives. Balancing can be undertaken both in terms of meaning (semantic) and in terms of rhythm. Several examples of parallel form come from a song collected in Sierra Leone about a woman's lot in life. The entire 'text' of "That is the Life that You Live" is provided later on in the chapter. Certain excerpts are supplied here to illustrate examples of parallelism.

The reader should note, for example, how oppositions are created between a woman and her husband in the third stanza with the line "Monkey do all the work: Baboons eating all the food," and again, "some are creating; some are destroying."

In spite of all that, it is a game of Monkey doing all the work,
    Baboon eating all the food.
That is the life that "You know who" lives.
Some are creating, some are destroying.

Later in the same narrative, oppositions are created between the faithful wife and the husband's many lovers. In the fourth and fifth stanzas, we will observe repetition in the redundant use of the word "leaves" that begins many lines. This is combined with excellent use of parallel form and clever use of names. The line "Leaves Gladys at home to find Sorrow outside the home" is rhythmically parallel, positionally parallel, and semantically parallel. (Sorrow and Gladys each have two syllables, a stressed followed by an unstressed; inside is in the opposite position to outside; Sorrow is the opposite of Gladys or Gladness).

Leaves Gladys at home to find Sorrow outside the home;
....
Leaves Alafiya (peaceful life) at home to procure "*Wahala*" (trouble, difficulty) outside.

The clever use of parallelism continues in the sixth and seventh stanzas.

Leaves Joy at home, to find Trouble outside;
....
You leave Beauty at home for Beasty outside;

You do not clock Blackie because you have to keep Yala (Yallow's) time all the time.[2]

....

You leave Nancy at home for "Kasi" (worries) outside; (Hinzen, James, Sorie, Tamu, 1987, p. 116–117).

"The Life That You Lead," obviously composed in English, demonstrates the remarkable ability of oral performers to create rhythmic and memorable turns of phrase. If many of the tales supplied in the last chapter appear less than musical or less than prone to rhythmic parallel, this is most likely because they have lost their musicality in translation from the indigenous African language in which they were first performed.

Piling

Oral bards also use a recitational device called piling that refers to the artist's ability to say the same thing in a number of different ways. The repetition is used to hook one line into the next, thereby aiding recall. This piling technique is used in this hunting song collected in Sierra Leone.

Now there was a hunter, Sori
    He had set out to hunt
He saw bush cows up a hill
The cow itself turned around looked
And it saw the hunter inside the town
The hunter said "I have seen bush cows"
The bush cow also said
"I have seen a hunter" (Hinzen, James, Sorie, and Tamu, 1987, p. 57).

Tonality

As noted earlier, while some of the narratives provided are merely spoken, others are chanted or sung. The use of tonal variation in African narratives can be compared to the chanting done between priests and people in some antiphonal singing which is part of the Catholic mass and other rituals.

The narrator can use tone much like the Catholic priest does, to produce a melodic effect. When the audience, the bard's apprentice or other assistant responds, they/he can use a different tone, thereby creating a tonal counterpoint.

The fact that African languages are tonal allows for additional clever play with the use of tone. The very tonal Yoruba language of Nigeria and Benin has been manipulated in performance with great effect. By using stylized formulary expressions, Yoruba bards can engage in simulated call and response interludes with a "talking drum," the drum itself recreating the tones of human speech. Al-

2. Yala (Yellow) is a reference to a light-skinned African woman. It may also imply that the woman has used skin lightening products.

ternatively, Yoruba bards can suggest reverence (or commonality) in a performance by using primarily high tones typically reserved to address a ruler, or by using largely low tones typically used to speak to a commoner.

Ideophones

African performance artists also employ ideophones in the creation of their art. An ideophone is a stylistic device that creates ideas in sound. It is like an onomatopoeia (the words "buzz," "purr," and "tweet" are examples) except that an ideophone has no life outside its created context, the oral performance in which it appears. Ideophones are often used repetitively in a chorus. They encourage group participation and add to the sense of communal delight of audiences.

An excellent example of the ideophone comes in the chorus from the tale "How Rabbit Married the Chief's Beautiful Daughter."

How Rabbit Married the Chief's Beautiful Daughter

One day Rabbit came to the chief and expressed his desire to marry his daughter. The chief willingly agreed to Rabbit's request, provided he would break all the palm kernels in his ten thousand stores with his teeth. Rabbit agreed, and asked the chief to open all the stores for him. Then he started breaking the kernels with his teeth, and singing at the same time. Actually Rabbit was not singing, but the sound of the palm kernels being broken by his teeth produced a nice melody like this:

Lead: Gbugula, gbugula
Chorus: Gbugula mugu nyamu-nyamu
Lead: Gbugula
Chorus: Gbugula mugu nyamu-nyamu
Lead: Gbugula
Chorus: Gbugula mugu nyamu-nyamu
Lead: Ku fuurr
Chorus: Gbugula mugu nyamu-nyamu
Lead: Ku Saarr
Chorus: Gbugula mugu nyamu-nyamu
Lead: Ku Feerr (Hinzen, James, Sorie, and Tamu, 1987, p. 291).

Songs and Chants

The present text has repeatedly noted the difficulty of classifying African performance genres. In the previous chapter, I presented narrative tales, for example, which were made up almost entirely of prose. I noted that although these tales are not rhymed, they are sometimes sung. And because prose is sometimes sung in African performance, or because spoken prose is often interspersed with song, it becomes difficult to distinguish between stories and other related genres such as chants and songs. In this chapter I maintain that distinction between the genres of story, chant, and song appears to be one of musicality. The tale is clearly the least musical; it is followed by the chant that occupies a medial position; and both are followed by song, which is clearly the most melodic. This section contains examples of African performance genres that clearly are rhymed and that clearly are meant to be chanted. Later in the chapter I will consider song as a separate genre.

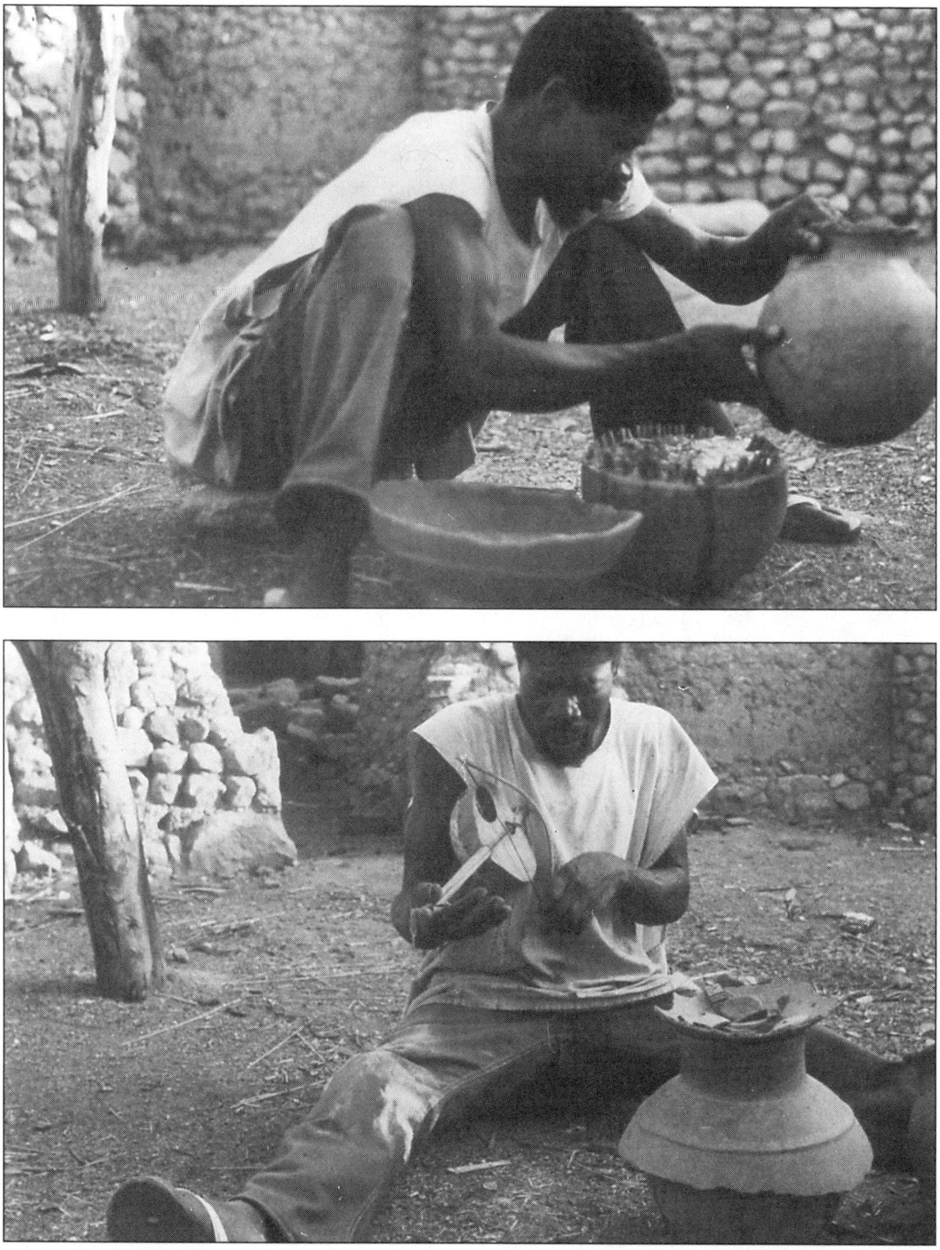

Figure 6-2. Divination Ceremony in northern Cameroon. Divination is usually accomplished with music, which is used to call the spirits.

Chants

As noted earlier, Western readers can understand African chanting performance by making reference to Catholic antiphonal call and response singing during the mass and during other rituals. Renditions of these performances use a more limited tonal range than does normal singing. Divination, involving the use of a specialist to communicate with the ancestors, gods, or other spirits, is widely practiced in sub-Saharan African societies. The practice usually involves some level of performance; the most important of which is chanting. The following example comes from the Yaka people of the Democratic Republic of the Congo (formerly Zaire).

In this instance, the diviner is trying to determine the cause of death of a woman named Suuta. According to Rene Devisch who studied Yaka divination rituals, Suuta's death is related to a hypocritical curse, with sorcery, and with the family's failure to perform appropriate rituals after Suuta's father's death (Devisch, 1991, p. 121). The diviner is in a trance when he pronounces the divination chant.

Diviner: (VERY HIGHLY STRUNG, HIS EYES STARING FROM THEIR SOCKETS): Where are the sorcerers hiding who want to make so many difficulties for me?
Where is Suuta? Where is Suuta? Where is Suuta? Where is Suuta? Where is Suuta? Didn't she die because you used the bridewealth wrongly [i.e., took it yourself after a hypocritical curse]? I see that Suuta went to Kinshasa. When she came back she was pregnant and very sick and she had a suitcase with her. You haven't opened her suitcase. Where are Koongu and Toonda? These are uterine [mother's side] forebearers who transmitted prohibitions. As if it were true!

Answer (BY ONE OF THE CLIENTS, SUUTA'S FAMILY): Indeed!

Diviner: I have just seen a curse. Listen: It is Mbela who uttered the curse. How did he withdraw the curse? What do I see in connection with this cursing? What have you done in connection for the bridewealth offered for our daughter Suuta? Have you thrown it on the edge of the village or what have you done with it? I see a woman called Meengi? How are you related to her? Has she got a husband or not?

Answer: Meengi is one of father's sisters. She is not married.

Diviner: Meengi is a sorcerer. And I see that you her brother Mbela [here present] went with Suuta to Kinshasa (Devisch, 1991. pp. 121–122).

Chanting tends to have an aura of sacredness about it. It is used in a good deal of court poetry, including the court praises (*izibongo)* recited by the Zulu court poet, the *imbongi*. In such chanted performance, the focus is on the human voice, usually that of the performer. The music is either very subdued, or it is absent. And audience participation is kept to a minimum. Brown describes the performance style of the *imbongi*.

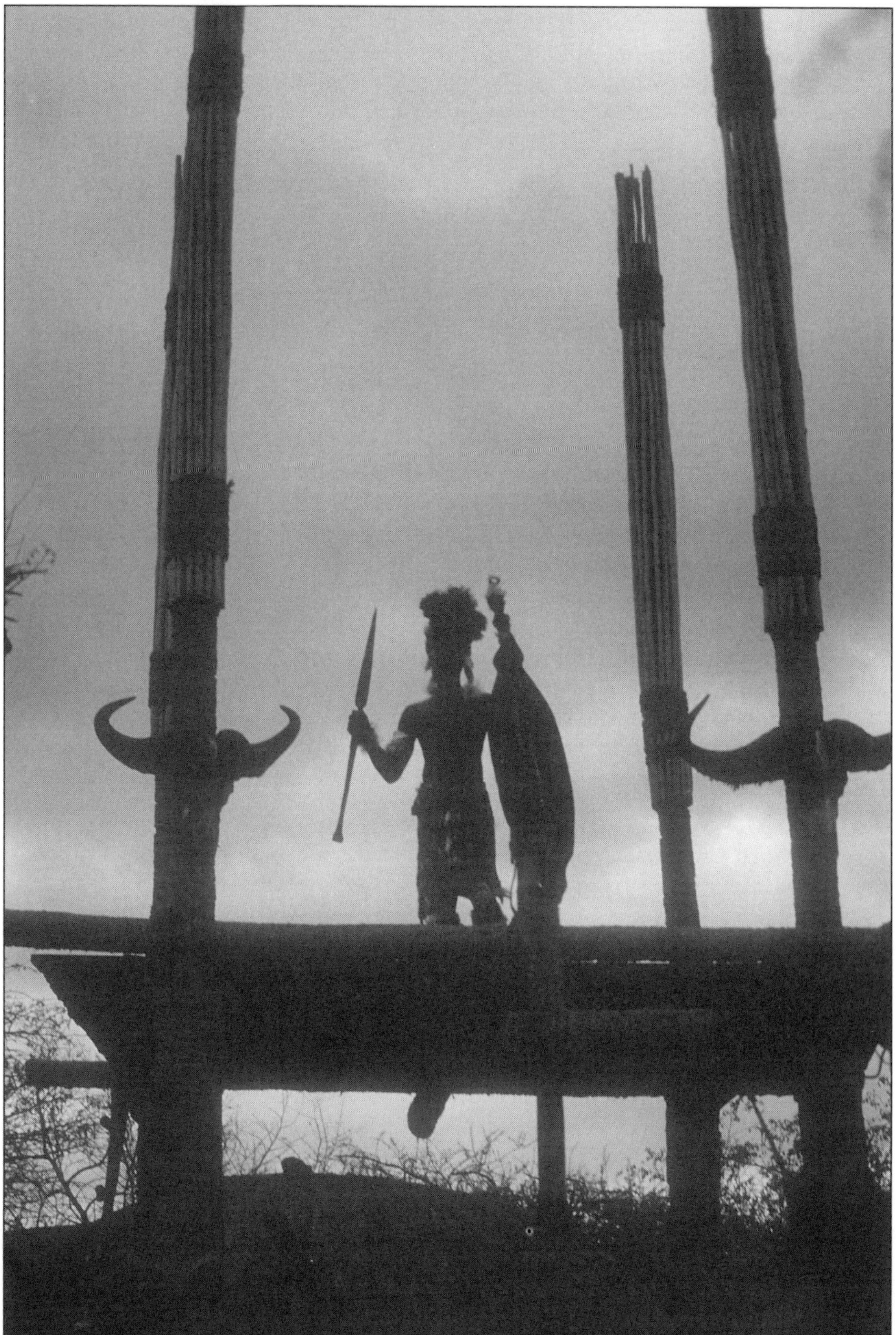

Figure 6-3. The Great King Shaka (1816–1828) united the Zulus and created a great warrior nation.

> *Izibongo* usually begin with an opening formula—a salute to the ruler, or the recitation of his clan praises—the primary function of which seems to be to attract attention of the crowd so as to create silence for the performance; and the poems generally end with a concluding sentence such as 'I disappear.' (1998, p. 97.)

One way to make contact with the dead, with ancestors, is to recite their praises. Opland argues that the *imbongi*, when performing praise poetry to the great King Shaka (1816–1828) and other past Zulu kings are acting in a spiritual capacity, almost as a vestigial shaman (1983, p. 72). Here is a section of Shaka taken from Cope.

> The beast that lowed at Mthonjanemi,
> All the tribes heard its wailing,
> It was heard by Dunjwa and the Yengweni kraal,
> It was heard by Mangcengeza of Khali's kraal.
> That burned the owls on the Dlebe hill,
> And eventually those on Madeblana also burned.
> He who travelled across to Ndima and Mgovu,
> And women who were with child gave birth easily;
> The newly planted crops they left still short,
> The seed they left amongst the maize-stalks,
> The old women were left in the abandoned sites,
> The old men were left along the tracks,
> The roots of trees looked up at the sky.
> He who reached the top of Bhuzane mountain,
> He came across a long line of buck,
> He passed by Mcombo as the cattle were leaving (Cope quoted in Brown, 1998, p. 86.)

© Oxford University Press 1968. Reprinted from **Izibongo: Zulu Praise Poems** collected by James Stuart, translated by Daniel Malcom, and edited with introductions and annotations by Trevor Cope (1968) by permission of Oxford University Press.

The following is a chant with a chorus created upon the Death of the late Premier of Northern Nigeria, Sir Ahmadu Bello, assassinated in the country's first coup in 1966. Here the court poet Alhaji Musa Dankwairo makes an appeal for calm. His recitation was said to have been somber and its mood subdued. Musa Dankawairo was chanting in the courtly tradition of the Hausa city states of northern Nigeria.

Eulogy for Sir Ahmadu Bello

Chorus: He doesn't tolerate insolence
No one can dare approach him with insolence
Amadu, the grandson of Bello, the brave warrior

Soloist: You are like the bone of an elephant
Of Alu, which cannot be swallowed
It alone can block up the throat.

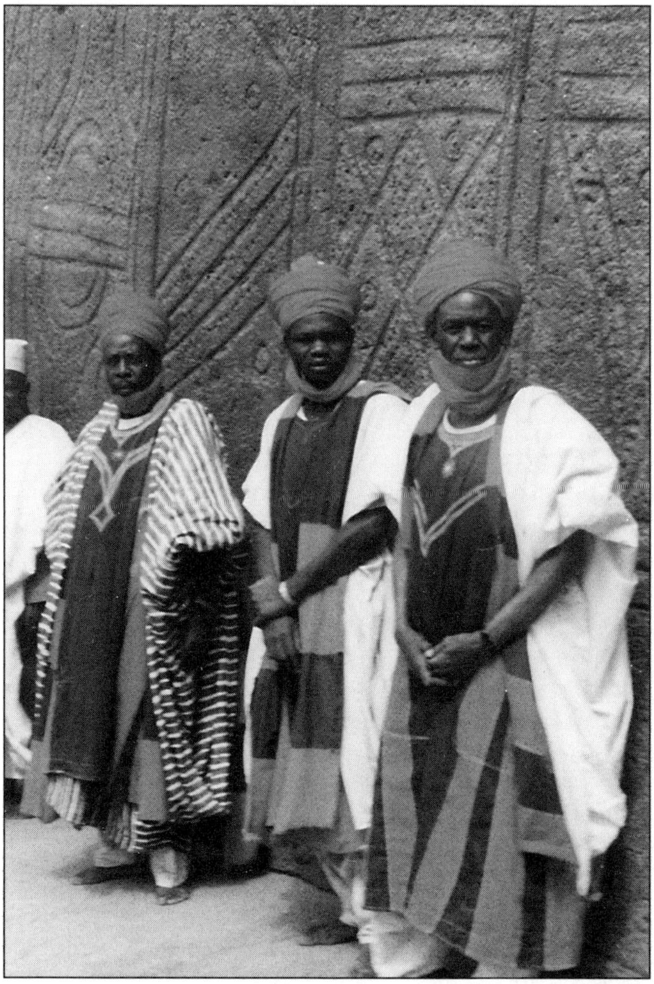

Figure 6-4. Courtiers at the Palace of the Emir of Kano. The courtly tradition in northern Nigeria dates back to the Middle Ages.

Chorus: He doesn't tolerate insolence
No one dare approach him with insolence,
Amadu, the grandson, the brave warrior.

Soloist: You Alhaji Musa Dankwairo,
Sing a song of meditation for Ahmadu Bello
Let us submit to the will of God,
That nobody will live beyond his day.
You know that none will live beyond his times.
When Amadu was ruling (administering)
He took good care of his people.
None of his followers went astray.
Even now his followers have not gone astray.
Amadu, the Premier of the North,
What did you do for Nigeria?

Will forever continue to be remembered,
Amadu, the grandson of a pious one,
You are brave, a trusted son.
May God pardon you.
Malam may Allah pardon you
Malam Ahmadu, may Allah grant you his pardon.
Now let us forget the past, and look
Forward to the future.
It remains for you now to find his replacement.
Let us forget the past, and look forward to the future.
You should next find his substitute.
He was fearless, and never gave up.
He demonstrated that he was the grandson of Shehu
(Usman Fodiyo)[3]
Ahmadu got all he wanted on earth,
And he showed his contentment by
Showing kindness, and taking good care of his brothers,
He took care of sons, and slaves,
He took care of servants and all his subjects.
But (alas), on a Friday, at 2:00 (a.m.)
Amadu was overpowered by a war.
I cried and commented bitterly,
But I soon remembered and congratulated him,
For rather than surrender (in such situations)
It is better for a Muslim to die a martyr
Which is not a blemish at all.

Chorus: He does not tolerate insolence
No one can dare approach him with insolence
Amadu, the grandson of Bello, the brave warrior.

Soloist: You are an ore-made wall, which does not sprout,
The brave one of Sir Kassim.
Bello the son of Hassan.
You have inherited the qualities of Dan Fodiyo
You have inherited the qualities of Abdullahi,
You have inherited the qualities of Muhwi,
And Atto, and Uwar Naje (Nana).
You have inherited the qualities of
Isan Kware, the last born child of Shehu.
You have inherited the qualities of
Ibrahim, the brave fighter,
The brave warrior, and a son of a brave warrior,
Your grandparents were true saints.
No iota of a joke at all.

---

3. Refers to Usman Dan Fodio the Fulani leader who came from the North and waged a Holy War for Islam in the 19th century, which led to the conversion of northern Nigeria to Islam.

Even in the next world we seek to be
Your right-hand ones (Dankwairo quoted in Yahiya, 1981, pp. 147–9).

The reader should note the courtly qualities of this recited lamentation. Replete with praise for a great man's bravery in battle and his ability to rule, it recounts his genealogy, taking care to trace his descent from a long line of warriors.

Not all chants recount the praises of court rulers or the deeds of slain leaders. Like most other genres, chants can be used in a variety of contexts. The following chant was used by an Efe Poet of the Gelede cult of Nigeria to protest the payment of a tax. The group was protesting the tax that ultimately was being collected on behalf of the colonial power, Great Britain. And it was objecting to the local ruler, a stand-in for the British government.

You are ringing the bell to remind us of tax payment.
You are ringing the bell to remind us of tax payment.
While we are demanding that we should have our own *oba* (ruler).
If you refuse to grant us our demand
We'll go round the world to air our grievances
You are ringing the bell to remind us of tax payment
(traditional bard quoted in Olabimtan, 1981, p. 160).

Beggars in many parts of West Africa also use chanting. The beggar will approach an individual and request a gift often in the name of Allah (God). If the person is generous, the beggar will compose a ***praise-prayer***. If the patron fails to give, the beggar may chant an insult. The form of the praise might begin something like the following.

In the name of God, the most generous
I intend to sing a new song
In praise of the beloved messenger
The savior of the Day of Judgment
Who loves him will never suffer (Na-Mangi quoted in Kofoworola, 1981, p. 301)

The rhythm of the above tune is identified as a *cagi*, and it is said to reconstitute that made by a mortar and pestle when yams are pounded or corn is ground (Kofoworola, 1981, p. 303). After this rather stylized opening shown above, the beggar will invent a praise-prayer appropriate for the patron. I myself have been the subject of Hausa praise poems that address my status as a *Baturia,* (a foreign or Caucasian woman), after giving gifts of coins to street beggars in Nigeria.

Chants can be used to taunt or to satirize individuals whose behavior is deemed unacceptable by a cultural group. The following chant was composed by a group of teenage Igbo (Nigeria) girls and was designed to chastise one of their age-mates that enjoyed the pleasures of sex and suffered its consequences. Its recitation was accompanied by lewd gestures designed to approximate the act of copulation.

Opening the waist is not the problem our children
Opening the waist is not the problem our children
Those about whom we are talking know themselves

A bottom once bitten by an ant gets wiser
Opening the waist is not the problem our children
The blood that splashed in the childbirth room.
Opening the waist is not the problem our children.
The screams from the Daughter-of-Mary in the childbirth room
"Take me in a car to the Aboh hospital!"
Opening the waist is not the problem young boys and girls
(Nwambara quoted in Nwoga, 1981, p. 234).

AIDS Chants

I have noted many many times in this volume that African oral literature is endlessly adaptable. The severity of the AIDS crisis on the continent has invited poets to comment upon it. The following two poem "*Mqothi Wembokodo Nesisekelo*" ("Annihilator") and "*Mthakatha Ndini Uyascbcka*," ("You Scary Sorcerer"), originally composed in Zulu by W. Lindani Cele, are written in the praise poetry style of the Zulu *imbongi*. Their appropriate presentation is in the *izibongo* chant form. Readers should be sensitive to the similarity in style between these poems and that of a section of the Shaka provided above.

Wembokodo Nesisekel (Annihilator)

We heard you grinding them overseas.
Still sunrise, you ground them again.
You annihilated.
Ground [them], then walked arrogantly with pride.
That is you,
Annihilator.

On televisions we saw them,
Disappearing whilst starring,
Disappearing like dew in the appearance of the sun.
In books we read about your works.
Blood terrifying works.

On radios, it has been you talked about;
All the sides, Ukhozi's,[4] Mandle Malakwante's[5]
All the sides, Metro's Glen Lewis[6]
Wo! Hhe!!! [SIGHS OF DESPAIR]
The list is endless.

---

4. Ukhozi is one of the South African Broadcasting Corporation's (SABC) powerful radio stations broadcasting in the Zulu language. Formerly known as Radio Zulu, the station was part of the official government apparatus of Apartheid or "separate development."

5. Mandla Malakwane was the Ukhozi's most popular presenter when the poem was written in 1998.

6. Metro is one of the SABC new commercial radio stations. It can be heard in all of South Africa's cities. Glen Lewis is a DJ there.

You are the most talked about, I'm telling you,
On busses, trains, and taxis.
That's you being talked about.

Even when sitting around the fireplace,
It's the same message: "No sex without condom."
I don't know what this means.[7]
In daily conferences, no solution.
Your presence is felt annihilator [BLUFFING].

You possess neither consciousness nor sympathy,
Despite some being respectful of you,
Four cardinal points of the world.
You don't stop.
That's annihilator.

You annihilate day and night.
Annihilate on the rainy and sunny days.
Let alone hail.

As I am talking the orphans are destitute.
Brothers and sisters, relatives: all in the Ancestral land.
That's because of you, annihilator.

Scientists and experts in knowledge
You left them frustrated and confused.
The Inyanga's[8] 'depleted' all forests,
Looking for herbs to counteract your frog-like stubbornness.
Let alone the church-people it's not a joke to pray on all God's days [WITH SARCASM]
'Satan get out of the way' has been a daily slogan.

Allow me to ask King of all kings,
Governor of heaven and Earth,
What sin did we commit?
Why such great anger?
For how long are we to endure this torture?
This endless torture... (Cele, n.d., translated by Ndlovu 2000).

Mthakathi Ndini Uyasclcka (You Scary Sorcerer)

You appear in the east,
Men's beard got frightened.
Appeared in the west,
Women screamed.
In the south and north,
Nothing would have stopped you from being there

7. This line appears in English in the original Zulu poem. This is why the next line reads, "I don't know what this means."
8. Zulu traditional herbalist.

Small kids get frightened of you like you were a snake.

Everyone blames the other because of you, Sorcerer
You a seed of dispute between lovers.
You ruin families of the entire Zulus.
You annihilate the Nation in general.
Everyone is so frightened to talk of you.

You frustrate without being biased.
The screams are in the east, west, south and the north.
You destroy Indians, Coloureds, Whites, Chinese, Blacks
The list is endless...

You care neither for the poor, nor the rich;
Neither for men nor women;
Not even for children. You destroy.
Not even before they are born.
You have no conscience, no sympathy.
You sorcerer.

We cried endlessly.
We mourned continuously.
They talked of you and never stopped.
Even now they are talking now about the solution.
Solution to counteract your witchcraft,
Sorcerer (Cele, n.d. translated by Ndlovu 2000).

Mr. Cele, a secondary school teacher, has founded a troupe of actors, who travel around KwaZulu-Natal province in South Africa and use his material in their performances. Mr. Cele is one of a number of amateur artists whose work on AIDS is performed in KwaZulu-Natal in South Africa. Health Ministry officials and non-governmental organizations readily use the performance media, including poetry recitation in the struggle against AIDS. Performances of such poetry is featured at AIDS awareness rallies; AIDS mural launchings; AIDS quilt displays; and other events designed to promote AIDS awareness. It is clear that these locally appreciated genres convey the sense of terror mixed with respect that is appropriate for a killer like AIDS.

Songs

The most melodic category of oral performance is that of song. Songs employ the full range of the human voice and are sung for just about any event or on any occasion. Okpewho, among others, notes the very prevalent use of song in African societies. Songs are used to calm a child and to celebrate his birth. Songs are used in rituals that accompany rites of passage, which transport human beings from one social stage in life to the next. Songs are used during work hours to lighten the burden of the task at hand. Songs are used in traditional ceremonies to celebrate the ancestors or the deities. And they are used in modern churches to revere the saints or the Christian god. Songs of praise are employed to raise up a person who is being honored by the community; songs of derision are used to chide a person who has dishonored the group. Songs are employed in politics to seek support for one camp; they are used in war to rally the troops against the opponent. Songs are used in play to entertain; songs are used in sorrow to mourn. This chapter provides just a few examples of songs and then proceeds to supply some of the songs that have been composed against AIDS. The discussion in this chapter liberally mixes songs sung acapella style, with songs accompanied by traditional and modern instruments. The accompanying compact disk shows the Diocesan choir of Kumasi, Ghana, singing songs of welcome to a group of visitors to the home of the Bishop. The second selection shows Africans singing in worship across a variety of congregations. Refer to Chants and Songs.

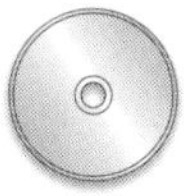

Video 1. Songs of Introduction and Welcome
Catholic Diocesan Choir, Kumasi, Ghana

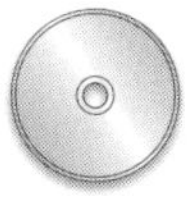

Video 2. 1. Shembe; 2. St. John's; 3. Durban Christian Centre; 4. International Central Gospel Church; 5. Diocesan Seminary Chapel
1., 2., 3. Durban, South Africa; 4. Accra, Ghana; 5. Kumasi, Ghana

Love is an important theme that has been the subject of song down through the ages. The following is a traditional Nigerian song of a son for his mother. It was popularized by Prince Nico Mbarga and Rocafil Jazz who released the juju tune in 1976. The tune combined the sounds of West African Highlife music with Mbarga's rumba guitar phrasing.

Sweet Mother[9]

So Sir,
Rocafil Jazz, sent to you sweet mother
Sweet Mother, I no go forget you
For this suffer whe you suffer for me
1
When I de cry
My mother go carry me

9. "Sweet Mother" is sung in West African Pidgin English. Done in highlife style, "Sweet Mother" is reported to have been the biggest selling African record of all time. Over 13 million copies had been sold by 1997!

She go say my pekin wettin you de cry-ye-eye
Stop, Stop! Stop Stop! Stop Stop!
Make you no cry again
2
When I waas sleep
My mother go pet me
She go lie me well for bed
She cover me cloth
Say make you sleep sleep my pekin-oh
3
When I de hungry my mother go run run madam
De find me something when I go chop-oh
Sweet mother a-a-a-ah
Sweet Mother o-o-o—h
So mama, sweet mother!
4
When I de sick
My mother go cry cry cry
She go say instead when I go die make,
She die-oh
She go beg God, God help me
God help me, my pekin oh-o-o-oh
5
If I no sleep, my mother no go sleep
If I no chop, my mother no go chop
She no de tire-a-a-a-, sweet mother
I no go forget this suffer whe you suffer
For me eh-eh-e-e-
Sweet mother a-a-a- Sweet mother o-oh
Aye Sweet mother
I can never forget you
You the suffer you suffer for me
And if I should forget you
Therefore, I forget my life
The air I believe in che-e-e- so so
And there all you man I beg
Never you forget your mother
Because if you forget your mother
You lost you life
Sweet mother I no go forget you
For this you suffer whe you suffer for me

Repeat 1, 2, 3, 4, 5
Sweet mother, you're the one who suffered for me
And I always keep that in mind
From the time I wanted to eat
You care for me, more! More! Suzie!
My sweet mother I no go forget you
My sweet mother, whe suffered for me

When I de cry, my mother go cry
She no no wettin to do.
You know well, na wettin de worry
You my pekin-oh!
You fit get another wife
You fit get another husband
But you fit get another mother?
Never-no-no-o-o-o-so ye!
My mother is great! Greater than the world

Repeat 2,3,5
Sweet mother ah-a-a-a- Sweet Mother
Oh-o-o (Prince Nico Mbarga & Rocafil Jazz 1991).

Social problems and people's misbehavior are often the subject of songs. The renowned Hausa bard Dan' Maraya Jos sings about forced marriage, the popular theme in patriarchal society where young girls are often given in marriage to older men. Here Dan' Maraya gives advice to parents especially fathers.

Father forced me to get married
Since it is against my wish
I will not be compelled to stay

If she marries whom she loves
You (parent) will be happy
She will be at ease,
The bridegroom will be happy,
On the day of naming ceremony,
Maraya and his kuntigi will be around
Will come and celebrate
There will be festivities
There will be prosperity (within the family)
(Jos quoted in Daba, 1981, p. 223)

Clearly human relationships and behavior between the sexes are powerful sources of inspiration for songs. Here is another love poem, a Somali song collected by Okot p'Betek.

When I see the beauty of my beloved's face,
I throw away the food in my hand;
Oh, sister of the young man, listen;
The beauty on my beloved's face.

Her neck is long, when I see it
I cannot sleep one wink;
Oh, the daughter of my mother-in-law,
Her neck is like the shaft of a spear.

When I touch the tattoos on her back,

I die;
Oh, sister of the young man, listen;
The tattoos on my beloved's back.

When I see the gap in my beloved's teeth,
Her teeth are white like dry season simsim;
Oh, daughter of my father-in-law, listen,
The gap in my beloved's teeth.

The daughter of the bull confuses my head,
I have to marry her;
True, sister of the young man, listen;
The suppleness of my beloved's waist.
(p'Bitek, quoted in Okpewho, 1992, pp. 139–140).

While there is a sub-text of sexual attraction in the romantic poem supplied above, no such high-mindedness exists in the following song of open sexuality, provided below. Recorded in 1970, "Come and Look at the Breasts," is a raunchy praise of rural women by Nigerian juju musician King Sunny Ade.

Come and Look at the Breasts

Come and look at the breasts of the married women that are washing clothes.
They wash in the day and the night.
It is for screwing, all of us, we bend down and screw
It is for screwing, their bottom is high [like a multi-storied building]
It is for screwing, their bottom is also fat
Come and look at the breasts of the married woman that are washing clothes
Wait a bit, I meet a baby with two breasts
And she's boasting me that if I paste my bottom on her, she'll paste her bottom on me (Sunny Ade and his Green Spots Band, quoted in Waterman, 1990, p. 133).

Women offer up a biting commentary on male sexual irresponsibility in this jeering satire against men, collected in Sierra Leone. The song "That is the Life that You Live" laments the female social position yet encourages women to accept their lot in life despite the misbehavior of their husbands.

That Is the Life That You Live

Ladies, stop sighing;
Stop grumbling and nagging about things
    That will bring you sorrow and leave you broken-hearted
Men are from the beginning deceitful, slippery and sly.
One foot on the sea, one on the land.
Men never fix their minds on one object!

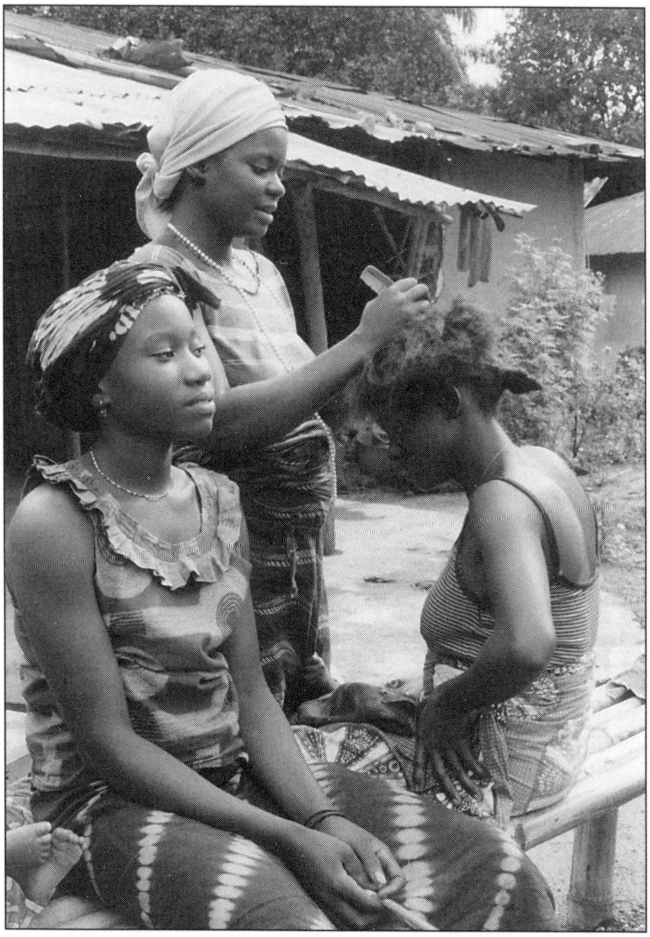

Figure 6-5. Group activities promote solidarity among African women and help them to withstand glaring gender disparities.

Ladies, do not despair.
Forget the men and listen to me for a few moments,
So that gladness will come to your hearts
And transform all your worrying to Hay Nomino.

One toothed man cannot chew corn.
Cockroach is a wonderful lawyer, he is always wearing his lawyer's gown.
But he will never appear in a court where Fowl is the Chief Justice.
Goat has many degrees from universities the world over,
But he will never lecture in Leopard's country.
No "Profession" in this world is as difficult as the Housewife Profession.
Twenty-four hours a day. Seven days a week, fifty two weeks a year...
No vacation leave, no increment, no pension.
All in one: she is a cook, nurse, washerwoman, painter, gardener, watchman, steward, teacher, lover, messenger, driver.
Tell me, what is there on earth that a housewife does not do?

In spite of all that, it is a game of Monkey doing all the work,
Baboon eating all the food.
That is the life that "You-know-who" lives.
Some are creating, some are destroying,
That is the life that you live!
Some help to gather, some are just there to scatter.
That is the life that you live!
Hastings[10] drinks, Waterloo[11] gets drunk
Kissy[12] harvests its mangoes, Freetown sells and eats them...
Another's husband is hidden in your room. Velvet foofoo[13] and Satin palava-sauce[14] are put on the table for him to eat.
In order to distract him from his wife and force him to abandon his home.
That is the life that you live.

Mister So-and-so's belly is protruding, several rings are appearing on his neck.
He is happy about it and calls it "Good Living,"
Little knowing that he had been given a charm to affect his rational thinking,
Which compels him to forsake Lily at home
And live with "Bajumor" (a big fat woman) out of home;
Leaves Gladys outside the home to find Sorrow outside of home,
Leaves Ella at home, to procure "Eleya" (problems) outside.
Leaves Lovet at home, to find "Bata" (beaten up) outside.
Leaves "Alafiya" (peaceful life) at home to procure "*Wahala*" (trouble, difficulty) outside.

Leaves Joy at home, to find trouble outside;
Comfort fills the parlour, he finds "Komandiya" (a commandeering woman) outside
Leaves Faith, to get stuck to Hopeless;
You leave Beauty at home for Beasty outside;
You leave Nancy at home for "Kasi" (worries) outside;
Leave Mazi for "Lord have Mercy."
You do not clock Blackie
Because you have to keep "Yala's" (Yellow's) all the time.
That is the life that you live!

---

10. Male Sierra Leonean name.

11. Male Sierra Leonean name.

12. Refers to the Kissy ethnic group in Sierra Leone, or more broadly to the ethnic natives of the country rather than to the urbanized Krios of Sierra Leone. It should be noted that the Krios are descended from a group of people who were destined for slavery in the New World, and whose ships were captured on the high seas by the English Navy in the mid 1800s. These captured Africans were brought to England where they lived for a time. Later they were deposited on the coast of Sierra Leone where they settled in Freetown, Sierra Leone's capital city.

13. A West African dish made of pounded yams or pounded plantain bananas.

14. Okra sauce. The teller of the tale refers to the fact that women use food to seduce men.

The leaves that taste sweet in a goat's mouth are the leaves that give it dysentery.
It is difficult to change a comma to a Full Stop.
Therefore a man who wants to prove that he is lettered, should know where to put a Full Stop.
That means—
You should avoid putting your spoon into every soup-pot,
Because some soups have gone sour (Hinzen, James, Sorie, and Tamu, 1987, 116–17).

"That is the Life that you Live" explains the customs and habits of men, and by mocking their foolish choices tries to relieve some of the suffering women must tolerate in a strongly patriarchal society. The reader should note the cleverness with which the narrator has set up oppositional categories using reassuring names for the wife at home to contrast with names of problem women sought after by straying husbands.

While some social comment focuses on the war of the sexes, much of it is frankly political. Chernoff notes that African song lyrics are especially concerned with moral and ethnical questions (1979, p. 70). In "Authority Stealing," the late Fela Anikulapo Ransome-Kuti lambastes the civilian government of Nigeria that governed the country during Nigeria's Second Republic (1979–1983). Fela, the originator of a highly original musical style known as Afro-Beat, was a long-time critic of successive Nigerian political regimes. Fela wrote many of his songs in pidgin English, the *lingua franca* of southern Nigeria, Ghana, and anglophone Cameroon. Known for his unconventional lifestyle that included heavy marijuana use, performing in bikini briefs, and sleeping with hundreds of women, he died of AIDS in 1997.

Authority Stealing

Instead of workers, we have officials
Instead of busses, dem dey ride motorcar
Instead of motorcycles, na helicopter
Instead of dem work, na worker to go waka for dem
Authority people dem go dey steal
Public contribute plenty money
Na him authority people dey steal
Authority man ne dey pick pocket
Na petty cash him go dey pick
Armed robber him need gun, Authority man him need pen
Pen get power, gun no get
If gun steal eighty thousand naira, pen go steal two billion naira
We Africans must do something about this nonsense! (Fela Kuti, quoted in Waterman, 1990, p. 226).

AIDS Songs

The tendency to engage in social comment in song has meant that the popular medium of song has been used in the fight against AIDS. In Uganda, where the AIDS epidemic first peaked on the African continent, a number of singers composed songs during the 1980s to help fight the epidemic. This one, composed by Ogwang Clipper, has a moral flavor. It is translated from the Swahili by Charles Okumu.

God Forbids Fornication

Please refrain from sins
God forbids fornication/adultery
If you fornicate, you spread slim (AIDS).

People must desist from fornication.
One of the symptoms is coughing.
Another is loss of weight.
That person is HIV positive.
Some with constant diarrhea
Someone with skin rash
People with itching skins
That person is HIV positive.

Someone with a coated mouth someone with thin legs
Someone who is weightless
That person is HIV positive.

Young men don't fornicate
Young girls don't fornicate
God forbids fornication
If you people sin
You invite death.

Elders don't commit adultery
Women don't commit adultery
If you sin you invite death (Clipper, quoted in Okumu, 1994, p. 341).

Another Ugandan song, this one by Jimmy Katumba, emerged during the same period. It told of the origins of the disease and warned people against it.

Slim (AIDS)

The new disease is deadly
The disease is called slim
We have never seen the like of slim
Slim came from overseas
It is here now
We have never seen the like of slim

Slim started spreading from Kampala[15]
NRA soldiers brought it here
We have never seen the like of slim
Slim is deadly
There is no medicine to cure it
It will kill us all.
It came from Nairobi[16] by train
It is now here
It came in the trailer from Nairobi.
NRA soldiers brought it here
We have never seen the like of slim (Katumba,
quoted in Okumu, 1994, pp. 340–341).

In many ways, these songs from the 1980s reflect the preoccupation of that decade. The song "God Forbids Fornication" necessarily describes the symptoms of the disease and warns about its spread through promiscuous and adulterous liaisons. The second song "Slim" is preoccupied with the question of the origin of the disease.

Zimbabwe's most famous popular song-writer, Oliver Mtukudzi wrote and produced the song "Stay with One Woman" in the 1988. It was produced by Development through Self Reliance, Inc., a company that creates edutainment products for distribution in the developing world. Mtukudsi's song gives advice on how to avoid contracting AIDS.

Stay with One Woman

Remember times are changing with every new day
While the sweet environment is fading
We have to move with the times
We live in a dangerous world
We can't pull back the hands of time
Our progress was through struggle
And we achieved our goals
But now there is a new disease called AIDS
And it's getting right out of control

(CHORUS) Stay with one woman
Keep to one woman
Stay with one woman
One woman
One woman for a man
Keep to one woman
Stay with one woman

With AIDS there is no cure
Prevention is the only way

15. Capital of Uganda.
16. Capital of Kenya.

Just stay with one woman
Just stay with one woman
We now live in a world of danger
Where people die of AIDS
Hundreds and thousands

(REPEAT THE LAST THREE LINES THREE TIMES)
CHORUS

Remember times are changing with every new day
While the sweet environment is fading
We have to move with the times
We live in a dangerous world
We can't pull back the hands of time

(CHORUS)
(CHORUS) (Mtukudzi 1988).

One of the most poignant singer-songwriters to compose an anthem about AIDS was Ugandan Philly Bongoley Lutaaya. After being diagnosed with the disease in the mid-1980s, Philly Lutaaya vowed to do something to try to stop the spread of HIV. One of the first public figures in Africa to go public with his disease, his story was documented by Frontline/WGBH TV Boston and aired on many PBS stations. Philly recorded an AIDS benefit cassette with the Swedish Red Cross. His original song, "Alone" addresses the social stigma of the disease and touches upon the loneliness caused by social isolation. Lutaaya calls for openness regarding the disease and he calls for social unity in the face of it. Unlike many of Philly's other songs, "Alone" was recorded in English. Lutaaya's concerts in the late 1980s were a watershed for the AIDS epidemic in Uganda.

Alone

Out there somewhere alone and frightened
Of the darkness, the days are long, oh
Life hiding no more making new contact
No more loving arms thrown around my neck
Take my hand now I am tired and lonely
Give love, give me hope
Don't desert me, don't reject me
All I need is love and understanding

CHORUS

Today its me, tomorrow someone else
It's me and you, we got to stand out and fight
We'll shed a light in the fight against AIDS
Let's come on out, let's stand together and fight AIDS.
In times of joy, in times of sorrow
Let's take a stand and fight on to the end
With open hearts, let us stand out
And speak out to the world—we'll save lives

Save the children of the world

Let's be open, advise the young ones
A new generation to protect and love
Hear them singing, playing, laughing,
Let's give them everything in truth and love

Take the message cross the frontiers
Break the barriers, we'll fight together
The doors are open, we'll lead the struggle
We won't bow down in defeat; we'll fight on
(Lutaaya n.d. Swedish Red Cross).

Unfortunately, there have been AIDS denial songs. Cameroonian *Bikutsi*[17] singer Bombardier produced a song in the early 1990s that spoofed the name SIDA, the French acronym for AIDS. It went something like this.

SIDA

S comme dans Slogan
I du mot Inventé
D comme dans Decourager
A comme dans Amour

Et moi le Bombardier,
Je dis: "SIDA, égale Slogan Inventé
pour décourager les Amoureux."

Laisse-moi vivre ma vie
Passe ton chemin, dis-je
La vie est comme une luciole
A peine se montre-t-elle que swiff
La voilà partie, à jamais
La vie est si belle
La vie est si courte
Tes dents sont-elles solides?
Alors croque-la avec plaisir
Mord dans la vie quand elle s'offre
On ne vit pas deux fois
Le vin, la femme
Voilà la vie, vieux frère
Laisse moi vivre ma vie, te dis-je
Comdom et puis quoi encore
On me refuse le full contact
On me veut faire à la manière
des chiens

S as in Slogan
I from the word Invented
D as in to Discourage
A as in Amour [Love]

And I, *Bombardier*
I say SIDA [AIDS] equals Slogan
Invented to Discourage Lovers

Let me live my life
Be on your way
Life is like a fire fly
It appears and then its gone
Gone forever
Life is so beautiful
Life is so short
Are your teeth not strong
So bite into life with relish
When it is offered to you
We only live once
Wine, women
That's life, old pal
I say to you, let me live my life
Condom and what again
They would deny me full contact
As in the manner of dogs

17. *Bikutsi* refers to a fast and furious song and dance genre popular in Central Africa. *Bikutsis* are often both pornographic and anticlerical. The French has been provided herein because the *Bikutsi* was originally produced in French.

SIDA, Oh malheur	AIDS, Oh misfortune
Slogan Inventé pour Décourager les Amoureux	Slogan Invented to Discourage Lovers
Je dis que la vie est belle	I say that life is beautiful
Il faut la croquer à belles dents	One must seize it in a single bite
Il faut la vivre quand il est encore temps	One must live it while there is still time
La femme est la vie	Women are life
Le vin c'est la vie	Wine is life
Laisse-moi vivre ma vie	Let me life my life
Passe ton chemin, vieux frère	Be on your way, old pal

(Bombardier, quoted in Doho, 1997, translation mine).

Such songs have emerged in some African countries within the context of AIDS denial. But generally as the epidemic spreads, these songs tend to disappear. Bombardier himself has changed his tune. By the late 1990s, he was still producing the ribald *bikutsi* genre, but now they warned about the dangers of AIDS. This genre seems particularly appropriate to the topic of HIV/AIDS for the *bikutsi* songs and dances are known for their potent mix of socio-political comment with frank discussion of sexuality, particularly from a female point of view. Here is a *bikutsi* for Prudence, a brand of condoms socially marketed in Cameroon.

Prudence, ma soeur	Prudence, my sister
Prudence, mon frère	Prudence, my brother
Prudence, petite soeur	Prudence, little sister
Ne lorgne pas si tôt du côté de l'homme	Don't have your eyes on a man
Quand son anaconda se balance,	When his anaconda hovers
Ferme très fortement les yeux.	Shut tight your eyes
Quand son serpent est nerveux	When his snake is agitated
Prends rapidement le large	Quickly take the wide path
Prudence ma soeur,	Prudence my sister, is the sister
est soeur de sagesse	of wisdom
Colle très fermement à ton homme	Stick tightly to your man
Comme une sangsue colle à la peau	Like a leech sticks to the skin
Et Prudence sera de ton côté	And Prudence will be at your side
Mais si d'avantage Anaconda te tente	And if Anaconda still tempts you
N'oublie jamais Prudence	Never forget Prudence
Qui t'assurera complète protection	Which will assure complete protection
Prudence est un véritable don	Prudence is a veritable gift
Comme condom égale vie	In that a condom equals life.

(Bombardier, quoted in Doho, 1997, translation mine).

Bombardier's paid announcement for Prudence Condoms together with the production of "Alone" by Lutaaya, and "Stay With One Woman" by Mtukudzi, raise the issue of artistic patronage in the context of the AIDS epidemic. It is clear that some African songwriters hope to attract the sponsorship of NGOs

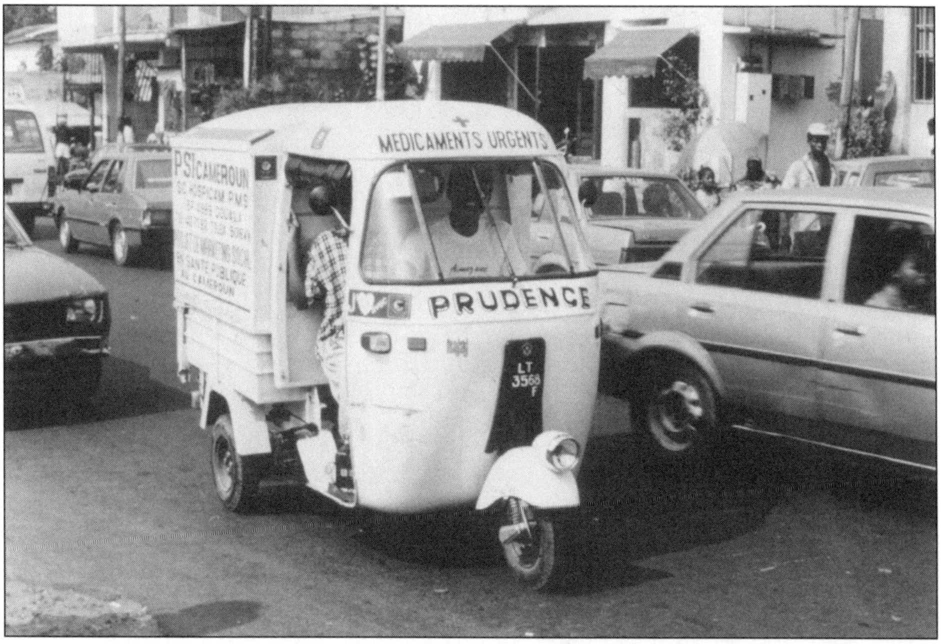

Figure 6-6. Prudence is a brand of condoms socially marketed in Cameroon. Photo courtesy of Population Services International.

when they produce anti-AIDS songs. And it is also evident that some songs have been produced at the behest of NGOs. But this detracts little from their power as social comment. Songwriter patronage is a time-tested tradition in many African societies, where independent popular music industries must struggle to survive. Indeed Chernoff notes that a person with a personal grievance or social issue may hire a song writer to air his complaints and invite community comment in a way that is not offensive (Chernoff, 1979, pp. 70–71). But as more and more African artists are discovered by new "World Music" labels, the topic of HIV/AIDS is likely to receive more airplay in the Western world. Zimbabwe's Oliver Mtukudzi, among others, has continued to address the AIDS issue in Zimbabwe and the rest of Southern Africa in CDs aimed at the commercial market. He re-released "Stay with One Woman" on a 1997 CD. And his 1999 Tuku Music CD, released on the Putamayo label, contains two songs about AIDS. The first, "*Todii?*" ("What Shall We Do?") addresses the stigma and hopeless surrounding HIV and AIDS. The second, "*Mabasa,*" ("Trouble") treats the horrendous death rate of young people in his country.

In South Africa, a country that does have an important recording industry, a variety of AIDS rallies and fairs are organized for purposes of AIDS awareness and AIDS education. Such events feature the talents of musicians, who perform gratis in the hopes of gaining exposure for a small fee. Budding rhythm and blues artists and performers such as Joel Zuma, M. Sibongiseni Mbambo, and Linda Hlongwane were performing at AIDS awareness fairs around Durban in KwaZulu-Natal in 1999. Zuma provided me with the words/translations to their songs. The first, a Zulu song, is "*Masibambisane,*" or "Let's Unite." The second, called "Come On," was composed in English. And a third entitled "If You Don't

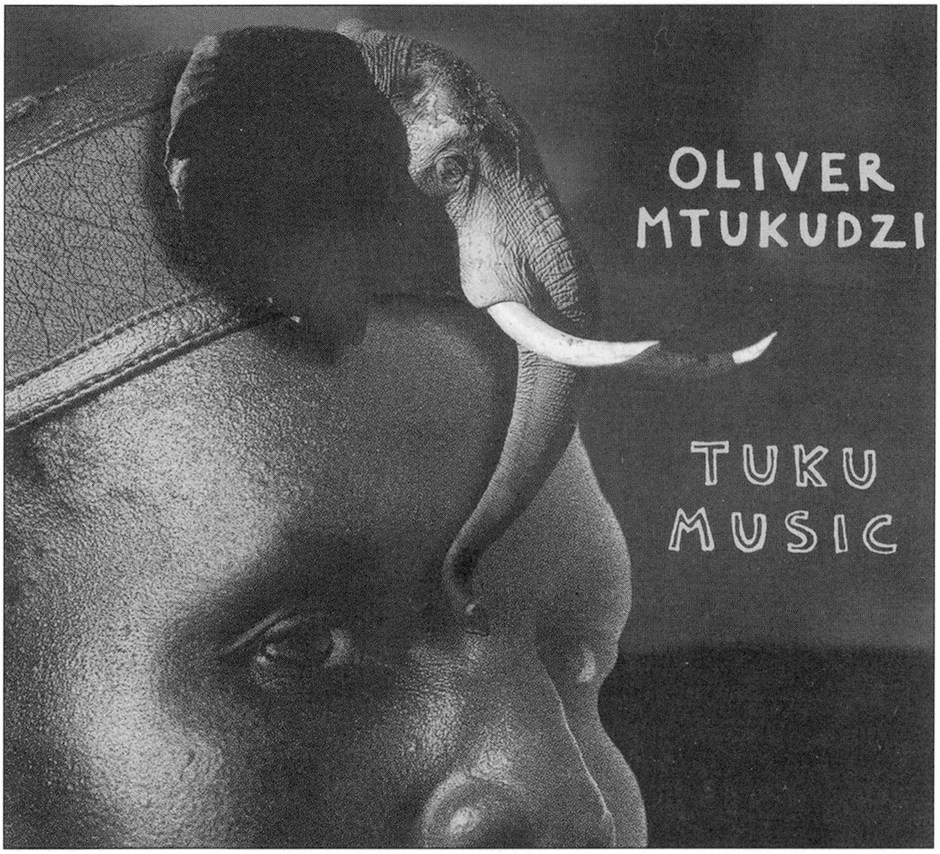

Figure 6-7. Through his music, Zimbabwe's popular bard Oliver Mtukudzi helps to raise awareness of issues surrounding HIV/AIDS.

Know AIDS by Now" appears to be a parody of a well-known pop tune. Excerpts of each of these can be seen and heard on the accompanying compact disk. The first song, *Masibambisane* ("Let's Unite") written by Zuma and Mbambo, is a general call for solidarity and positive thinking. It is sometimes sung in English, sometimes in Zulu, and sometimes in a mixture of both. A rapped chorus may be substituted for the rhythm and blues style chorus provided here.

Masibambisane (Let's Unite)

Now is the time, to work together
Let's all stand, and fight against AIDS

BRIDGE
People have been dying enough, killed by AIDS
Now is the time, to stop this dying.

We've been fighting [for so long], often fighting unnecessary fights
Now is the time, to fight a good fight
BRIDGE

We are facing a python, we are facing a lion
But if we stand together they won't defeat us.

CHORUS
Let's work together
And make our land a better place
Let's work together
And make our land a better place
Let's work together
And make our land a better place

It is very easy to break one stick
But it is impossible, to break a bundle
AIDS won't conquer us, if we work together
But if we separate, it will sweep us away.

Doctors, and herbalists, and nurses
Are not able to cure AIDS alone
But if we, work hand and hand with them
We can find, the cure of AIDS.

Let's work together
And make our land a better place
Let's work together
And make our land a better place
Let's work together and make our land a better place
(Zuma and Mbambo 1999, translation supplied by Zuma 1999).

Refer to Chants and Songs.

Video 3. AIDS Ryhthm & Blues and Rap
Joel Zuma and Sibongiseni Mbambo and Linda Hlongwe at AIDS Summit and Edu-Fair, South Africa

The Song "Come On" picks up the now familiar theme encouraging the care and support for AIDS patients. "Come On" is intended for singing by three singers. A lone singer sing-chants or raps the verses, and two others sing the chorus.

Come On

Brothers and Sisters
There's something that worries me all the time
I have been around
Watching what's happening
The only thing I noticed
Is that people distance themselves
They don't wanna know

What' s happening, what's going on
Around the place we're living in?

CHORUS
Come on, let's take initiatives
Come on, let's all be involved
Lets care for those people with AIDS
Let's keep them strong, and looked after
Come on
Come on

For now it's them,
And tomorrow it might be you
No matter who you are
No matter how charming you are,
The serpent is around
And it strikes everyone
We don't really know
What's happening, what's going on
Around the place we are living in

Come On
Come On
Everybody X 8 (Zuma 1999)

"If You Don't Know AIDS by Now" is an AIDS awareness song that promotes condom use. It can be heard on the compact disk that accompanies the text. Refer to Chants and Songs.

If You Don't Know AIDS by Now

All the things, you've been told
You should understand, and make use of them
You must know the difference, between right and wrong
So you don't do anything silly
But you'd rather say no.

Oh no, don't get too excited
And do unplanned things
Because one mistake you make
You've ruined your life forever

CHORUS
If you don't know AIDS by now
You will never, never, never know.
If you don't know AIDS by now
You will never, never, never know.

You know what people do
They die now and then
Because they jeopardize their lives

I'm gonna tell why they do
They wanna be in fashion,
They wanna be in style
So they don't wanna use condoms
But AIDS is around

If you wanna live longer
And live a long time
Please do as you are always told
Because AIDS is around

CHORUS
If you don't know AIDS by now
You will never, never, never know it
If you don't know AIDS by now
You will never, never, never know it.
If you don't. . . . .(REPEAT TILL FADE OUT) (Zuma 1999)

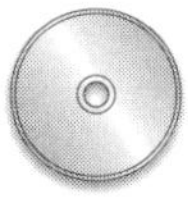

Video 4. AIDS Ballad
Joel Zuma and Sibongiseni Mbambo, AIDS Edu-Fair, South Africa

Singing in a much more traditional mode, Griotte Teme Dembélé of Bamako, Mali, has composed a song on the kora, the 21 stringed harp-lute. Dembélé's song was composed in French, the official language of Mali. Teme's song is a plea for social solidarity, care for the sick, and a warning about the terrible scourge of AIDS. Parts of her performance can be seen and heard on the accompanying compact disk. Refer to Chants and Songs.

AIDS *(SIDA)*

Africans!
Sickness has become incomprehensible
Discussions over tea in the hang-outs
Talk of AIDS
Young girls in the kitchen
Surrounding the cooking pot
Talk of AIDS
Oh people! Whence does the disease come?

This disease kills slowly
Infidelity, prostitution
This disease is new
But it has taken
First place in the news.

If all people join hands
We can conquer AIDS.

This disease has no mother,
No father
No home
It's the latest great plague
A disease which
Boggles the mind
AIDS is the disease
Of Modern Times
It makes thousands
Of widows, of orphans, of widowers,
The world empties itself
Oh Brother!
Help your brother,
Your father, or your infected son.

One day you will be wiped out AIDS
AIDS, the scourge of modern times (Dembélé n.d., translated by Ly and Bourgault 1999).

Video 5. SIDA, AIDS Song
Griotte Teme Dembélé, Bamako, Mali

Teme Dembélé, whose father is a renowned Bamako griot, has won a prize from Malian national television for best upcoming talent in Mali. Her entry "SIDA" was featured on RTM's (Radio-Télévision Malienne) "Top Etoile" ("Top Star") program, a program which features young talent.

A number of Mali's griots are now creating AIDS songs. Griotte Naïni Diabaté has produced an AIDS song in Bambara. The song was recorded privately and circulates in Mali and neighboring countries of the Mande diaspora.

SIDA/AIDS

CHORUS

AIDS is a serious sickness
AIDS is a serious sickness
I'm speaking to everybody

CHORUS

AIDS is not good
AIDS is not good

When someone has AIDS, do not exclude them

When someone has AIDS, do not exclude them

Hey Hey, everybody. Take care of people with AIDS.
Take care of yourselves. Age well!

CHORUS

AIDS is a serious sickness that is not good.
AAAAAAIDS.
Take care of yourselves. Age well!

A bad parent is not bad
A bad brother is not bad
A bad friend is not bad
It's a bad sickness that is our enemy
Let us fight against AIDS

CHORUS

AIDS is bad
AAAAAids
The disease of AIDS is bad
AAAAAAIDS.

AIDS is the most dangerous sickness on earth.
All the doctors of the world know science.
But there is nothing to do, no solution without condoms,
condoms protectors[18] (a brand name), *capote,*[19] *foukoulan nafama* (beneficial hats),[20] or fidelity.

CHORUS

AIDS is a serious sickness that is not good.
AAAAAAIDS.

Some believe that this is propaganda.
Do not listen to them. AIDS exists.
Others think it's a lie.
Do not listen to them. AIDS is with us well and good.

CHORUS

AIDS is bad.
AAAAAAIDS.

Ho! Men be faithful
Ho! Women be faithful.

---

18. 'Protector' Condoms is the brand name for American-made condoms that have been widely marketed in Mali through the efforts of Population Services International (PSI). The name "condom protector" is often used in Mali as the generic term for condom.

19. Capotes is the French word for condom and is often used in Bambara.

20. A Bambara euphemism for condom that means "beneficial cap."

Ha! Fidelity.

CHORUS

AIDS is bad.
AAAAAAIDS.

(Diabaté n.d., translated by Keita and Bourgault 2001)

At least one other Mande griot, Amadou Couibaly has an AIDS song. So does griotte Assetou Kanouté. Besides these griot songs, AIDS has inspired at least a dozen other recording artists in Mali alone.

Some of the artists that have produced AIDS pop songs include Tom Diakité, Ami Element Système, Mama Diabaté, Oumar Koïta, Mamadou Sesse Doumbia, Djeneba Diakité, les Escrocs, and les Zotto Boys. The genres they produce vary from the traditional griot songs already cited through to Malian reggae, blues style crooning, Wassoulou style[21] pop, and even rap. The songs give warnings and advice, telling young people to be careful. Most affirm that AIDS is real, not Western propaganda as some have alleged. They recommend fidelity, or failing that, condom use. They encourage young people not to be embarrassed about condoms, as condoms might save their lives. They urge caution in the use of blades and scissors. They also encourage the healthy not to reject the unwell. They advocate care and support for those who are ill with AIDS. They call on doctors of the world to find a cure for AIDS. Would-be pop stars, such as Abubakar Kouyaté,[22] sound engineer at the recording studio of World Music singer songwriter Salif Keita, has an AIDS song he shared with readers of this volume.[23] Refer to Chants and Songs.

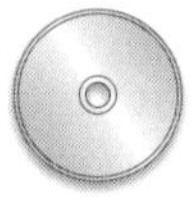

Video 6. AIDS Rap
Abubakar Kouyaté, Wanda Records, Mali

Amy Element Système, a pop singer who died of a wasting disease of unknown cause, produced an interesting selection entitled "Bluess Don." The song actually recreates an urban male-female flirt/sexual encounter where the protago-

21. A style of Malian music that has become very popular in Mali since the 1980s. Popularized by Oumou Sangaré, the music makes use of the *kamelan ngoni*, the young man's ngoni, or five stringed lute.

22. Aboubakar Kouyaté's father is the griot of Salif Keita's father.

23. Mali's recording industry is underdeveloped and Malian recording artists suffer from an industry that is poorly policed. Many of the Malian songs that have appeared in this volume can be found in the markets of Bamako where bootlegged copies of excellent music abound. Mali's only official distributor of registered labels is Mali Casette. And Mali is home to only two professional recording studios, Studio Balafon and Wanda Records, the latter owned by Malian superstar Salif Keita. Salif operates this studio so that budding Malian musicians may have the opportunity to make professional recordings of their music.

nists address one another seductively in French[24] and in which the female negotiates condom use in the most suggestive of ways. The chorus urges women to beware, to be careful and to take care of their men.

It is clear that chants and song are excellent repositories of culture, powerful forces for social solidarity, and emotionally charged calls to action. Chants and songs are portable, that is, they are capable of being carried inside the head (as well as in a walkman or other portable playing device) long after they have been performed. NGOs continue to encourage the production of AIDS pop-songs, all as part of organized campaigns against this terrible scourge. But apart from that, African artists and musicians feel compelled to make music about an epidemic that touches their lives in a myriad of ways. Together, they will continue to bring issues surrounding HIV/AIDS to the attention of popular music worldwide.

In the New Millennium popular music artists continue to release new music addressing the subject of the AIDS Pandemic.

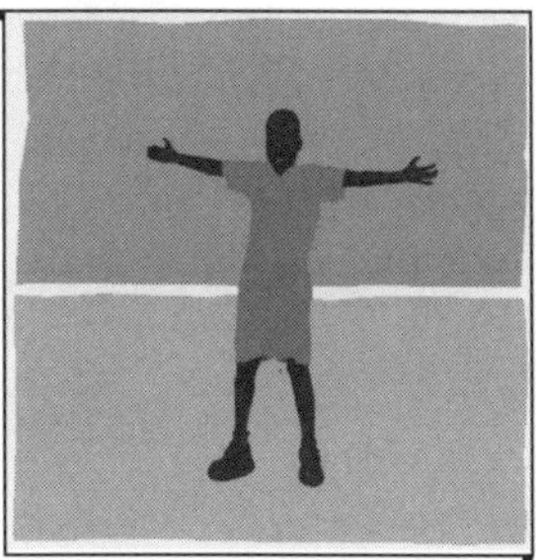

Today, the AIDS pandemic has a clear place on the World Music scene. The World Music Network, in conjunction with Oxfam United Kingdom and the New Internationalist, produced in 2001"Africa-Dance Rhythms from Algeria to Zimbabwe." A portion of the proceeds from that CD will be contributed to Oxfam projects. The CD contains a track by Mabulu, a new group from Mozambique, entitled "AIDS." In 2001, the Mercury Phoenix Trust released "Spirit of Africa" on Peter Gabriel's Real World Records label. That CD features a collection of AIDS musical arrangements by a number of African artists and is designed to focus global attention on the AIDS pandemic. The following artists and their songs are included: Papa Wemba, (Democratic Republic of the Congo) "If You Go Away;" Maryam Mursal (Somalia) "Somalia, Don't Shame Yourself;" Omar Pene & Super Dianomo de Dakar (Senegal) "AIDS the Devil;" Youssou N'Dour (Senegal) "Our Young People," Mzwakhe Mbuli (South Africa) "It's Sad in this World," Tama and Assitan Mama Keita (Guinea Bissau/Mali) "Long Life;" Ayub Ogada (Kenya) "Spirit Mix;" and Hamid Baroudi (Algeria) "Baraka;" Bernard Kabanda (Uganda) "The Firewood collection;" Remmy Ongala (Tanzania) "Things with Socks;" Dr. Hukwe Zawose & Michael Brook (Tanzania and Canada) "The Bedbugs Bite;" Imbizo (Zimbabwe) "Heaven is My Home;" The Taso Choir (Uganda) and "AIDS the Disease." The "Spirit of Africa" also contains and extract of traditional drumming from Burundi. The Mercury Phoenix Trust, a charity established in the wake of the death of Freddie Mercury, has donated over seven million British pounds (about $14 million) to AIDS projects in 100 countries.

In 2002, the Ghetto Ruff label, South Africa, produced "Steps-Tracks from the STEPS documentaries and music inspired by the films." "Steps" is a documentary series commissioned and funded by the cultural ministry of Finland and the Scandinavian television systems. The series contains sixteen films produced by filmmakers in southern Africa that show people living positively with HIV/AIDS.

Figure 6-8. "Spirit of Africa" CD released by Mercury Phoenix Trust and Real World Records 2001.

24. The fact that they are speaking in French is a sign they have adopted Western standards of morality (or amorality), and Western dating styles, are urban dwellers, and participate in their way in a global popular culture.

Review Questions

1. What stylistic devices do oral performers use in Africa to help them to remember long narratives in prose and in song? What effects do these stylistic devices have on the nature of the narratives?
2. How does "orature" work to foster community spirit? In which ways can communal energies be especially powerful in the fight against HIV/AIDS?
3. What themes have African AIDS songs tackled? Why are these themes important? What other issues surrounding HIV/AIDS would you like to see treated by African singers and poets.

Chapter 7

Dance

The subject of African dance is a vast one, one that merits treatment in depth in a separate work. Dance is a key component to just about any African performance and it figures prominently in AIDS awareness activities on the African continent. This chapter provides an overview of African dance and should serve to whet the appetite of the reader new to the subject. The chapter will discuss some of the adaptations of existing dance forms to the struggle against AIDS. Chapter 7 concludes with a short segment on AIDS awareness rallies and parades. Many of the dance and performance genres discussed in this chapter can be seen on the accompanying compact disk.

As noted in Chapter 4, Africans are generally spiritually minded people. The spiritual realm is never far from the material in African social life and in African consciousness. Ancestors and spirits participate in the everyday world of the people and interact with people's lives. Spirit and matter mingle freely in society and in the individual in Africa. The operation of the spiritual realm is not only a matter of the mind or the brain or the "soul" as it is for the Westerner. Reality on the African continent is thought to generate out of a competition of a number of spiritual and material forces all acting upon one another in a rather complex way. This is true for individual personhood, and it is true for the larger community. These interactions are dynamic, they are fluid, and they are brought about through action, through performance. Music and performance help a person to be, to manifest those competing forces rhythmically.

According to African musicologist Francis Bebey, "Music [in Africa] is a necessity—a vital function. Music is the outward and audible manifestation of inward biological functions; it is the support and realization of their metaphysical purpose" (1969, p. 132–134). Music and dance are thus needed for psychological, sociological, and cosmological well balance.

The reader should note that the world view of most of Africa's people is bereft of the "mind/body dichotomy" that has long been a part of Western culture at least since the time of Descartes.[1] And they have largely been spared the alienating effect of Anglo-Saxon or puritan avoidance of physical pleasure together with the Western distrust of things corporeal, including the dancing human form. Indeed there is an old adage that says African religion is danced out rather than thought out, that it is something to do, preferably before an audience, rather than something to abide by (van Beek and Blakey, 1994, pp. 12–13).

---

1. René Descartes a 17th century French rationalist philosopher who argued that the only thing that could not be doubted was doubt itself. He is known for his celebrated dictum, "I think, therefore I am."

Dance is also important in Africa because, like music, it is a necessary accompaniment to all social occasions. In contrast with the West, music and its inseparable companion dance, are integral parts of all aspects of life in Africa. The famous African musicologist Francis Bebey also wrote "A village that has an unorganized music [scene] or neglects community singing, drumming, or dancing is said to be dead" (Nketia, 1966, p. 33). This is because, as we noted in Chapter 4, Africans live in oral societies whose history and whose belief systems are not so much written down as they are performed. A village that no longer (or does not yet) organize itself to tell its history is a village without a history. Independent of records, that history cannot exist unless someone tells it or someone performs it. A village that does not organize its members to demonstrate dramatically (to enact) their relationships with one another must have (as yet) no social relationships. And a village that cannot organize its members to replay their relationship to common ancestors must have no common ancestors. The purpose of performance is at once a creation and a presentation. It is at once both constitutive and representative.

The aesthetics of any performance, including dance in Africa, revolve around the promotion of sociability and the reinforcement of group interconnectedness to place, to people, and to the ancestors. A musical group in Africa that does not get people to dance will be considered a failure. For dance is the natural complement of music. And people are expected to dance in order to play their part in the reenactment of group harmony and the enjoyment of a public aesthetic experience. A dancer who calls attention to himself or herself through exaggerated movements is a dancer who has gotten out of balance with the musicians. Such a person is not appreciated and will be gently mocked by the community. But this does not mean that Africans cannot distinguish themselves on the dance floor. On the contrary, virtuosity in African dance is very much appreciated. A skilled dancer is one that can use his/her steps to create an additional rhythm, dancing to the spaces in the music. Such a skill is seen as a demonstration of dancer's heightened involvement with the music and with the musicians. Indeed, African dance expresses the values of harmony and balance in a meta-communicative style.

John Miller Chernoff, who has studied African drumming in Ghana provides the following valuable comparison of Western and African dance as communication.

> A Western dancer uses the body for expression: a movement or a posture conveys a feeling or an idea through representation within the vocabulary of dance, as in pantomime.... A modern dancer can communicate abstract conceptions like anxiety by putting the parts of the body at disjointed angles, isolation by slowly drawing the body into itself, serenity by gracefulness, doubt by random movements and pauses. Western dance is basically imitative and iconographic, and it is no wonder that many people have suggested that an African dancer, through the certainty of feet placed squarely on the ground, knees slightly bent, weight moving downward, is communicating unambiguous tribal life. The sense of rootedness and security is there, of course, but if we understand the music, we know that the rootedness to the drums, and that the confidence of a foot is the placing of communicative certainty into a context of rhythmic ambiguity (1979, p. 144).

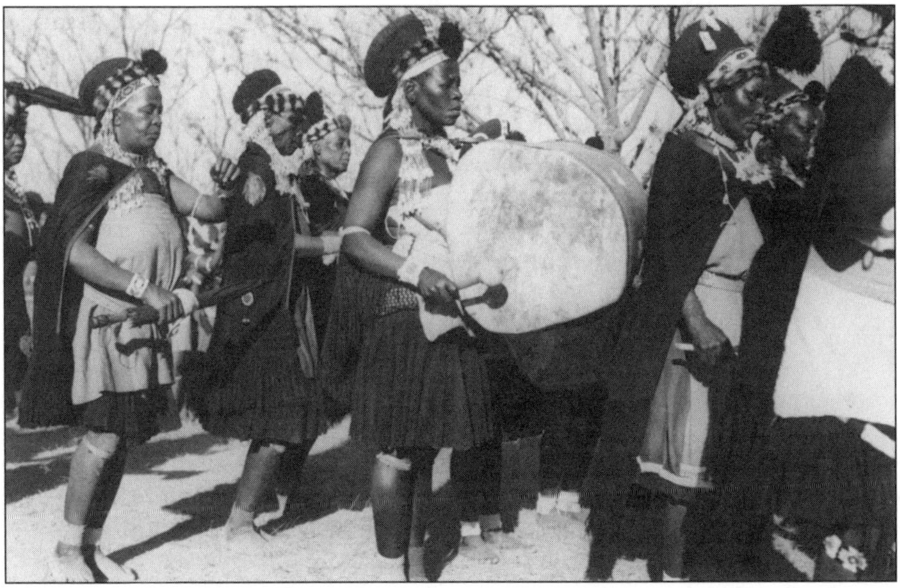

Figure 7-1. Women followers of Shembe, a syncretic African religion that combines Christianity with elements of Zulu culture. Photo courtesy of the Killie Campbell Collection.

For aesthetics in African music and dance mirror the values of social life. And Africans value the ability of human beings to negotiate between conflicting forces, competing interests, rival kin, and even jealous ancestors. This is the essence of "keeping it all together" which Black people throughout the African Diaspora greatly admire.

Dance has been defined as "1) purposeful, 2) intentionally rhythmical, and 3) culturally patterned sequences of 4a) non-verbal body movements 4b) other than ordinary motor activities, 4c) the motion having inherent and aesthetic value" (Hanna, 1987, p. 21). Purpose in dance may be something as simple as "to create movement" or as complex as to appease the gods, or to introduce a play. The concept of purpose is included in the definition so as to exclude patterned movements which might seem like dance, such as the gingerly stepping movements of a shaman walking on coals, or the multi-step response of a person who has just stubbed his toe.

The notion of intentional rhythm is included here because it makes requisite the consciousness of the dancer or the choreographer in the design/execution of the dance. Intentionality must also be highlighted so as to exclude from the definition of dance such behaviors as physical work (stamping of grapes, smoothing of mud floors), or rhythmic sports and games, such as jogging, or table tennis.

Cultural patterning refers to the fact those non-verbal movements, gestures, and sequences in dance have meaning within the specific cultural contexts in which they have arisen. A movement that implies a supplication to the gods in one culture, may look simply like a plea for erotic attention in another. Again these movements are symbolic rather than purely motor so that such activities as barrel rolling or "hula-hooping," however rhythmic, would be excluded from the definition of dance. Inherent or aesthetic value implies that the dance can be performed and appreciated on its own terms, i.e., for its own sake and that it conforms to some notion of beauty or appropriateness in performers or audiences.

Dance is believed to have originated deep in pre-history when human ancestors expressed their emotion—delight, or perhaps fear with some feat of movement reminiscent of apes at play. The movement would then have become stylized or ritualized and performed in conjunction with similar events (Langer, 1976, p. 130). A dance or movement expressed as pantomime performed just as a rainstorm began, for example, would have evolved over time into a rain dance. As Langer notes, ritual (in non-Western societies) often accompanies or completes an event rather than causes it.

It is often difficult for Westerners to appreciate the connection between dance and religious ritual. This is because Western Christianity, after the Protestant Reformation of the 1500s, took on a decidedly verbal and non-ritual bent. Indeed much Christian religious practice and dogma has focused on elevating the mind and taming the body. As we shall see, this penchant for promoting the mind-body dichotomy has not squared well with the holistic African world-view. It has led, for example, to the development of the African Independent Churches, churches who practice syncretistic blends of Western Christianity and African tradition, churches who generally incorporate dance in their worship services.

Chapter 1, the African overview, discussed in general terms the impact of colonialism on African societies. As noted in that chapter, colonizing European societies introduced a very alien way of life on Africa's peoples. Europeans introduced a literate, capitalistic world, organized for the production of goods for profit. The European world was a world in which the sacred and the secular existed in two different planes of reality. Western humankind entered the spiritual realm periodically as the need arose. This compartmentalized world of the European was very different from the holistic world of the African where the secular and the sacred coexisted side by side, where spirits and deceased ancestors coexisted with the living and mingled freely with the affairs of people. Because the world-view Europeans brought to Africa from the 1500s onward was so alien to the world of pre-contact Africa, it caused radical cultural and social changes. Authors and scholars treating African history and social phenomena have tended to divide their discussions into two categories: pre-colonial or pre-contact (so-called "traditional") African history and social processes; and post-contact (so called "modern") African history and social processes. This is a convenience for authors and readers alike. It can be an acceptable way of presenting very complex reality provided several factors are noted. First, comparatively less is known about pre-contact Africa than post-contact Africa because of the shortage of written records from that period. Thus authors treating these periods are summarizing broad swaths of history. Second, African civilizations were not static before the arrival of Europeans in Africa. African societies underwent continued change through migration and through interaction with neighboring groups.

The above caveats aside, this book takes the view that pre-contact forms have persisted in rural parts of Africa to a great degree well into the 21st century albeit with some modification. These forms will simply be referred to in this chapter as "traditional" or "ethnic" forms. Those that evolved in urban or peri-urban areas after contact with the West, will be referred to as "contemporary" or "modern" social forms. The reader will note that most of the dance forms listed as contemporary could equally be considered fine examples of popular dance culture.

A cardinal principle of this book has been that the African way of life is a holistic one, one that is not easily deconstructed into component parts. This holistic principle, applied to dance, simply means that it is difficult to talk of dance without talking of related forms, drumming, singing, mime, puppetry, and so on. Indeed, in many African languages, the word that most corresponds with the English word "dance" may include other meanings. For the Igbo of Nigeria, for example, the word for dance also implies a play-like performance accompanied by a drum (Hanna, 1987, p. 18). For the Tiv of Nigeria, the word for dance also encompasses several other performing arts including game playing and gambling (Hanna, 1987, p. 18). For the Akan of Ghana and Côte d'Ivoire, the Efik of Nigeria, the Azande of the Sudan, and the Kamba of Kenya, the word dance also implies both song and musical instruments (Hanna, 1987, p. 18).

Despite the above claim, it is possible to talk about prescribed stylistic elements required in a given performance. It is also possible to identify movement sequences wherein the way the body moves is of more importance than the music or any other elements or contextual details that energize these movements. Thus it is worthwhile to consider dance in isolation.

Traditional or "Ethnic" Dance

A commonly held belief, as noted above, is that dance originated in primordial times, in religious ritual. From these rituals, in which ancient peoples including African peoples worshipped their gods, came a whole range of uses of dance. Felix Bergho provides a schema useful in mapping out the traditional African dance scene. The different types of dance, according to Begho's typology include Sacred Dances, Ceremonial Dances, Entertainment Dances, and Recreational Dances (Begho, 1996, p. 164). I have provided an elaboration of each of Begho's four categories below.

Traditional Sacred Dances

Sacred dances are dances performed in the main for honoring and communing with gods or ancestors. Sacred dances reflect the collective religious sentiments of the groups who perform them. They may include dances of worship performed by an entire community, cult dances performed by specialized cult members dedicated to specific spirits, and ritual dances performed in conjunction with a sacred rite, either by specialists or by the entire community.

The religious dances performed at the Orisa-Nla festival by the Yoruba of southwestern Nigeria and Benin provide an excellent example of sacred dances that are dances of worship. The Orisa-Nla is a nine-day festival that reenacts the story of the creation according to Yoruba mythology. Within the festival are four religious dances. The first is the Invocation dance which uses dance movements [of supplication] to invite the gods to be present at the festival. The

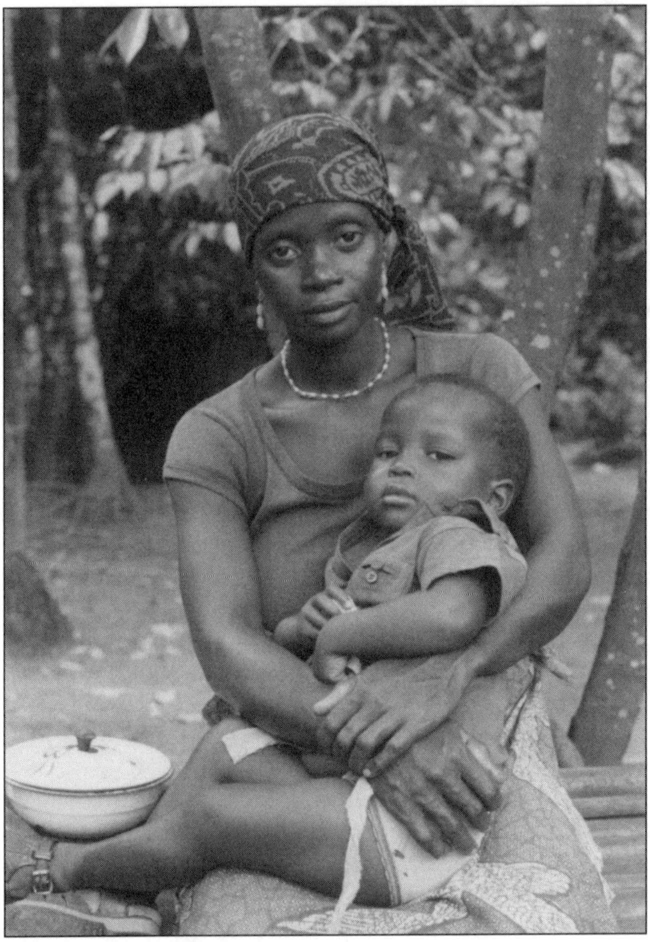

Figure 7-2. A member of a secret dancing cult in her day-to-day garb, Mawah, Liberia.

second sacred dance is the War dance that signifies through whirling movement the universe in chaos as two gods Obàtálà and Odùduwà feud. (Obàtálà is said to have started the creation of the world and Odùduwà is said to have finished it). A third traditional sacred dance is the Sacrifice dance performed at the festival as the god Obàtálà and his followers plot to return to Ife, the home of origin of the Yoruba. Here a goat is sacrificed, probably in ritual enactment of the battle that would take place between the followers of Odùduwà and Obàtálà. The fourth sacred dance is the Obàtálà dance with its smooth and harmonious movements said to represent the reintegration of Obàtálà's followers with those of Odùduwà in a now peaceful Yorubaland (Ajayi, 1998, pp. 43–75).

It is noteworthy that the Yoruba deities (the *orisha*), like many of the African deities and ancestors, have human foibles and failings. They appreciate dances in which they are imitated. They can be vain and pretentious. And like living beings, they can lash out if they are ignored. So during festival time, a time when the Yoruba gods should be honored, Yorubas take great pains to pay deep respect to the god ancestors through a display of good dancing. Under appropriate circumstances, the ancestors may return through possession of a member of the living to participate in the dance proceedings.

Another category of sacred dances includes cult dances. Cult dances are dances performed by members of secret dancing societies who use the performing arts of musical chants and dancing to appease social and spiritual forces. Serving in the maintenance of power of a certain temporal or spiritual group, these dances may be done in secret locations so as to better guard the secrets of the society. In some cases, even the membership of these dance society cult members is kept secret from the community.[2] The Kpelle and Gola of Liberia have dancing cults in which the secret of membership is kept even from the dancers' own family members (Bourgault 1989). This is because these cult dancers are believed to have important ritual power. Power in such societies is diffused through a range of secret groups who then serve as checks and balances to one another.

Ruth Stone, who has studied music and dance forms of the Kpelle of Liberia, notes that among the Kpelle, true virtuosity in performance is believed to come from the ancestors (1994, p. 397). Musicians call out to ancestors asking them to join them in performance. When a musician is really firing, when he/she is really "on" (when there is *flow*), the ancestors are said to have arrived. A pedestrian event, according to Stone, becomes an aesthetic one through the presence of the spirits (1994, p. 392). Sometimes they take over the body of a dancer or a drummer. Stone also notes that music and dance among the Kpelle is multi-vocal. It may be religious and entertaining at the same time. "A ritual accent does not negate the entertainment value nor does the entertainment accent negate the ritual value" (1994, p. 397). Again it is worth noting that categorizations of dance provided herein represent tendencies or weightings of life-ways whose descriptions defy hard and fast Western categorizations.

Ritual dances are sacred dances that may be performed to supplicate the gods for answers to community or individual problems through divination rites. The traditional healer, the *Isangoma* of the Zulu and related groups of Southern Africa performs a dance that is part of the ritual used in diagnosing illness. The dance is used to invite spirits to participate in the diagnosis and cure of sickness (Janzen, 1994, pp. 161–182; Campbell 1998). A *sangoma* divination dance, a dance of the Zulu diviner, is provided on the accompanying compact disk. Refer to Dance.

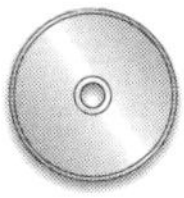

Video 1. Sangoma Divination Dance
Shakaland, South Africa

2. The subject of secrecy in traditional African society is a complex one. Beryl Bellman (1984) who studied the concept of secrecy among the Kpelle of Liberia and argues that secrecy generally refers to information which may not be discussed.

In some cultures, ritual dance that mimics life and health is used metonymically to chase witches and other evil spirits believed to be responsible for sickness and death. Here life, and by extension health, are represented by the act of dancing. And the Tiv of Nigeria actually recreate danced images of sickness, dropsy and elephantiasis, which they attempt to cure through iconographic representation and metonymy (Hanna, 1987, p. 111).

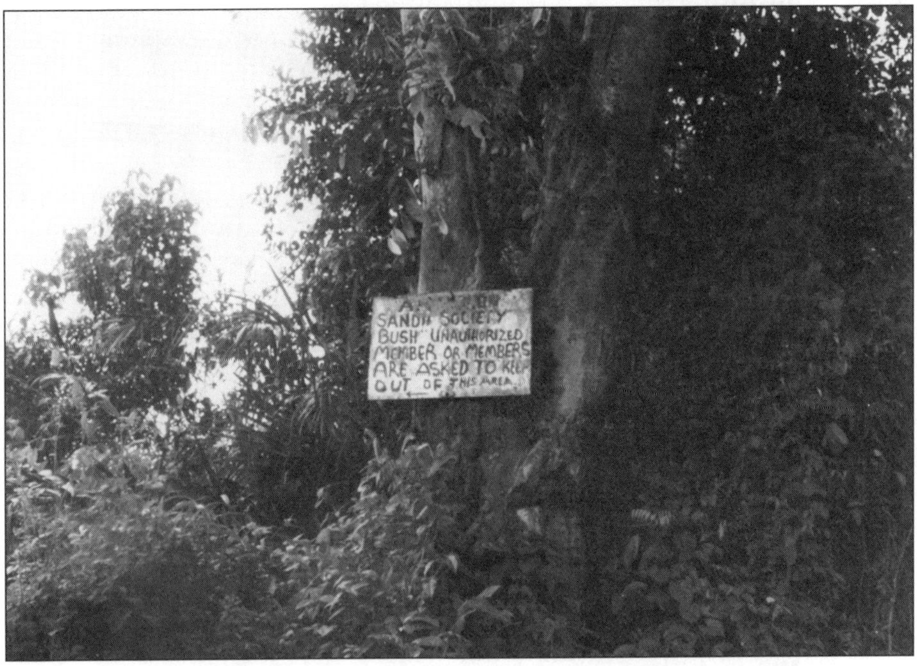

Figure 7-3. A sign demarcating a section of the rain forest in central Liberia reserved for activities of the Sande, the women's secret society.

Traditional Ceremonial Dances

Ceremonial dances are so classified because they are especially intended to mark or to honor some earthly event. And although the ceremonial dances are not devoid of spiritual intent and spiritual significance, their primary focus is on the living. Ceremonial dances may be performed only by specific dance sects, in which they would be classified as Ceremonial Sectarian. Alternatively, if the entire community performs dances, they would be classified as Ceremonial Communal dances.

Ceremonial Sectarian dances include Age and Sex Group dances that typically celebrate the passage of a group of young boys or young girls from one stage of life to another. This can be understood (by Westerners) as a sort of a cross between a graduation and a [Christian] religious Confirmation when graduates demonstrate their new adult status with special dances. Among the Bemba of Zambia, female initiates, according to anthropologist Audrey Richard, were actually "danced" from one age group to the next. The women in charge of them actually believed they were enacting supernatural changes in the initiates (Hanna, 1987, p. 112).

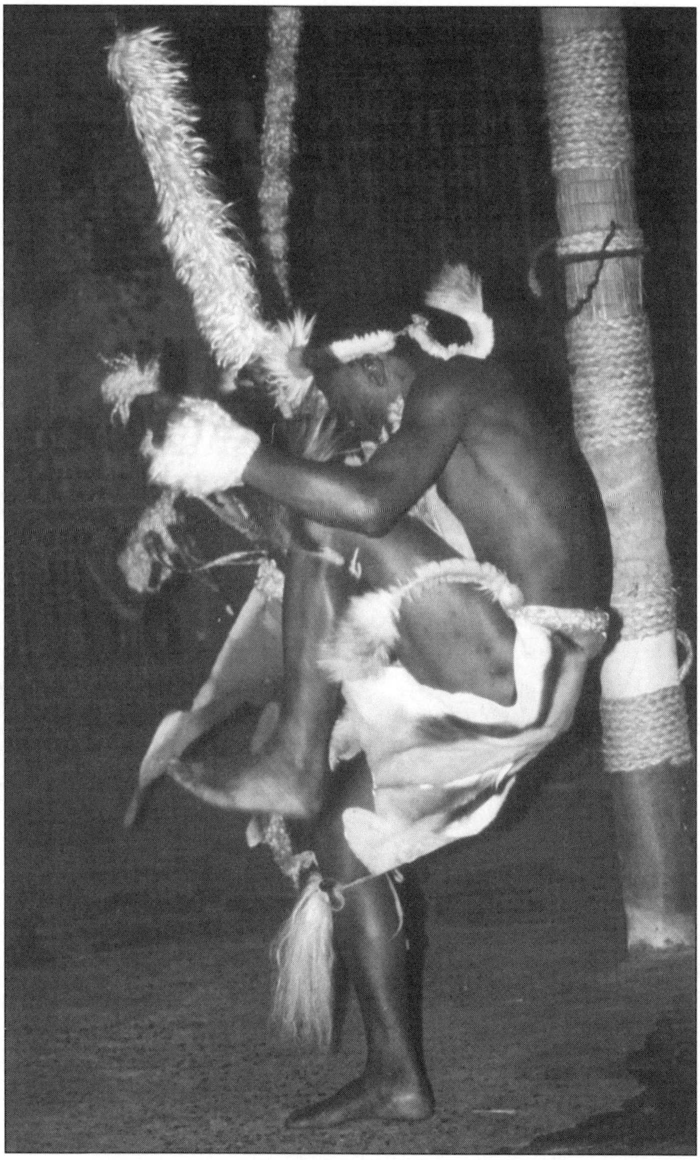

Figure 7-4. Zulu males perform dances that celebrate heroic feats and the warrior tradition. Photo courtesy of Neil Cumberlidge.

Among the Mende of Sierra Leone and the Gola of Liberia, the rite of passage to adulthood involves attending the female Sande school. Sande school represents the liminal phase (see Chapter 9) of the rite wherein girls learn the secrets of adulthood and undergo excision (female genital cutting) procedures. After their period of exclusion, they dance in demonstration of their newfound status as adults, in a dance wearing the celebrated Bundu helmet mask. The Bundu dances and the masks celebrate the ideals of Gola and Mende womanhood, i.e., demure quietness and calm beauty. Gola and Mende dances represent rare instances of women donning masks of any kind in West Africa. Generally throughout West Africa where mask dancing is common, this practice is restricted to men. Other ceremonial dances may include wedding dances, naming ceremony dances, and funerals.

Traditional ceremonial dances include cyclical events such as harvest festival dances where people give thanks to earth gods or goddesses for successful crops, and where sacrifices may be offered to the land/land spirits to promote continued good growth. Equally important are dance ceremonies that beseech gods or spirits to provide bountiful harvests. In Tanzania, the Sandawe perform erotic *phek'umo* dances by moonlight symbolically recalling a woman's menstrual cycle and the sexuality of human beings in an attempt to acquire fertility of the land (Hanna, 1987, p. 111).

The Bamana (Bambara) of Mali perform a dance to a god of agriculture. The Tyi Wara mask, an antelope headdress, represents a supernatural being, half man/half animal that first instructed humans in the cultivation of the lands. The dance is still performed (among animist Bamana) as an invocation to the spirit for blessings for a good agricultural season in this poor and harsh savanna land (Hanna, 1987, p. 122).

Heroic Dances, also included within the ceremonial dance category, are dances that celebrate the exploits of war and victory. Dance steps are designed to make the dancers look fearsome and to prepare them for battle. Warrior groups such as the Zulu of South Africa have a number of these dances. Some were danced with the *assegai,* a light six-foot (almost two meters) throwing spear and some were danced with the *ixhwa*, the short stabbing spear developed by Shaka for close combat. These dances were clearly designed to rehearse Zulu warriors for bloody battle. Other warrior dance variants, including the well-known *ukugiya,* use sticks in place of spears to prove that the men are merely engaging in mock combat. Clearly these dances celebrate aggressive masculinity, the bravery of warriors, and militaristic values of society. Today these dances are sometimes adapted and used in the fight against AIDS in South Africa. Zulu choirs have been known to urge young men of warrior age to "*guya*" with a condom, a not so veiled reference to the phallocentric symbolism of this dance. Both the traditional *ukugiya* and the adaptation at an AIDS awareness event can be highly stylized, the clanking of sticks in mock combat creating the rhythm of the dance. A demonstration of *ukugiya* is provided on the accompanying compact disk. Refer to Dance.

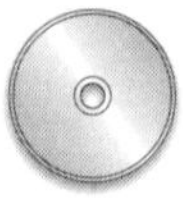

Video 2. Zulu Stick Fight
Shakaland, South Africa

Funeral Dances represent another type of ceremonial dance. The Ubakala of Nigeria perform the Nkwa Uko and Nkwe Ese dance-plays in order to accompany the deceased to the land of the ancestors. Before the performance of the dances, the spirits exist in a netherworld or limbo between the world of the living and the world of the dead. The processual metaphor puts a visceral meaning on death and helps to dissipate tension associated with it (Hanna, 1987, p. 113).

The Nyakyusa of Tanzania use funeral dances to mediate between the immediate grief at the death of a kinsmen and the new social order where the kinsmen is absent. The funeral dance begins with a violent expression of anger and eventually transforms into motions of peaceful acceptance as the dancer expends his energy and his anguish in dance (Hanna, 1987, p. 113). In this case, the dance serves as a rite, transforming mourners from a group that is angry at a loss of a community member, into a group with a newfound equilibrium.

Among warrior groups, such as the Nguni of Southern Africa, funeral dances might involve stylized accounts in dance of the deceased in battle. Generally speaking, with regard to funeral dance and other funerary preparations, the more important the person, the more complex the ceremony and the more lengthy the event. Here the dance functions at the funeral more in a commemorative capacity than in the transformative capacity of the funeral rites of the Nyakyusa. Still it is possible to regard the entire Nguni funeral as a ritual event that socially transforms the deceased from a member of the community of the living to a member of the community of the ancestors.

Bebcy notes that non-Africans are often shocked by the tumult and the apparent gaiety of an African funeral. But he urges readers not to assume that because there is dancing there is no sadness. Rather, Bebey says, the African responds to the incomprehensibility of death with the rhythms and the music of life (1969, p. 126).

Special ceremonial dancing may also mark coronations and traditional title taking designed to convey status on the recipient of the award. The Dagomba people of Ghana have a drum-dance (a dance cum drumming arrangement) they call *Zhem*. The *Zehm* is played and danced when a new chief is officially recognized. And it commemorates the installation of the first paramount chief of the Dagomba people. *Zhem* is also played when a chief dies. So sacred is *Zhem* that Chernoff's Ghanaian drumming teacher waited four years before showing his American ethnomusicology student the *Zhem* drum. And the instructor required Chernoff to perform sacrifices and undergo ritual and moral teaching before this important musical lesson (Chernoff, 1979, pp. 46; 83).

Traditional Entertainment Dancing

Entertainment dances are performed by specialized performers chiefly for the purpose of amusing others in the community. They may involve the charging of fees. Entertainment dances may include entertainment masquerades, acrobats, and puppets.

Many societies in West Africa have entertainment masquerades that feature masks that may be seen by all members of the community. Such societies may have parallel hidden masks used in secret ritual contexts. (See Chapter 8, discussion of the Grassfields of Cameroon). In other cases, the entertainment masquerades may have completely supplanted the ritual use of masks that have since lost their sacred significance. The Dan of southwestern Liberia and east central Côte d'Ivoire are well known for their versatile use of masks in dancing. And even though the dancers may no longer represent spirits, this does not mean they are insignificant. Masked dances may imitate members of the community whose behavior has violated social norms of the group. Through mime, the masked dancers will poke gentle fun at these persons thereby amusing the village and serving as a means of social control. Because many of these masquerade dances require special skill, and because not everyone engages in masquerade,[3] this form of dance has been classified herein as an entertainment dance.

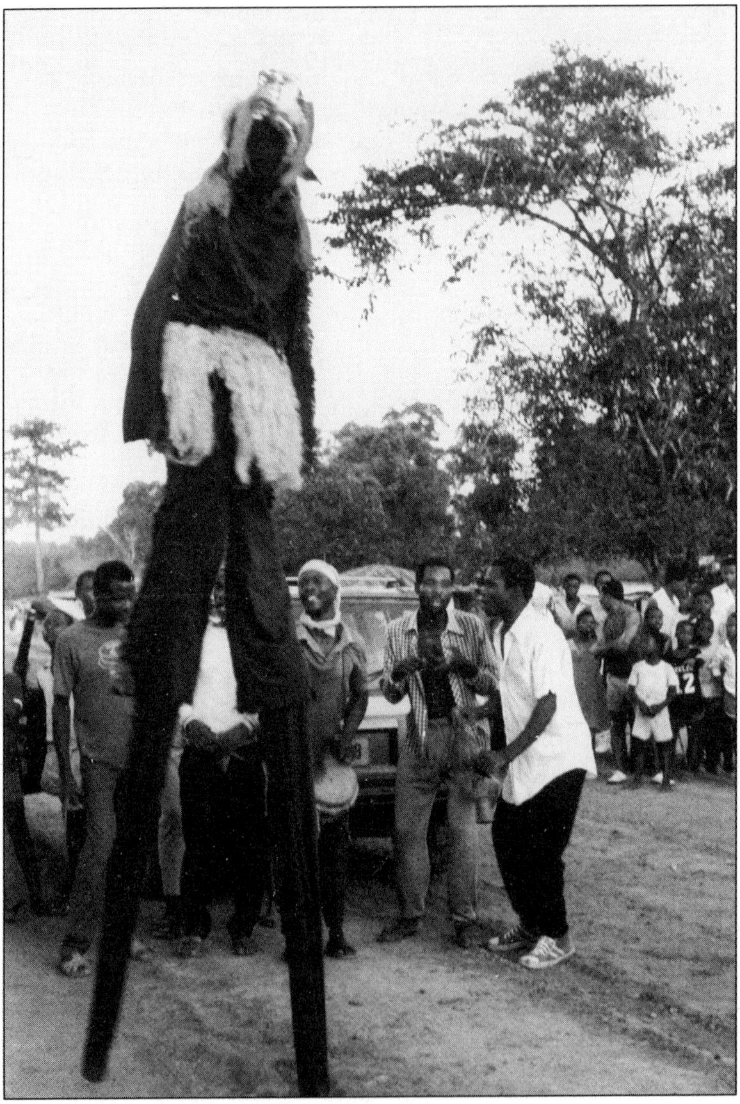

Figure 7-5. Dan masked stilt dancers in Liberia and Côte d'Ivoire entertain the public and correct social transgressions.

3. Women are generally excluded from performing masquerades.

Acrobatic dances are dances that also display particular virtuosity. Some examples might include stilt dancers of the Dan of Liberia and Côte d'Ivoire and the Bambara life-sized puppet dancers (*marionettes habitables*) that perform such feats as summersaults or expansion in size. A dancer wearing an expandable bird costume performs the entertaining *Kono* or Bird Dance of the Bamana in the accompanying compact disk. Refer to Dance.

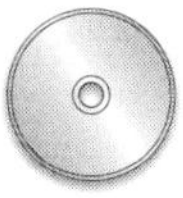

Video 3. Life-Sized Puppet Masquerade
Sologon Marionette Theatre, Mali

Traditional Recreational Dancing

Begho's fourth dance category, Traditional Recreational Dancing includes dances representing no more than community play involving all members of society. Recreational dances include the sub-categories of dances in children's games and tales, fraternal social club dancing, and communal village dancing at village celebrations.

The International Encyclopedia of Dance maintains that dance in Africa has long been the most popular form of recreation (1998, p. 14). Recreational Dancing is a category that includes dance for the simple pleasure of it. And because dance may occur spontaneously at any moment as an expression of happiness, it is important to include it here. Two categories include children's games and tales, and adult dancing just for the fun of it.

Children or youth, segregated into their own age grade societies, organize dances games and storytelling sessions to amuse themselves. The dance games may include most forms of dances their parents do plus stylized game activities akin to what Westerners call "jump rope," "Double Dutch," "Chinese jump rope," ("cat's cradle" for the feet). There are also games that involve rhythmic clapping combined with dance-like steps and turn taking. One of them in "*damatiso*" practiced in Black communities in South Africa.

A children's rhythmic dance game is demonstrated in the accompanying compact disk. Refer to Dance.

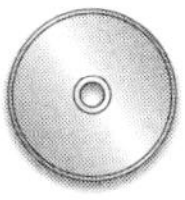

Video 4. Children's Rhythm Dance Game
DramAide Warm Up-Exercise, South Africa

Adult recreational dancing, even in villages, is often organized into fraternal dance organizations, wherein people engage in friendly competition so to develop new dances for the amusement of the people in the locality. As Ruth Stone notes, "to be an adult person in Africa is to perform with some degree of proficiency in song and dance" (Stone 1995, p. 265).

Contemporary or Modern Dances

Contemporary dances can be looked upon as dances of the 20th century. The contemporary dance is marked by a preponderance of entertainment forms. As noted above, and in Chapter 1, Western civilization introduced to Africa the dichotomous division of life into sacred and secular. Today the vast majority of modern African dances should be classified as entertainment. This speaks volumes to the way modern contact has secularized performance and secularized life in Africa.

According to Begho, there are four main types of modern dance: Contemporary Religious Dances, Cultural Revival Dance Shows, Entertainment Dances, and Contemporary Recreational and Party Dances.

Contemporary Religious Dances

Dance that was once used to honor the pagan gods of old has been reworked into the framework of Christianity. Indeed the so-called African Independent churches or the African syncretistic churches represent a collection of Christian churches founded in, or evolved on, the African continent. Such churches typically focus on those aspects of religion important to Africans, such as physical healing, exorcism, and prophecy. They tend to feature worship styles more attuned to African needs than the European Missionary churches. Robert F. Thompson described African religions as "dancing faiths" (1973, p. 85). As noted above, dance movements express biological rhythms, and they demonstrate social values of plurality, of harmony or sociability, and of balance. The circularity of many African dances is also said to express African cosmology, one which stresses consistently repeating patterns rather than a Western linear progression (Smith, 1997, p. 324).

One South African Christian group with clear African roots is the Shembe. Shembe worship services are held outdoors. Men are allowed to practice polygamy and the married males among them don leopard head rings denoting adult male Zulu status. The Shembe regularly perform sacred dances in sexually segregated groups. Carrying shields, Zulu men of warrior age dance in slow and ponderous movements dancing in a double row and moving in a counterclockwise direction. Shembe dances are demonstrated on the accompanying compact disk. Refer to Dance.

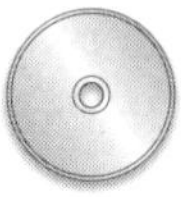

Video 5. Shembe Dance Demonstration & Worship Dance
Eager Artists of South Africa in Michigan & Shembe Service, South Africa

Owing to their particular Euro-American traditions, some African Independent churches, among them the Zionists and related groups of Southern Africa, still forbid dancing. In many of these, a kind of ecstatic jump-shout-shuffle and a vigorous circular processional march have developed (Smith, 1997, p. 323). Both of these pseudo-dance styles are accompanied by rigorous hand clapping. These forms of "dance substitution" are common in the Apostolic Faith churches of Southern Africa whose European roots are in Methodism, and in the South African Zionist groups who trace their origins to American Pentecostalism. Refer to Dance.

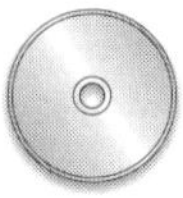

Video 6. "Jump Shuffle,' a Replacement for Dance
Saint John's Apostolic Faith Church, South Africa

The Aladura Movement of Nigeria, the Celestial Church of Christ, and the Cherubim and Seraphim Society, all based in Nigeria in West Africa, also incorporate dance into their worship styles as does the Harrist Church Movement of Liberia and Côte d'Ivoire.

Modern Christian churches, aligned with global neo-Pentecostalism are open to dance in worship style. The Durban Christian Center, without actually featuring dance, encourages exuberant dance like movements. In Ghana, where a Christian neo-Pentecostal revival was in full swing at the turn of the third millennium, the International Central Gospel Church in Accra encourages exuberant modern dancing. Modern Christian church dances are provided on the accompanying compact disk. Refer to Dance.

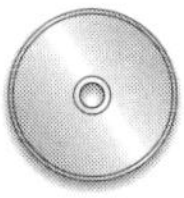

Video 7. Neo-Pentecostalism in Africa
Durban Christian Center, South Africa; International Central Gospel Church, Ghana

Contemporary Cultural Revival Dance Shows

A second category of contemporary dance involves the Cultural Revival Dance Shows. Such organized performances are the products of African governments in the post-colonial period that wished to revive the traditional rural dances of the past, by performing them in urban settings for large audiences at festivals or similar venues. In the late 1960s, Presidents Leopold Senghor of Senegal, Sekou Touré of Guinea, and Modibo Keita of Mali all founded "*ballets nationales*" in an attempt to keep African musical traditions alive. Guinea's *Ballets Africains* toured internationally, acquainting foreign audiences with a smorgas-

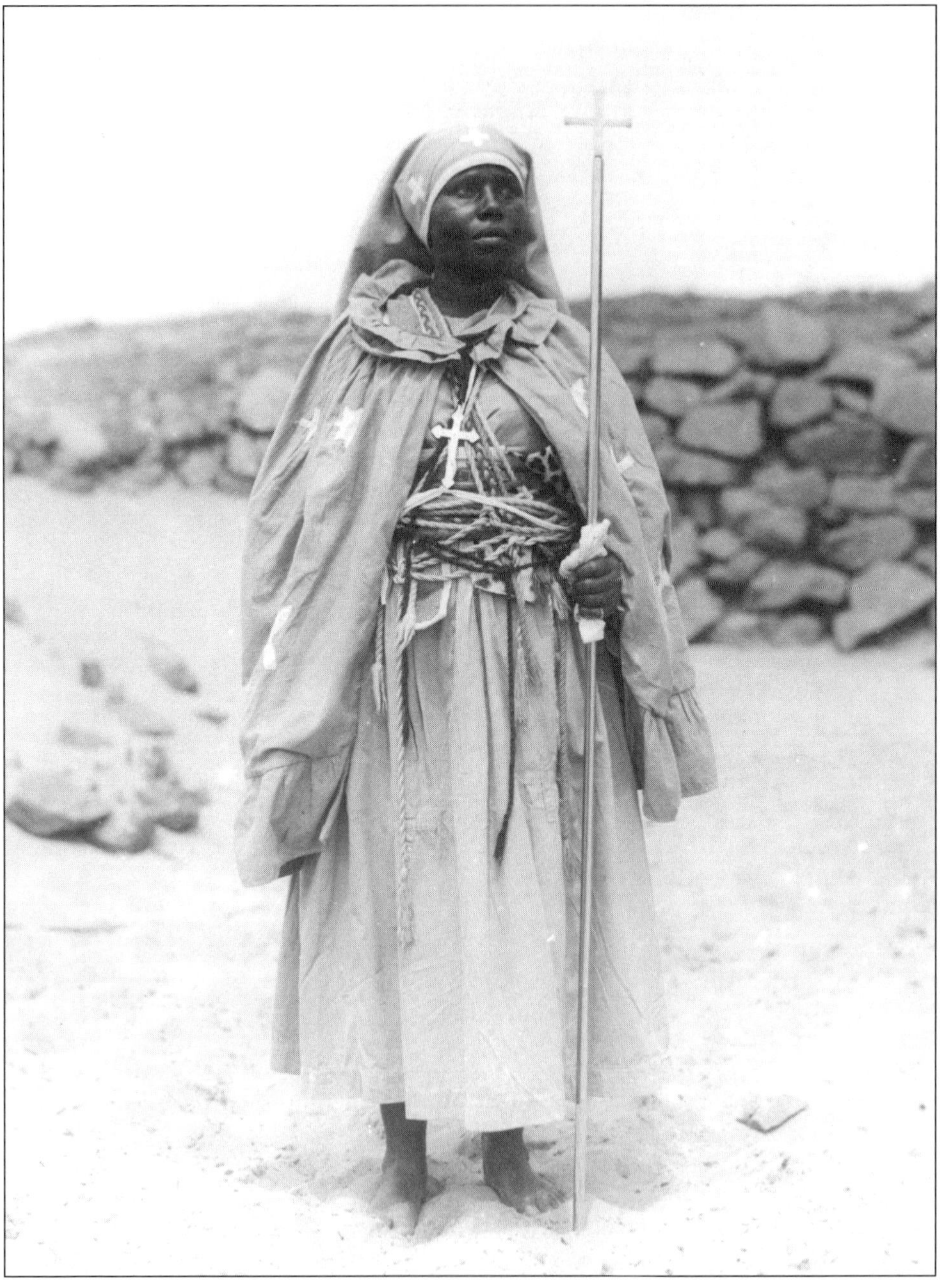

Figure 7-6. A member of a South African Zionist sect. Zionists typically do not allow dancing during religious services. They may substitute jump-shout-shuffle for dance. Photo courtesy of the Killie Campbell Collection.

bord of traditional dances from a range of Guinean ethnic groups. And in Nigeria, the celebrated FESTAC was held in 1977 in an attempt to promote the arts of the continent. Far from serving as repositories of ancient music, these modern national dance troupes and festivals tend to promote musical hybridization. Try as they might, contemporary musicians and dancers working indoors in an urban setting are unable to recreate the village past, the context for so many of the traditional dances (Charry, 2000, p. 211–213).

In places where there is a good deal of tourism, so-called traditional dancing, a poor cousin to the national dance troupes, is featured at hotels and resorts. This is true of the many beach resorts along the Gulf of Guinea and the Atlantic beach resorts of West Africa. In East Africa, the Bomas of Kenya, a folkloric center outside the Nairobi National Park, features troupes performing an array of folkloric dances for paying customers.

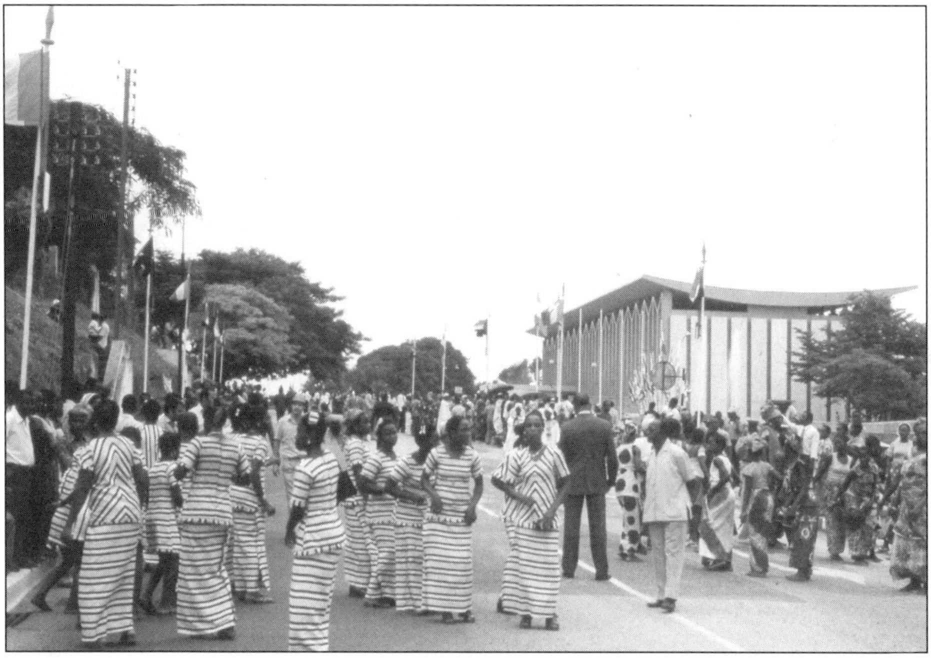

Figure 7-7. Ivorian dance troupes prepare to welcome a visiting dignitary in front of the headquarters of the *Partie Démocratique de la Côte d'Ivoire* (PDCI), Abidjan.

Contemporary Entertainment Dances

Entertainment dance represents a third category of contemporary dances. Dr. Begho identifies several types of contemporary dance or urban African dance. First there is a group of dances called metropolitan neo-traditional dances because they are performed today for urban dwellers by rural dancers newly arrived from the hinterland. Typically they are performed in vacant lots or in roped off areas of African cities. The dancers adapt their performances to urban schedules, dancing for example on Sundays and holidays. They dance for coins or for bills pressed on their foreheads by appreciative audience members. Many of these urban dancers eventually join ethnic dance organizations, thereby formalizing their role in preserving the dances of their own particular ethnic groups. Such groups have regular dance uniforms, pay dues, enjoy scheduled dance rehearsals,

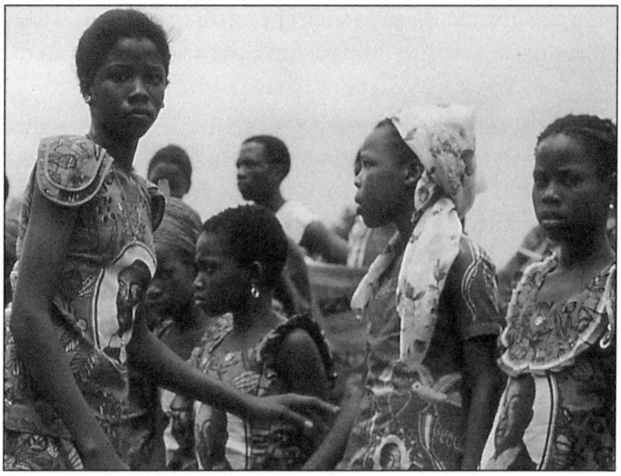

Figure 7-8. African dance troupes often sport colorful costumes that feature the image of their president in the material. Côte d'Ivoire's long-serving President Félix Houphouët-Boigny (1960–1993) is featured on the attire of these dancers.

and act as support networks for one another in a variety of ways. Ethnic dance groups are also often called upon to provide entertainment for weddings, naming-ceremonies, or other social events. And they may be asked to provide street entertainment for national holidays or for the passing motorcades of visiting dignitaries.

Ethnic dance groups may also be called upon to liven up a political rally. For example, ethnic dance groups are frequently called out as welcoming parties for visiting dignitaries in African countries. They perform at national airports for distinguished international visitors. In francophone countries this sort of group dancing in honor of personalities is called "*animation.*" *Animation* is sometimes used to honor homegrown dignitaries of ruling parties as well as foreign ones. In many African polities, particularly in the 1970s and 1980s, *animation* was used to create a sense of pseudo-traditional pomp for party élites in one-party states.[4] In this case party operatives would encourage folk groups to dance and to enliven crowds. Typically, the dancers would dress in colorful costumes of wax prints bearing the image of the nation's head of state printed into the fabric. But *animation* could also be used to surreptitiously bring a politician to ridicule. Mbembe describes how Togolese would use subtle and clever and shifts in the Eve tonal language to make crude remarks about the long-standing ruler President Eyadema. Insults delivered in rapid-fire Eve within the context of *animation* would easily elude all non-first language Eve speakers[5] (Mbembe, 1992, pp. 7–8;

4. Most of these governments were voted out of office in the early 1990s, so that this sort of "animation" is currently out of favor.

5. President Eyadema is from the Kabré ethnic group. He and most of his party operatives would have spoken Eve as a second language.

Dubuch, 1985, pp. 44–53). A clever musician who recreates tonal language with a "talking drum" may do the same, encouraging dancers to join in and punctuate a group insult.

A second type of entertainment dance is the drama dance or a dance within a play. In better plays, dance is well integrated into the story-line and is used to advance the plot. The renowned Nigerian playwright Wole Soyinka used dance in his plays "A Dance of the Forest," and "The Lion and the Jewel" incorporating them within their narrative structures.

Mbongeni Ngema's musical "Sarafina" made use of drama dance. "Sarafina" is the renowned musical that became the emblem theatre piece for the dismantling of Apartheid. The play tells a story of a young girl who dreams of playing Mandela in a school play. She dreams of Mandela, is cast for the part, and actually gets to play him *for* him as he is (fictitiously) released from Robbin Island in time to see her performance. The musical played on the London stage just prior to Mandela's release and came to symbolize the heady South African period of change of the late 1980s.

Dance is an integral part of theatre for Eager Artists of Durban, South Africa. The troupe performs an original musical "My Voice My Life," written by Tu Noque and Jerry Pooe, the latter being the troupe's founder and director. "My Voice My Life" tells the story of Patty Nokwe (Tu's mother) who because of racial barriers, had to struggle most of her life to become a professional singer. When the play wants to establish that Patty is exploited as a domestic in the home of the relative, Patty's character performs a sad stylized pantomime of domestic chores. And when Patty tells of her life as a frightened young girl in a South African city, the players recreate a shebeen scene replete with the edgy tension of fast-paced jive dancing. The choreography of the performance exercises discipline so that the dances are not ends in themselves but clearly add to the audience's understanding of the story. Eager Artists' AIDS awareness play, "One Life to Live," equally uses song and dance in ways that satisfy a taste for South African Black musical performance without overpowering the important message of the play. A drama-dance from "One Life to Live" is provided on the accompanying compact disk. Refer to Dance.

Video 8. Drama Dance from "One Life to Live"
Eager Artists of South Africa in Michigan

In productions of lesser quality, dance is simply used as an interlude between scenes, a kind of mildly amusing break between message-laden content. Mali's arsenal of AIDS information media products includes video-tapes for use in rural primary health care and AIDS information sessions. Most of these have been commissioned by International Non-Governmental Organizations working with local NGO partners. Many of these videos are deliberately produced with musical interludes that serve as natural breaks in the story.

The breaks are used to provide a moment at which a facilitator can interrupt a video presentation in order to hold an AIDS awareness discussion. It is clear the dances are considered secondary by both the amateur drama troupe and the INGO sponsors who have commissioned these tapes.

Night Club Show dances represent a third type of contemporary entertainment dance and resemble their counterparts in the West. Typically they feature scantily clad performers dancing to the beat of a club orchestra. Probably the most famous of these nightclub show dances in all of Africa was held at the Shrine of the infamous Fela Anikulapo-Kuti of Nigeria. A huge ensemble of thirty music and dance performers performed Fela's original *afro-beat* music.[6] The dancers in Fela's group consisted of a bevy of bare-breasted teenage dancing girls whose frantically paced rhythmic movement appeared to put them in a sweaty trance. Night Club Show dances are an important part of any number of contemporary African popular music performances from that of Nigeria's King Sunny Ade to those of Congo's Kanda Bongo Man. Such shows have become much more common since the rise in popularity of World Music in the late 1980s.

Traveling street musicians and dancers form another group of modern or contemporary dance entertainment. Often these dancers perform fantastic feats, such as body contortions, snake charming, or fire eating. Alternatively, traveling street musicians and dancers, particularly in West Africa, may perform on stilts, or atop long posts, or even on top of motorcycles. Traveling street musicians, unlike masquerades, wear no masks, and draw little or no inspiration from traditional African village cultures.

The South African pop scene features a kind of music derived from township jive (*mapantsula*) and updated with a rapping lyrical style and a techno beat. The genre is called Kwaito and it is usually sung or chanted by teen or pre-teen aged boys. Typically, the music is danced more or less in the manner of U.S. street rappers who perform, sometimes for tips, on the sidewalks of U.S. cities. Kwaito enjoys a high degree of improvisation and is constantly adapted so as to comment on contemporary situations. Kwaito music and dance are typical features of AIDS awareness rallies. The words are typically shouted out; they can be quite redundant. Kwaito is sung in several indigenous languages of South Africa as well as English.

Examples of these words are provided below.

Watch out! Watch Out!
You will say he has been poisoned
But it's AIDS

Use a Raincoat [condom]

---

6. Fela was known for his eccentric lifestyle which included sharing of a household with dozens of wives and concubines and their children. His shrine was a steamy Lagos nightclub that occupied most of a Lagos street. Open 24 hours a day, it was a haven for *dagga* and liquor. Openly critical in his music of Nigeria's authorities, Fela was arrested periodically for his outspokenness. And apart from Nelson Mandela he was Africa's most famous political prisoner. Fela acquired his candor from his mother who pioneered the movement for women's rights in Nigeria. Fela was frank about most things, including his appetite for sex. And although the name Anikulapo means "having control over death" in Yoruba, he died of AIDS in 1997.

Otherwise you're going to border [cross over the border between life and death]

Watch out! Watch out! (Lyrics to Kwaito song recorded at a Youth Correctional Facility AIDS Rally. Translation from original Zulu language provided by Musa Ndlovu, October 1999).

Two demonstrations of Kwaito dancing are provided on the accompanying compact disk. Refer to Dance.

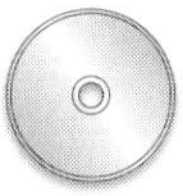

Video 9. Kwaito-1
Juvenile Offenders AIDS Awareness Day, South Africa

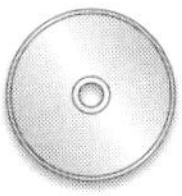

Video 10. Kwaito-2
M. L Sultan Technikon AIDS Edu-Fair, South Africa

Puppet Theatre Dance shows are identified by Begho as another type of contemporary entertainment dance. Relatively common in West Africa, puppet theatre tends to draw on folk tales in its effort to dramatize contemporary issues. The Tiv peoples of Plateau State in Central Nigeria have a puppet theatre called *Kwagh-Hir*. These puppets have often been used to lampoon politicians and to comment on political issues. The puppets are life-sized and they alter their shapes and heights to add to the sense of drama as they dance with other musicians and entertainers in the course of a *Kwagh-Hir* performance.

Mali's Sologon puppet theatre uses stick puppets, marionettes, hand puppets, as well as the heretofore mentioned traditional "living puppets" (costumed life-sized puppets known as *marionettes habitables*) to treat contemporary issues. Some of the issues tackled have included the importance of education, the significance of community, and the dangers of arrogance.

In the 1990s, the Sologon puppets began to speak about the AIDS issue. Like many people today, Sologon's producer-director and chief puppeteer Yaya Coulibaly thinks of AIDS as the ultimate social disorganizer. He conceives of AIDS as the disease that breaks up families, both literally and psychologically. He compares the promiscuous and mischievous monkey with its disorderly sexual relations to AIDS. Some of this notion of social disorder is displayed in puppet shows he has produced for AIDS awareness in Mali.[7] A demonstration of the

---

7. The notion that AIDS in Africa has been brought about by social disorder engendered through Westernization has considerable currency. See Gausset and Mogensen, 1996, pp. 455–476.

Sologon Marionette Theatre monkey marionette is provided in the accompanying compact disk. Refer to Dance.

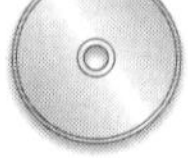

Video 11. AIDS Awareness Puppets
Yaya Coulibaly, Sologon Marionette Theatre, Mali

Contemporary creative dance is a category of African contemporary entertainment dance that comes from a fusion of styles and movements originating in different African ethnic groups within a given country or region. Contemporary creative dance has developed in African urban areas, where dance clubs and competitions have encouraged experimentation and improvisation in dance.

South Africa is particularly rich in contemporary creative dance forms because the country has long been a magnet for migrant labor from a broad region. Different men from all over East and Southern Africa have traveled to South Africa to work in South African mines and other industries. In the men's hostels[8] in South Africa, Nguni speaking men[9] all representing cattle rearing groups, developed the cattle dance. This helped the men to pass the time, and to get over their homesickness for the rural areas and their cattle herds.

Team dancing is common in South Africa, and dates at least as far back as the early 1800s, when the troupes of Shaka the great Zulu warrior were gathered together in military camps to prepare for war. The dancers, always men, raise their legs high, and stamp downward in perfect unison. Such dances, not unlike the Beni and the Kalila performances (described in the next chapter) have long been popular among Nguni speaking peoples who have strong militaristic traditions. Traditionally, these team dances recreate the sense of mock combat. It is probably for this reason that these dances were unaccompanied by instruments. Music for these dances is supplied by singing voices and clapping, those of the dancers or those of the audiences themselves. As we shall see below, many of these contemporary creative dance traditions have been adapted and co-opted into the fight against AIDS.

Dance traditions grew up around the townships in urban South Africa. The famous gum boot dance was a dance developed about 100 years ago by mine workers in the Witwatersrand, near Johannesburg. The name was derived from the footwear worn by the dancers. Gumboot dancers create complex rhythms by the slapping, clapping, and stomping of hands and rubber booted feet. Until well

8. Throughout the history of modern South Africa, Black workers have come to the cities of South Africa to work in factories or mines. Considered aliens in these White urban enclaves, they were usually unable to obtain housing of their own or to bring their families. Such workers were housed in very crowded single-sex barracks known as hostels adjacent to their place of employment.

9. Nguni speaking ethnic groups in South Africa include the Zulu, the Xhosa, the Ndebele, the Swazi, and others.

into the 1990s, gumboot dancing was exclusively the purview of males in South Africa. But the new constitution guarantees equal rights for women, and the new legal thrust in South Africa is clearly skewed in the direction of gender equality. The struggle for gender blindness is a very significant part of the New South Africa, and this is reflected in the arts. Today, young teenaged girls can be seen performing the gumboot dance, kicking their legs and their modesty high in the air. The thrust of this new liberation is also related to the efforts on the part of the South African Ministry of Health to encourage female assertiveness in the wake of the horrifying AIDS epidemic. Indeed, females performing gumboot dances has emerged in the context of AIDS awareness performances. Girls performing these dances at AIDS awareness festivals and school open days have even explained their behavior to researchers saying, "This body belongs to me" (Seidel, 1995, p. 157). Such pronouncements are encouraging for South African AIDS activists who hope their work will help erode some of the enormous gender disparities that help fuel the epidemic in South Africa. Two demonstrations of South African gumboot dancing are provided on the accompanying compact disk. Refer to Dance.

Video 12. Gumboot Dance
Eager Artists of South Africa in Michigan; Esikhawini AIDS Mural Launch, South Africa

Never short of improvisational techniques, facilitators from the South African DramAide project (see Chapters 3 and 8) involved in HIV/AIDS awareness performances have devised a modified Gumboot dance number called the "Fruiti-Tooti HIV/AIDS and Rights Abuse Prevention Pack." The dance features a group of dancers holding up various fruits denoting sexual responses. Spectators are enjoined to partake of the "abstinence apple," "strawberry kisses," or failing that, not "comrade banana" but rather "condom banana." A condom-wearing two foot cardboard banana is obviously the star visual aid, particularly when one the female dancers instructs spectators on the timing of the condom application. A demonstration of the Fruiti-Tooti modified gumboot dance is provided on the accompanying compact disk. Refer to Dance.

Video 13. HIV Prevention Dance
DramAide Troupe, South Africa

Another contemporary creative dance is *Isicathamiya*. *Isicathamiya* is a singing and dance tradition that employs both Western and traditional Zulu forms. *Iscathamiya* is probably best known outside South Africa through the work of Ladysmith Black Mbazo. *Iscathamiya* uses a lead singer, known in Zulu as *Izugu* who calls out to his troupe who respond with song and dance steps. This acappella style of song and dance developed in the 1930s in South Africa's men's hostels where eight to 12 industrial workers lived cramped in a single room. The industries for which these men worked sponsored competitions as a way of keeping their men occupied, entertained, and out of trouble. Because the hostels were so crowded, it is said there was little space to dance. And because the dancers needed to be quiet so as not to rouse the police or even sleeping men in the neighboring hostel, they developed the hushed singing and movement styles of *Iscathamiya. Isicathamiya* dancers typically dress in black trousers, white shirts, red bow ties, and white gloves. *Isicathamiya* remains very popular in South Africa today, especially in KwaZulu-Natal province. Durban's City Playhouse holds an annual *Isicathamiya* contest where several troupes from around the region compete for prizes.

Like so much else of the popular culture in South Africa, *Isicathamiya* dances have been incorporated into the fight against AIDS. It is rare that a public festival or an AIDS related function can occur in KwaZulu-Natal Province without there being some kind of AIDS *Iscathamiya* dance. The words of the song encourage the dance and the dancers to move forward.

These words were sung during an *Isicathamiya* performance at an AIDS rally held in July 1999 at the juvenile division of a South African Correctional facility.

We can conquer it
If we talk to each other
If we stop undermining each other
If you do sex, use a condom

This disease is difficult to heal
It's difficult for doctors
And for *Inyangas* (traditional herbalists)
It kills the young
It kills the old ones
It kills Whites
It kills Blacks (Translation from the original
Zulu version by Musa Ndlovu, October 1999).

Isicathamiya is an adaptable form. It builds its messages through call and response, overlapping harmonies, and repetition. An *Isicathamiya* dance was performed at the launch of the South African AIDS Memorial Quilt Project on the University of Zululand campus in August 1999. This was one of the many activities of the South African Beyond Awareness 2 Campaign.

You mothers and fathers
You have to learn to
Teach your children
About this Disease (Translated from the original
Zulu version by Musa Ndlovu, October 1999).

REPEAT SEVERAL TIMES

A demonstration of *Isicathamiya* dance performed at the South African AIDS memorial quilt launch is provided on the accompanying compact disk. Refer to Dance.

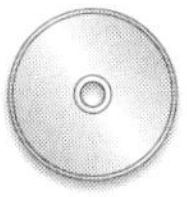

Video 14. Isicathamiya
1999 AIDS Memorial Quilt Launch, South Africa

Another South African contemporary creative dance is the *toyi-toyi.* The *toyi-toyi* originated in the guerrilla camps of the African National Congress (ANC) which supported the struggle for the liberation of South Africa. It is therefore related to the heroic dance classification listed among the traditional communal dances earlier in this chapter. *Toyi-toyi* was clearly evident in the Soweto children's marches of 1976 and it featured prominently as a war dance of the 1980s performed during marches protesting the racist Apartheid regime. The dance was immortalized in the South African Black liberation musicals of the 1980s. When performed in the context of a musical, it can be considered an "entertainment" dance.

Today, the *toyi-toyi* dance, with its characteristic Black Power Salute, has been appropriated by the AIDS struggle. Indeed *toyi-toyi* is a dance performed by people who wish to fortify themselves for collective struggle. Popular South African singer Mbongeni Ngema produced an Anti-AIDS hit release in the *toyi-toyi* song-dance style. *Toyi-toyi* has appeared in "open-day" school events as part of organized performances against AIDS. And it can emerge spontaneously as it was said to have done during the Soweto demonstrations. In contemporary South Africa young people focussing on an issue or a cause will often burst spontaneously into a *toyi-toyi.* At the University of Fort Hare, for example, I witnessed student activists who had participated in an afternoon of AIDS memorial quilt making, burst into a *toyi-toyi* dance when they came upon their art student colleagues producing an AIDS awareness mural on their campus. Outbursts of *toyi-toyi* dancing often occur at AIDS awareness activities and rallies. The dancing symbolizes the willingness of young people to join in a community or a national struggle.

The issues of AIDS and gender violence are particularly salient sources of inspirations for the *toyi-toyi.* The DramAide troupe uses the *toyi-toyi* to energize young university students to fight gender abuse and other violations of human rights. Three demonstrations of *toyi-toyi* dancing are presented on the accompanying compact disk. Refer to Dance.

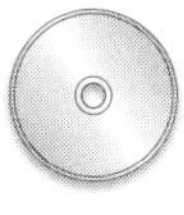

Video 15. Toyi-Toyi Rally Dance
Eager Artists of South Africa in Michigan; Students, University of Fort Hare, South Africa; DramAide-South Africa

Contemporary Recreational and Party Dances

A final category of contemporary dance in the Begho dance classification includes recreational and party dances. These are so termed because they represent fun-seeking and unconscious abandon. Once popular High Life dance music of the 1950s and 1960s in Nigeria has given rise to the more popular fuji, jùjú, and Afro-jùjú styles in that country. And soukous in the francophone countries of Africa has given way to faster track party music from the Congo, and the newer sounds of such West African superstars Youssou N'dour of Senegal and Salif Keita of Mali. Again, since the World Music phenomenon of the nineties made African music popular world wide, there has been a growing cross-pollination of Western with African music. Africans dancing in clubs and at parties to these sounds are engaged in contemporary recreational dancing.

As noted in the previous sub-section, Kwaito music is the current rage in much of South Africa. Kwaito is often performed by rappers who can also dance in a sort of electronic Michael Jackson "moon walk" style. But the crowd, with considerable less virtuosity, dances to Kwaito with the characteristic partnerless, autonomous moves of global rock and pop culture.

It should be abundantly clear that music, and by extension dance, are present at just about all public events in Africa, both modern or traditional.

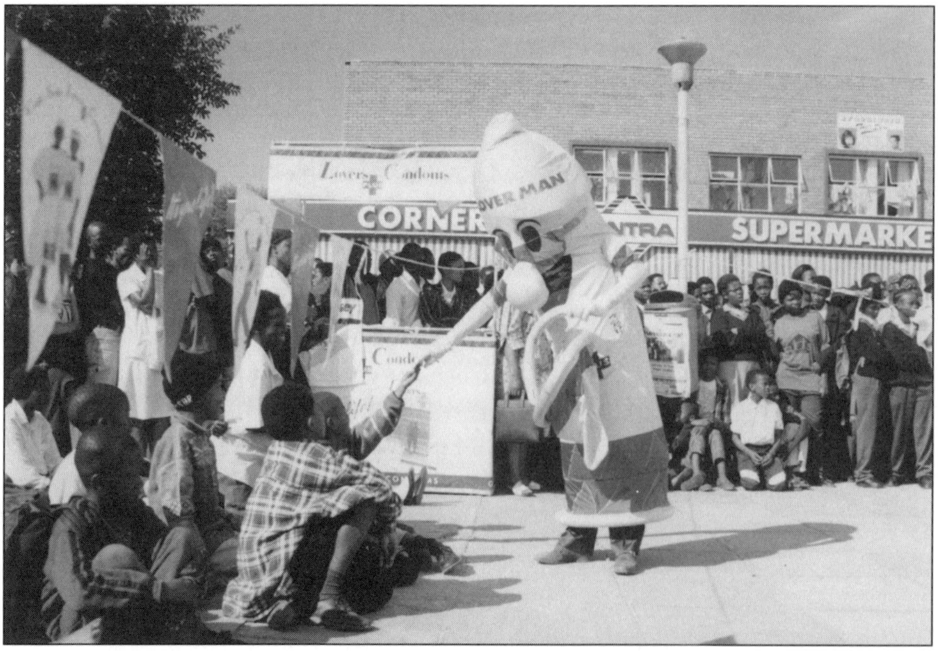

Figure 7-9. Condom Man appears at AIDS rallies in Southern Africa. Photo courtesy of Population Services International.

AIDS Rallies

This chapter has referred repeatedly to AIDS events of various types. These events, well worthy of elaboration, are discussed herein. AIDS fairs, expositions, or rallies have become a common part of edutainment and participatory communication strategies used in the fight against HIV and AIDS. In South Africa, Schools and Tertiary institutions (universities and technikons) regularly feature such events. AIDS Edu-Fairs provide an opportunity to distribute literature on HIV/AIDS and related issues, such as STDs, gender abuse, risk behaviors, and so on. Edu-Fairs are staffed by guidance counselors and medical personnel who are on hand to answer questions and to quietly encourage HIV testing for those needing or requesting it.

The Edu-Fairs also provide and encourage the celebration of a new and more open sexuality, women's-empowerment, and a fun and free culture of safer sex. Edu-Fairs attract youth through the presentation of plays, skits, and songs on HIV. Some of them can be quite graphic in their descriptions of alternatives to penetrative sexual intercourse. Attendees are encouraged to join into the sense of play of the fair, and especially to participate in the singing and dancing. And they are also urged to help themselves to condoms that are gleefully distributed in an atmosphere of celebration. Through these means, organizers believe that students as the leaders and shapers of the mores of their generation will internalize a more honest, more open, and more egalitarian culture of safe sex. AIDS rallies/parades also feature imaginative student-decorated floats peopled by genial condom men[10] and other symbols of safe sex.

In South Africa, the Beyond Awareness 2 AIDS Mural project executed by DramAide provided opportunities for community celebration. When murals were officially "launched" the host community would gather around for a kind of group ritual performance. These would typically include opening prayers and speeches, followed again by AIDS songs, AIDS dramas, and AIDS dances. And the launching of the South African AIDS Memorial Quilt Project, the first official public exhibitions of the South African quilts was celebrated in a similar, albeit more subdued manner as is fitting for a commemorations of the dead.[11]

Mali also uses public processions and public forums to demonstrate the severity of the threat of HIV and AIDS and to rally the public, especially the young into a posture of self-defense. Mali's CNIECS (*Centre National d'Information, Education, et Communication pour la Santé*) has organized whistle-stop HIV/AIDS rallies along the train line that links Mali's capital Bamako with the Senegalese capital of Dakar. The train has brought performers and information to local communities who contribute to the general carnival atmosphere with speechmaking, songs, music and other performative additions of their own. The

10. There are still far too few "Condom Women or Condom Girls," as one would hope for given the desire to promote female empowerment as a way to combat the spread of HIV/AIDS.

11. This celebration was held in August 1999 at the University of Zululand in KwaZulu-Natal. It was organized by the DramAide project.

title theme of one of Mali's train rallies was "*Le SIDA ne passsera pas par moi*!" or "I will not be the one to transmit AIDS!"

Mali also celebrates World AIDS day in December with an exposition wherein educational materials, health brochures, photo-novels, AIDS comics, HIV games, AIDS cassettes and videotapes, and of course condoms are distributed. The event provides an opportunity for a good deal of spontaneous recreational or party dancing. Malian youth even danced around a condom application lesson at the World AIDS Day commemoration in 1999. The lesson was provided by an NGO physician brandishing a carved life-size wooden phallus. Drums invite young people to dance at such events, and eventually to process into an auditorium to hear prayers and speeches about the importance of safe sex, wise choices, and so on. Recreational dancing and a condom lesson is provided on the accompanying compact disk. Refer to Dance.

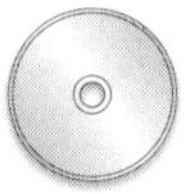

Video 16. Dancing for AIDS Awareness
1999 World AIDS Day, Bamako, Mali

The notion of fun in the context of an AIDS rally may seem peculiar to the Western mind-set. Part of the use of fun in these contexts is to attract youth, the next likely targets of HIV/AIDS, youth who might otherwise shun a more serious event. The entertaining atmosphere also helps to destigmatize the virus, thereby attenuating denial. Edu-Fairs and rallies also make it possible to "out" the virus, to speak of it in a safe, public, and a non-threatening atmosphere. On the subject of fun and death, however, it is also worth reminding Western readers, that African youth, particularly those from the poorest of countries are generally far more acquainted with death than their Western counterparts. In Mali, for example, well over 10% of babies die before their fifth birthday, and life expectancy is 47 years of age.

Hanna, moreover, argues that dancing is done in Africa as an affirmation of life, as a way to defy the incomprehensible. This she explains, is one of the many reasons Africans dance at funerals. Given these considerations, dancing even joyously in the face of the AIDS epidemic becomes understandable (Hanna, 1987, pp. 111–114).

It is clear that dance is an adaptive form of expression. Africans use dance to show an incredible range of emotion. They dance in grief; they dance in joy. They dance in worship, and they dance to recreate history. They dance to support politicians, or to comment ironically on their misdoings. They dance to pass from one stage of life to the next, and to mark the changing of seasons. They dance to honor the ancestors, to diagnose an illness and to heal the sick. They dance to seduce the opposite sex, and to celebrate the unification to two families. They dance to prepare for war or to calm down a tense social situation. With dance, they can praise their hosts, and flatter their patrons. They can use dance to announce danger and to rally for change. They dance to amuse and to entertain, to warn and to gently correct.

Unlike the West, music and dance performances in Africa are not exceptional events to be enjoyed only within the carefully bounded periods of time set aside for recreation. Rather, music and dance in Africa is part of how people learn, how people socialize, and how people communicate spirit in the face of destiny.

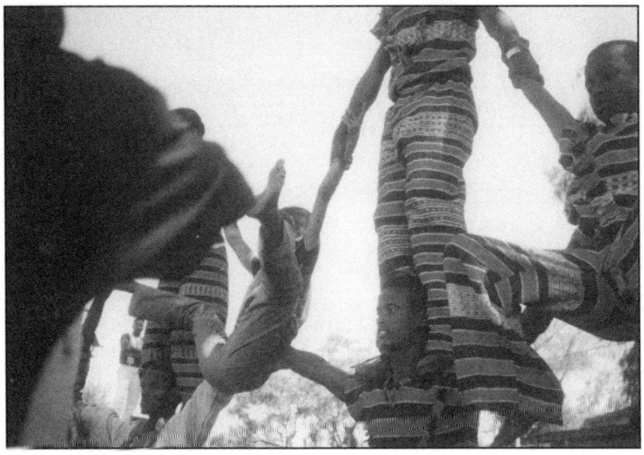

Figure 7-10. Debub Nigat AIDS education Circus, Awassa, Southern Ethiopia. Photo courtesy of David Schein, Awassa Children's Project.

Review Questions

1. What is the role of dance in African social life? How does dance express African social values?
2. What social and historical processes have made African traditional dances different from African contemporary dances? What processes have helped to diminish the role of the spirits in today's world?
3. What is an AIDS rally? What is an AIDS Edu-Fair? How and why is dance incorporated into these events?

Chapter 8

Drama

This chapter provides an overview of drama on the African continent beginning with a theory of the origin of drama. It discusses pre-colonial, colonial, and post-colonial theatre in Africa. At the end of the chapter the AIDS issue is introduced and the uses of theatre in the AIDS struggle are discussed in the national contexts of South Africa and Mali. The award-winning South African television series, Soul City is also presented within the context of South African AIDS drama.

Ritual Roots of Drama

Scholars who study African theatre usually expend some energy discussing the source of theatre in Africa. In this context, the subject of ritual generally arises. Because ritual in Africa is so suffused with drama, and because drama can seem so ritualistic it can be difficult to distinguish theatre from ritual.

Anthony Graham-White argues that the basic distinction between ritual and drama is the belief that ritual will have consequences beyond itself. Graham-White adopts the position that the effects of a dramatic performance stop when the drama ends, while those of ritual continue (Graham-White, 1974, p. 17). Graham White's formulation preceded the discussions of postmodern performance theorists as Richard Schechner and Jerry Growtowski whose work investigates the use of theatre in social change and personal growth movements (Schechner, 1988, 106–152).

David Kerr's distinction between ritual and theatre focuses not on the expectations of the "audience" or the participants but rather on the purpose and the targets of the performance. Kerr argues that ritual is an action that is performed to praise, to request, or in some way to intercede with super-natural forces. He points out that these behaviors may or may not involve dramatic acts or performing arts of any kind. His definition of ritual moreover, tends to highlight the repetitive as opposed to the performative nature of ritual. Kerr's definition of drama includes a set of actions that tell a story with an element of suspense to an audience (Kerr, 1995, p. 1). His definition of drama tends to spotlight the performative, as opposed to the repetitive nature of drama even though stock stories from folklore contain few surprises. For Kerr, the ritual is directed primarily at spiritual forces, and the drama is directed primarily at a human audience.

The distinctions made by both Graham-White and Kerr, while comfortable at face value, are contestable by scholars of ritual and scholars of theatre. Anthony Graham-White's conception of theatre or drama is a narrow entertainment-oriented view of this art form. It excludes "Theatre for Development," urban guerilla theatre, and other theatres for social change including Western medieval and mystery plays.

Kerr's distinction is based upon target audiences gives short shrift to the social or communal rites such as Yoruba rituals that re-enact foundation myths (see below) or performances that re-enact Biblical stories.[1] His contention that stories (drama) are enacted for human audiences, fails to take into account the fact that the dead (the spirit world) in Africa live on, both through their descendents and exist as ever-present ancestors. Indeed, as I have noted in previous chapters, performers often call upon the spirit of dead performers to aid them in drumming, dancing, or mime. Oftentimes, moreover, living performers often ascribe the quality of a performance to the presence or absence of a given ancestor.

A brief examination of the operation of secret societies also reveals the way ritual and theatre were conflated in many traditional African societies. The kindgoms of the Grassfields of northwestern Cameroon were governed through reticulate systems of secret societies. Even today, these traditional systems wield considerable power at the local level of governance in Cameroon. Each of these secret societies has a totem animal, and members who join these secret societies acquire a "double," a mystical totem animal into which they are transformed. In the Grassfields, a human "turns into" his "double" through a dance that takes place in the sacred forest. Here, non-initiates are banned under pain of death or serious retribution. These transformed mystical beings, part human, and part spirit, then help the king to govern.

Each of the secret societies in the Grassfields has its own orchestra and its own specific dance performances, dances they perform at specific key events such as the installation of a new king. Other secret societies make their appearance only at the burial and the mourning of a deceased chief, the beginning and the end of a reign. One of the most important of these societies is the *Kwi'ifo*, the kings' sacred orchestra and his chief militia. At the installation of a new king the *Kwi'ifo* performs a dance in a clockwise direction. This performance signifies that things are returning to normal in the community after a change of leadership. This clockwise movement runs counter to the dances of the other secret societies, dances that are usually performed in an anti-clockwise direction. The *Kwi'ifo* dance features performers who are dressed in costumes of leopard, buffalo, lion, and elephant. These animals signify the "double lives" practiced by members of the secret societies that help the king with governance. A failure of the *Kwi'ifo* to appear at the installation ceremony would indicate he did not have the approval of the secret societies. Without the support of these secret societies, a king in the Grassfields would be powerless and would be unable to govern.

What is important to understand in this discussion of the *Kwi'ifo* is that the rituals involved are constitutive. An initiate becomes a member of a secret society and acquires a "double" through performance, a performance that connects the cosmic, the spirit world, with the earthly body of the initiate. And a king is in-

1. In Latin America and in Mediterranean countries, the passion of Christ, complete with the way of the cross is reenacted on Good Friday in a procession that clearly contains both elements of religious ritual and elements of entertaining performance.

stalled through performances by secret societies whose members are dressed in regalia suggesting the presence of non-human cosmic "doubles" of these society members (Doho 1989; Doho n.d.).

The above presentation on secret societies serves only to highlight some of the difficulties bound up in trying to differentiate ritual from theatre. And it highlights the fact that these two performative genres are closely related. Indeed, scholars from Aristotle through to an early twentieth century group of anthropologists known as the Cambridge Group, believed that theatre descended from ritual as societies secularized (Schechner, 1988, pp. 1–5; Graham-White, 1974. p. 17). (We will return to this contention in Chapter 9). Describing the process among the Dogon peoples of Mali, Graham-White notes, "Little by little, from being attentive to the rite, the crowd becomes attentive to the spectacle"(1974, p. 19).

African Pre-Colonial Theatre

Most of what we know best about African drama comes from genres and forms developed after colonial contact in Africa. It is important nevertheless to examine pre-colonial forms of drama. Important among these are the masquerade[2] and the *Kòtèba.*

Masquerades seem to have been widespread in pre-colonial West Africa. The term masquerade refers to masked dances that often include mime, acrobatics, and pantomime. Many of us are familiar with African masks that we have seen in art galleries, but these masks form only part of the masquerade regalia. The masks are worn with costumes of cloth, raffia, and sometimes feathers. These costumes are attached to the mask and typically hide the entire body of the masquerader, making it easier for the audience to forget the human agency in the masked dance. The carved mask may be worn over the face or on top of the head facing the gods. Masquerades in the Grassfields of northwest Cameroon, the "public face" of secret society dancing described above, use wooden masks heavily decorated with beads, cowry shells, and feathers.

Masquerades are exciting events. Surrounded by drummers and singers, the dancers appear well after the crowd has long awaited their arrival. Sometimes young boys accompany the masquerades shaking sticks to menace the crowd when they crush in on the dancers. As noted above, in some of the societies of West and Central Africa that feature masquerades, the performances are the public manifestation of a parallel spiritual world. In other cases, these masquerades are little more than the secular entertainment vestiges of what was once a deeply spiritual practice. But in many societies in West Africa, masquerades remain a bit of both, an entertainment form that still contains elements of the sacred.

A good example of a masquerade is the Yoruba *Egungun* masquerade that is performed at the *Egungun* festivals that honor the corporate spirit of Yoruba

2. The fact that masquerades are classified as dance by some scholars and as theatre by others is indicative of the polyvalent nature of African performing arts.

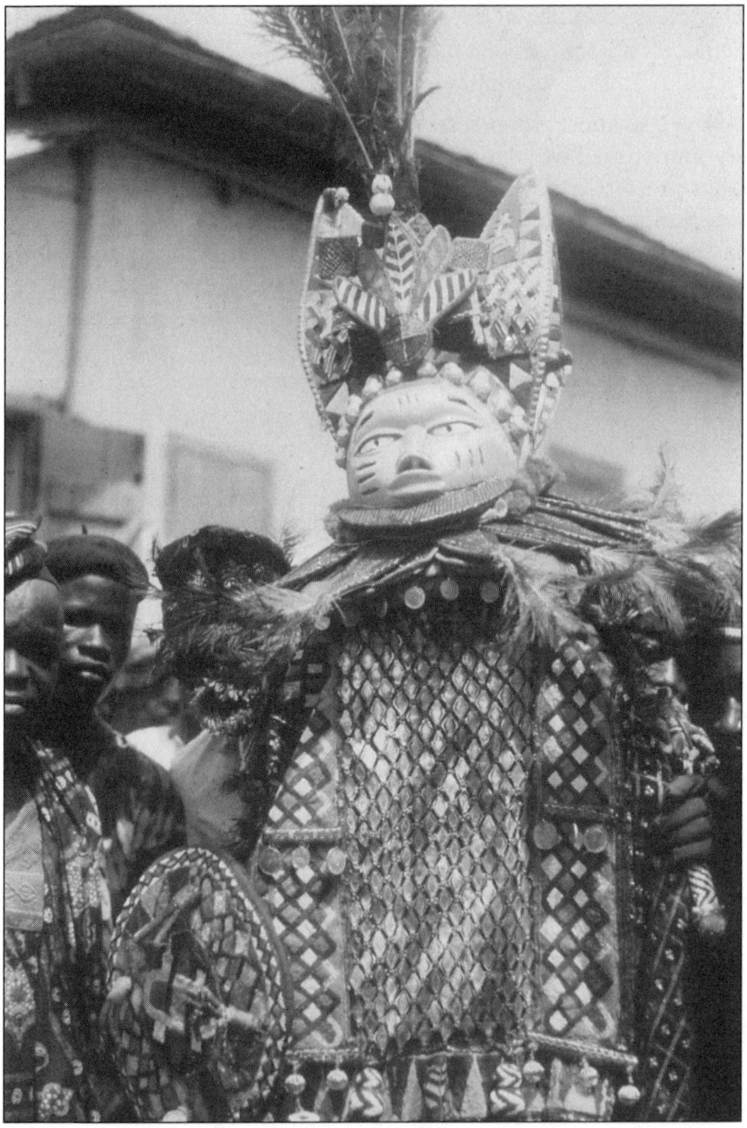

Figure 8-1. Egungun masquerade dancer.
Photo courtesy of Norma Wolff.

dead. *Egungun* masquerades also make their appearance in Yorubaland at the second burial celebration for a deceased relative[3] (Perani, 1998, p. 148). The origin of the *Egungun* is obscure, but most think it derived from ancestor worship cults from different parts of West Africa. According to Kerr, semi-secular Yoruba theatre emerged about 500 years ago as the Yoruba peoples gained in power and importance in what is today southwestern and south central Nigeria. By the 19th

3. In many parts of Africa it is common to hold more than one funerary rite to honor a dead relative or an ancestor. These are held at specific time intervals following the person's death.

century, *Egungun* became quite secularized (Kerr, 1995, pp. 13–14; Hackett, 1996, p. 54).

There is a great deal of variety of masks, performance behaviors, and characters represented in the *Egungun* cults. They may include the trickster *Egungun*, the *onidan* (miracle worker) and the *olokiti* or tumblers. They sing, dance, mime, and pantomime, often mocking village members who have displayed anti-social behavior or violated other social norms. They may speak in low growling voices of the dead or make animal noises.

Sometimes, and in some contexts, the *Egungun* cult dancers perform just for fun; sometimes they perform death rituals or help to celebrate an important festival in the Yoruba religious cycle. Sometimes their role is in combating outbreaks of witchcraft (Apter, 1993, p. 115).

Another pre-colonial theatrical form is the *Kòtèba* theatre of the Bamana, a Mande people of central Mali. The *Kòtèba* refers to a satiric theatre performed without masks, originally by all male cast members. The Bamana (also known as Bambara), Mali's main ethnic group, are a hierarchical society organized into two main caste lines that include the *horon* and the *nyamakala*. The *honon*, are the nobility who farm, govern, defend, and conquer and the *nyamakala* are the craftspeople who work with metal, wood, clay, words, and certain music. These materials are considered to hold spiritual power. These social divisions are what remains of the 14th and 15th century feudal Bamana kingdoms, groupings that once included slaves. Five hundred or more years ago, elaborate masked rituals appear to have emerged to support this system, a system that subordinated youths to the elders. Within this strongly patriarchal system whose contours echo throughout much of the continent, *Kòtèba* developed. At that time, the *Kòtèba* was also performed by a secret society.

Today, *Kòtèba* is a secular unmasked drama that functions to maintain social equilibrium. It does this by holding up to ridicule anti-social elements of society, thereby mocking those who would violate codes of social justice and basic human rights as defined by the Bamana people (Sissoko, 1995, p. 7). Like much traditional theatre in Africa, *Kòtèba* uses several common stereotypes in its performances. These include "unfaithful [female] lovers, cowards, greedy persons, morons, arrogant, wicked or lazy farmers" (Kerr, 1995, pp. 4–5). The *Kòtèba* uses ribald humor to satirize a society in which a system of polygynous marriage and bride price payment tends to keep young men sexually frustrated bachelors and forces young women into coupling with older powerful men.

Kòtèba theatre is performed by the *kòtèton*. The word *Kote* means "satiric speech" and the word "*ton*" designates youth age grade. "The *kòtèton* is in fact a satirical theatre group restricted to young men who have been given some leeway in the gentle lampooning of their elders. The *Kòtèba* traditionally included skits presented by age sets—young boys, teenaged boys, and men in their twenties. Once a man became an elder, he no longer participated in *Kòtèba*, becoming instead a victim of its humor. Artists including actors in Bamana society enjoyed privileged though marginal status. They were feared for their *nyakaro* [comic relief] and their ability to mock and mimic (Kerr, 1995, p. 6). Already secularized and not particularly subversive to the social order, *Kòtèba* was allowed to persist through colonial days.

Like many African art forms, the early dramas, semi-secular masquerades such as the *Egungun* described above succumbed to the pressures of colonialism. Christianity discouraged the practice of sacred ritual through masquerade. In so doing it promoted the desacralization of ritual objects (masks and costumes), and of ritual performance (dances and plays), and the transformation of these objects and genres into entertainment.

Colonialism also encouraged secularization by luring young men who participated in masquerades away from their village home base. The demands of paid employment kept them from rehearsals needed to put on complex ritual performances (Graham-White, 1974, p. 57). And the same forces of colonialism encouraged the performance of ritual for monetary gain, i.e., the performance of formerly sacred events as spectacle in decontextualized urban spaces by detribalized multi-ethnic performance groups. Anthony Graham-White summarized the situation well.

> The influence of the colonial period upon traditional African drama can be summarized by saying that while it contributed to the decline of traditional performances, it also suggested new directions in which the drama might develop as well, of course, as providing new subject matter (1974, p. 59).

He adds further.

> The real contribution of colonialism was to provide models for the development of literary drama.

Drama in the Colonial Period

Colonizing Europeans introduced two forms of drama in Africa: theatre designed by and for the European community and dramatic forms designed to 'domesticate' and socialize Africans. Apart from the inappropriately named 'African Theatre' in Cape Town (South Africa), colonizers typically built "little theatres" which were attached to sports clubs. This was especially true in places where there was a large European settler population such as in the east and central-southern African colonies of Kenya, Southern Rhodesia [now Zimbabwe], Northern Rhodesia [now Zambia], and of course in South Africa.

The colonial sports clubs maintained exclusive membership roles making them targets for and badges of acceptance and advancement for working class European settlers in the colonies. Racism was the order of the day in these clubs, whose social function was to isolate the colonized from the colonizers and demonstrate the superiority of the latter group. The plays performed in these venues tended to be of two types: either high blown classical fare; or safe, bland, middle class domestic drama which appealed to aspiring upwardly mobile Europeans of the era.

Drama designed to domesticate Africans came in the form of school drama, mission drama, and imperial propaganda. Catholic missionaries often organized elaborate festivals and ritual performances around saints' days. This was particularly true in the Portuguese colonies of Mozambique, Angola, and Guinea-Bissau.

Missionaries in anglophone and francophone Africa encouraged the dramatization of Old and New Testament stories: the creation, the crucifixion, David,

Saul, the prodigal son, and so on (Kerr, 1995, p. 33). In schools, students performed bits of Shakespeare in the English colonies, and the works of 18th century French classical authors such as Racine, Corneille, and Molière in the colonies of France (Kerr, 1995, p. 34). And colonial schools also performed their task of domestication through teaching of European theatre and dance. The William Ponty School in Senegal promoted the adaptation of traditional folktales into written French plays. Here, a generation of native civil servants for the French colonies was trained. The theatrical adaptation process was a double-edged cultural sword, both serving to preserve African traditions while at the same time helping to critically distance the students from them.

During the colonial period, the colonizers held festivals and ceremonies designed to display the power of the motherland. This included such events as coronations, jubilees and other celebrations of European rule, together with investitures and turbanning of local rulers collaborating with the colonizers. Such events were marked by military parades featuring brass bands and other regalia from the home countries. Other types of imperial propaganda included Boy Scout jamborees and concerts. The pomp displayed at these events would shape the development of syncretic entertainment genres on the African continent.

Syncretic Theatrical Genres

Dramatic forms that combine traditional African elements with European performance styles are known in the literature as syncretic popular theatre. Two broad types have been identified: militaristic mime and concert parties.

Militaristic Mime

Militaristic mime developed in East Africa using the indigenous *ngoma* dance forms for the basic movements and grafting on more Western elements to the performance. Dancers used a mixture of traditional and Western instruments and more or less imitated military bands. Kerr describes the Beni Dance Society of East Africa.

> Beni was an entertainment dance in which the participants often dressed in smart military style uniforms, and danced in regular and ordered columns with sticks imitating guns or batons. The Beni dances featured a hierarchy of roles that included a king, officers and subordinate ranks. The dance parodied British military stratification with its bugle music, its flutes, its side-drums, its neat uniforms, and its regular marching steps. All of this suggested the important influence of colonial marching bands (Kerr, 1995, p. 60).

Sometimes the dance appeared as a parade, sometimes a procession. At other times it would appear as a march past or as a drill step. Beni dance teams engaged in competitions in which representative teams symbolized rival social groups. Competition between these groups was believed to have functioned in ironing out the social order (Gunderson, 2000, p. 9). Terrence Ranger who studied the Beni extensively says the genre was replaced in East Africa by the rise of urban jazz groups in the 1960s (1975, p. 2).

The *Kalela* dances of Northern Rhodesia (now Zambia), like the Beni of Kenya and Tanzania (then Tanganyika), also drew from the British military whom they admired. The *Kalela* could boast a similar hierarchy complete with governors, officers, nurses, and privates. These *Kalela* dancers dressed in crisp well-pressed uniforms, shiny shoes, and immaculate handkerchiefs (Kerr, 1995, p. 65).

Militaristic mimes evolved and were adapted by different societies for different purposes. In some localities they went out of fashion as early as the post World War I period. In Tanzania, they remained popular until after World War II when they were superceded by modern dance band music (Ranger 1975). In Northern Rhodesia [now Zambia] a militaristic march called the *mganda* was used to parody colonial policemen in the 1950s. Kerr remarks that as late as the 1980s, the militaristic mimes were alive and well on Likoma Island in Zambia (Kerr, 1995, p. 70)).

Ranger quotes an informant who claimed the *Mganda* originated in northern Malawi and explained how the genre came about.

> This is how it all started. In 1914 during the First World War, people from Usisya [Malawi] saw soldiers marching. While marching they sang songs and played trumpets. They all marched with the same step. When war was ended the soldiers left, so the people of Usisya tried to do what the soldiers were doing.... After some time they discovered the idea of using gourds for trumpets.... When they made the trumpets those who had deep voices played bass and those with soft voices played the tenor. They tried very hard to make a drum that would look like the soldiers' until finally they made it (quoted in Nyoni, 2000, p. 235–236).

Nyoni describes a militaristic mime called the *mganda-wa-kinkachi* that is practiced in Tanzania today. The genre includes militaristic dance movements, dramatic skits, magic tricks, masks, and songs. Notably, in recent years, the songs have dealt increasingly with deaths from AIDS (Nyoni, 2000, pp. 50–51).

It is interesting that many of the churches in Southern Africa have appropriated militaristic dance music. Brass bands form a part of the pageantry of the African Independent Churches, often leading processionals used in the energetic worship styles found therein. Brass bands constituted some of the Christian mystique that helped win converts to Christianity in Southern Africa during the 19th and early 20th centuries. Indeed Pauline Dlamini, a member of Zulu King Cetsweyo's *Isigodlo* (harem) describes in her memoirs how Zulu people wanted to convert to Christianity when they heard the strange and otherworldly sound of trumpets which they had never before heard (Filter, 1986, p. 89). The Salvation Army used brass bands near to South African gold mines to attract workers to listen to Christian sermons (Maloka, 1997, p. 245). Many of the African Independent Churches have their own congregational brass bands. One such band, belonging to Saint John's Apostolic Faith Church of Durban, South Africa is seen on the accompanying compact disk. Refer to Drama.

Video 1. Brass Band, African Independent Church
Saint John's Apostolic Faith Church Band, South Africa

Concert Parties

Another syncretic African performance genre is the concert party. The name concert party seems to have derived from concerts performed on Empire Day[4] or at the end of the school term. These concert party performances much resembled vaudeville acts and contained comic sketches, mime, and song. Concert party performers came equipped to performances with bags of costumes, make-up including false beards and mustaches, and even blackface minstrel style make up (Kerr, 1995, p. 74).

The concert party genre developed in the 1920, in West Africa and drew from many Western sources. These included religious plays and hymns from Christian missions; rag-time songs, tap dancing, and stand-up comedy traditions (which had developed in southern Black America and returned to Africa by way of Liberia;[5] and Hollywood movies of the 1920s and 1930s, especially those of Charlie Chaplin (Kerr, 1995, p. 74).

Concert parties provided a way for recently urbanized Africans to enjoy their newfound urban status. Some of the mimes took gentle jabs at local and national politics of the day. They became especially popular in the 1950s when they added "highlife" music[6] to their repertoires. By the early 1970s, there were over 40 concert party troupes in Ghana (Graham-White, 1974, p. 147). By this time, many of the highlife bands were using the concert party genre to supplement their incomes. In the new millennium the concert party genre had almost disappeared in the face of new competition from the indigenous video-film industry (Braun 2000).

Much like the *Kòtèba*, West African concert party sketches used stock or stereotypical characters. And like the *Kòtèba*, they saw the world through men's eyes. The stock characters created for these newly urbanized audiences were the long-suffering wife, the naïve and victimized husband, and the rapaciously fashionable urbanized girlfriend.

Here in the concert party tradition, like the *Kòtèba*, the performances were carried out by a small troupe who played multiple roles, including all male casts playing the female roles. And as with the *Kòtèba* and with most other African

4. Empire Day represented the day in which all of the colonies of the British Empire celebrated their common governance under the British.

5. A group of returned American slaves settled in 1822 off the coast of what would become Liberia. In 1847 they declared themselves a Republic and thus founded Black Africa's first independent and sovereign nation.

6. A syncretistic popular music form which developed in West Africa but which was inspired by both the Big Band sound and military marches, and used modern brass instruments and African polyrhythmic beats.

performance, concert party audiences would participate actively in the spectacle, booing, hissing, jeering, and exhorting the players, and even pressing money upon an actor whose behavior they admired (Graham-White, 1974, p. 148). And because African theatre is highly didactic, there was always a moral lesson to be had from the performance.

Yoruba Opera

Similar to the concert parties was a genre called the Yoruba Opera, which developed in southern Nigeria in the 1940s. Yoruba opera was a kind of quasi-religious multi-media performance spectacle that drew upon religious elements from *Egungun* masquerades and African independent churches. Some of the early open-air operas featured Christian plots. The action of the players in these spectacles was commented upon by a cast choir swaying from side to side, clapping, and singing continuously to organ or to drumbeat.

It should be noted that there are about 40 million Yoruba speaking peoples packed into the southwestern and south-central region of Nigeria and the southern half of neighboring Benin. This makes it possible to produce popular performances in the Yoruba language and to find a ready audience.

One of the best known composers of Yoruba opera was Herbert Ogunde. As a child, Ogunde was exposed to *Egungun* cult masquerades and hoped one day to lead his own troupe. As an adult, Ogunde became a policeman and a choirmaster in the Church of the Lord, an African Independent church in Lagos, Nigeria. Ogunde's early operas treated the syncretic worship traditions that had been evolving in the early 20th century in many parts of Africa. One early work, "Africa and God" (1944) depicted Yoruba life before the arrival of Europeans in Africa. Most of his other titles from the 1940s reflected Biblical themes: Israel in Egypt (1945); King Solomon (1945); and Journey to Heaven (1947).

In the 1950s, Ogunde's operas became more secular and more political. Adding highlife music and scantily dressed dancers, his Yoruba operas merged into a genre rather similar to that of the concert party. The genre featured Yoruba oratory, music, and dance within a broadly defined framework of European musical.

Other Yoruba Operas continued to draw from the vast and complex repertoire of Yoruba mythology. Another Yoruba opera troupe leader, Obutunde Ijimere wrote and produced an opera called "The Imprisonment of Obatala," which deals with the ancient conflict between Shango, God of Thunder and Obatala, god of creation and King of the Yoruba city of Ife (Graham-White, 1974, p. 154).

Literary Drama

About 100 years ago, literary drama slowly began to unfold in Africa. A new genre, different from the concert parties and Yoruba operas, began to emerge. These plays were products of, and for, a new literate class of Africans. In contemplative and intellectual ways, these newly educated writers treated their own personal dilemmas and those of their contemporaries. Typically such authors explored the themes surrounding cultural clashes between communal African culture and the more individually oriented European one. Indeed this has been a central preoccupation of much African literature, even to this day.

The earliest surviving literary text of a play from Black Africa is Kobina Senyi's "The Blinkards" from 1915, written in a mixture of English and Fanti. Senyi's work, accessible to popular urban audiences, would not reemerge until the 1950s with Amos Tuotola's publication of *The Palm-Wine Drinkard*. Other examples of early literary drama genre emerged sporadically during the first half of the 20th century. In 1935, for example, South African playwright Herbert I. E. Dhlomo wrote in Zulu, "The Girl who Killed to Save," a play which treats the conquest of southern Africa by the Europeans. Five years later, J. B. Danquah, from the Gold Coast (now Ghana), produced "The Third Woman." Nobel prize-winning Nigerian playwright Wole Soyinka explored themes of cultural clash in two of his early plays, "The Lion and the Jewel," and "The Swamp Dwellers" in the 1950s.

Literary drama might have grown more rapidly in Africa before World War II had the cinema not siphoned off potential audiences. The first film projectors arrived on the continent around the turn of the century, much the same time they made their appearance in other parts of the world. And by the late 1920s and 1930s, according to David Kerr, "a significant sector of urbanized Africans were very interested in [Hollywood] feature films" (1995, p. 25).

But French and British colonial policies of the 1920s and 1930s to increase African education did pay off in literary terms within a generation or so. By the 1950s and 1960s, Africa could boast a respectable number of African playwrights. Much of the literature from the period bears the particular marks of that era. And the theme of culture wars, Western versus African, remains a predominant preoccupation of much of written literature from African even at present. Many of the writers whose careers seemed to blossom around the time of independence cut their teeth in playwriting by writing for the BBC.

The British Broadcasting Corporation played in important role in promoting a literate theatre tradition. It sponsored the African Theatre Competition between 1962 and 1969, accepting radio play script entries written in English from its colonies and former colonies. Most well known English speaking playwrights from the era had their works performed over the air (Amankulor citing Owomoyela, 1993, p. 149). Some famous names from the period include Ngugi wa Thiong'o (formerly James Ngugi) and Kudlip Sondhi (Kenya); John Pepper Clark [Bekederemo], Femi Euba, and Obi Egbuna (Nigeria); Pat Maddy (Sierra Leone); Guillaume Onoyo-Mbia (Cameroon); and Chewanda Kutse and Bloke Mondisane (South Africa). J. Ndukaku Amankulor aptly notes that it is fair to say that the BBC's "African Theatre" series stamped an indelible mark on the development of African drama in English (Amankulor, 1993, p. 149). Since 1970, the BBC World Service has been running the Africa Performance Play competition. This serves to attract scripts from budding young playwrights.

The British Council and the French Cultural Center have also promoted the development of literary drama by providing rehearsal space and other logistical

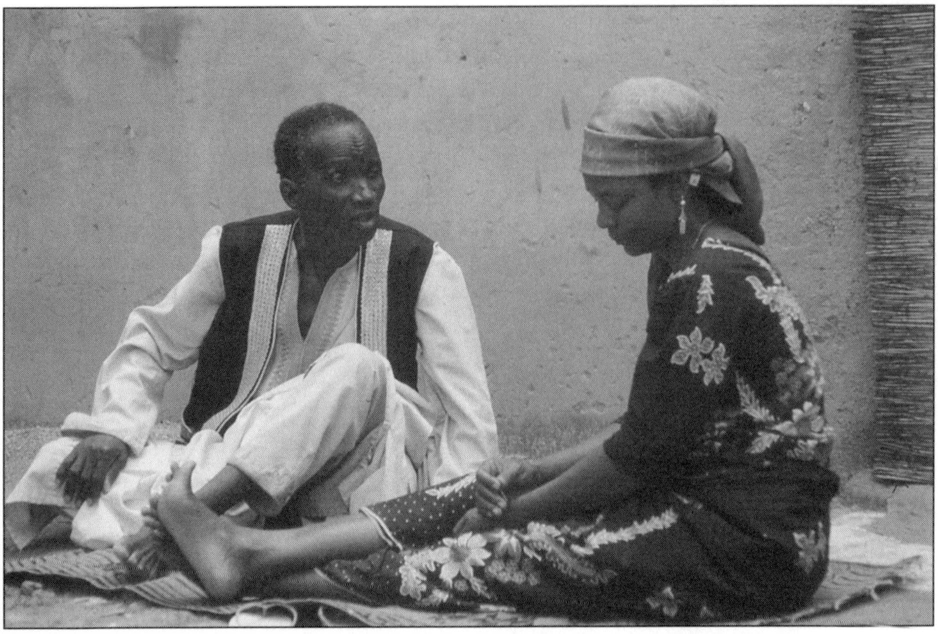

Figure 8-2. Traveling Hausa drama groups have long entertained rural publics in northern Nigeria with live performances. In the second half of the twentieth century, many of these dramas were adapted for television.

support to African playwrights, especially those writing or producing in the language of the colonizers.

Around independence in the early 1960s in most countries in Africa, drama and theatre continued to evolve stylistically along the lines already established. There was urban-based "art theatre," delivered in the colonial language, and supported by university or foreign radio patronage. And there was the traveling troupe tradition of popular theatre (such as *Kotèbà*), rendered in indigenous languages and supported by the African proletariat. A third strain of drama combined elements of both lines. This was a form called Theatre for Development.

Theatre for Development

Theatre for Development refers to performances conducted in aid of specific development projects. A government promoting a vaccination campaign, a family planning initiative, or the planting of high-yield rice seeds, for example, may use indigenous theatrical styles to promote its aims. This use of Theatre for Development was actually pioneered in the 1930s during the African colonial period. The British used "story films" (films which told stories about Africans) to show the benefits of taxation, modern banking, and the like (Kerr, 1995, p. 26). The British productions, entitled, *Tax* and *Post Office Savings Bank* illustrate an important point about performances planned by distant governments for local people. Often such a message is very "top down," imposing an idea that benefits the government far more than it benefits the people. This type of Theatre for Development is sometimes called the propaganda model of popular theatre because it seeks to impose the will of ruling élites on the masses.

There is a another type of Theatre for Development, one in which there is genuine participation of the populace. This second type, the type influenced by Augusto Boal (1979) and Paulo Friere (1974), has been used on and off on the African continent with varying degrees of success. True Theatre for Development, as we have seen in Chapter 4, aims at raising the consciousness of the downtrodden. Such theatrical activity, because it is political, has incurred the wrath of authorities. During the 1970s, a number of African artists and playwrights were imprisoned or went into exile after having produced consciousness-raising theatre. The most renowned were Ngugi wa Thiongo and Ngugi wa Mirii and their colleagues whose 1976 Kamiriithu theatre produced a genuine people's response to neo-colonial oppression in Kenya. Kamiriithu was banned in 1977 and Ngugi wa Thiongo was detained in a Kenyan maximum-security prison. In 1982, three truckloads of policemen burned Kamiriithu to the ground. Eventually all the theatre professionals associated with Kamiriithu went into exile.

Ever since the 1970s, there have been experiments in Theatre for Development that have attempted to skirt the built-in political contradictions involved in doing true populist theatre. Here I am referring to the use of revolutionary methodology, one that raises popular expectations, in politically authoritarian countries where rulers expect to govern unchecked. But attempting to negotiate these contradictions can prove unsatisfying. In theory, the participatory theatre genre would provide a voice for the least empowered. In practice, it is usually quite difficult to prevent the dominant from dominating. The more socially enfranchised have a way of controlling theatre workshops for social change, so that the core issues of the people remain untouched. It the end, it is the ideas of the wealthier classes whose agendas are followed. It was these contradictions, the contradictions of trying to empower African poor in the face of unresponsive, undemocratic governments that prompted Ross Kidd to despair. Here was a committed expatriate who tried to use the techniques of Theatre for Social Change in Africa and then rejected the methodology. In a soulful admission of angst, he wrote that such theatre workshops only raised false hopes of the African people who were bound to be disappointed by unresponsive political systems (Kidd 1979; Kidd and Byram 1981). But today many African theatre practitioners, more adept at living with contradiction, still advocate and support theatre for Social Change. The way to skirt around the contradictions, Hansel Eyoh of Cameroon once argued, is to do it half-way, to "tread softly" in matters political (1984 n.p.).

Contradictions and purist arguments notwithstanding, Theatre for Development has attempted since the 1980s to be more democratic. Expatriate-funded projects as we have seen in Chapter 3, have become far more sensitive to grassroots needs and initiatives. And meanwhile a whole new generation of African theatre professionals has become conscientized into the value of people's theatre. Very often, it is these African theatre professionals who work with audiences on people's theatre projects. Often they organize their own local development NGOs or else they are funded through NGOs (Doho and Julien, in press).

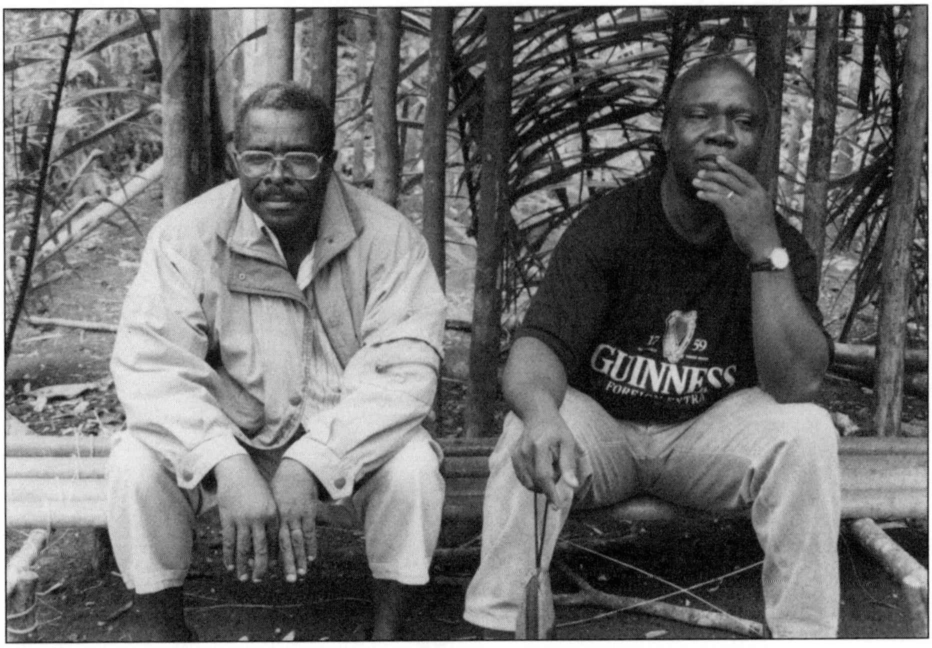

Figure 8-3. Gilbert Doho (left) and Bole Butake (right), two Theatre for Social Change dramatists from Cameroon. Photo courtesy of Gilbert Doho.

Operating in the indigenous languages of the people, African popular theatre professionals use a variety of techniques to engage rural peoples in the process of their own empowerment. Such theatre professionals might work with extension workers to organize people politically to demand change—from their local landowner, from their immediate supervisors, or from their local governments. As popular theatre advocate, Gilbert Doho notes, "popular theatre conceived as an instrument of self criticism, of conscientization, of reading of one's environment, leaves little room for deception" (Doho, 2000, p. 6, translation mine).

Again, Theatre for Development is sensitive to role-playing theory that allows powerless individuals to establish control over their lives by rehearsing behaviors that will lead to their liberation. And role-playing aspects in Theater for Development have been particularly effective in projects where gender is an important factor such as in family planning initiatives. The women in Burkina Faso practiced negotiating birth spacing techniques and the use of birth control through the theatre project entitled Atelier Burkinabe (Morrison, 1991, pp. 29–40).

In its purest form Theater for Development represents a whole process of change. Change begins with consciousness-raising theatre techniques. South Africa's DramAide project has developed an entire war chest of games and exercises designed to help laypersons to physically process and express social problems and to work in and through groups to arrive at solutions. (See Chapter 3). These are linked to role-playing exercises for empowerment. Empowerment leads people to the formation of strategic action plans. All of these are refined and reenergized through constant theatrical interaction. South Africa has used Theater for Development in its struggle against the spread of AIDS. These initiatives will be discussed in more detail after a brief review of South Africa's theatre history, a review which helps to shed light on contemporary theatre practices in South Africa.

Drama in South Africa

After the turn of the century, vaudeville shows in South Africa developed more or less along the lines of the West African concert parties. These vaudeville performances featured stock township characters: prostitutes, new immigrants, cruel policemen, and so on. These productions, like their counterparts in West Africa, drew from African as well as Western traditions, providing entertainment for a newly urbanized proletariat.

Later, (i.e., after 1948), more serious indigenous Black African theatre development was impeded by a series of laws designed to bolster the racist system of Apartheid. There was for example, the 1950 Suppression of Communism Act which forbade the quoting of banned authors,[7] and the Public Safety Act of 1953 which forbade any activity the Ministry of Justice felt might help to undermine the South African State (Kerr, 1995, p. 216). Despite these and many other restrictions, a genre known as township musicals developed in South Africa in the second half of the twentieth century.

A first in the business of Black township musicals was Gibsen Kente. Kente had worked for a White-owned record company during the 1950s. Longing to have his own business, he wrote and staged a first township musical "Manana, the Jazz Prophet" in the early 1960s. A second musical, "Sikalo," made him a modest success and launched a South African Black township musical tradition (Kerr, 1995, p. 219). Kente's musicals were popular and escapist, featuring the usual stereotypical township characters. Indeed Shebeen queens,[8] *tsotsis* (thugs),[9] sellout Black policemen, and stupid and brutish White ones appeared in sketches with loosely woven plots strung together with songs, poems, and dances. By the 1970s Kente was a noteworthy commercial success with a large and varied group

---

7. Banning was a technique used by the South African Apartheid regime to silence critics of the regime. Persons banned by the government could not be with more than two persons at one time. It was a crime to quote any statements or writings of banned persons even those works or words stated before the banning order.

8. A shebeen refers to an illegal purveyor of alcohol in the Black townships of South Africa. Shebeens were in fact tolerated by the South African authorities as a means to allow Black Africans to "blow off steam" in the townships. The fact that they were officially illegal only made it easier for police to raid them capriciously. Many of the owners of shebeens were women. They were known for being tough businesswomen, capable of confrontations with both White authority figures and drunk and unruly Black customers. Many were also known as great hostesses, accommodating customers from among the downtrodden. These are the women who would be known as Shebeen Queens.

9. The term *tsotsi* refers to a South African hoodlum or gang member. See Henry Nxumalo's "The Birth of a Tsotsi," which appeared in *Drum Magazine in 1951*.

of performers. Eschewing politics, Kente's plays were highly moralistic. South African activists criticized Kente's works, and other escapist township musicals, for lacking political edge. Kente's real contribution to South African arts was to the popularization of Black aesthetics. Indeed these musicals raised the stature of improvisational (Black) performance, and began to erode the bias in favor of literary (European) forms of theatre.

By the 1970s, particularly in the wake of the Soweto riots of 1976,[10] theatre in South Africa became more politicized. Peterson aptly describes the subject matter of these performances.

> The most frequent depictions have been those of pass arrests, the humiliating experience at the medical examinations conducted at the labour bureaux, petty bureaucracy, police violence, prison conditions, examples of racial discrimination, struggles of migrant workers, conditions in the hostel compounds, and the breakdown of moral and cultural values in the town ships (Peterson, 1994, p. 44).

And following international trends in experimental theatre, South African performers began to develop plays in workshop settings. The workshop approach resonated with the communal spirit of doing things that is typical of Black South African culture and it operated in parallel with African performance traditions which are open to audience involvement. These plays, moreover, were more difficult to censor than anything that had come previously. This is because they lacked a single author and very often lacked a complete script. The plays were topical, treating the themes of Black oppression in the townships. They were produced in a variety of styles described again by Peterson.

> Forms as diverse as dialogue and mime, song and tableau, sounds and dance are combined into striking and aesthetically appealing total performance. The language used is equally syncretic and in a single performance can shift from indigenous languages to Afrikaans and English or a mixture of all of them in township slang (1994, p. 44).

By the mid-1970s, there was considerable change on the drama scene in South Africa. The Black Consciousness movement was decidedly affecting all aspects of Black cultural life. The growing popular interest in experimental theatre helped nurture the work of a number of South African performance artists including Athol Fugard, John Kani, and Winston Ntshona. Workshopping of plays, and indeed the umbrella notion of art for social change was promoted by the African National Congress[11] and supported by a number of financial supporters, especially the Scandinavian countries. Workshopping of improvisational per-

10. The Soweto uprisings began on the 16 June 1976 as a protest by school children over the enforcement of a long held educational policy to teach half the subjects taught in Black South African schools in the Afrikaans language. Most Black South Africans viewed the Afrikaans language as the language of the oppressor. They also viewed Afrikaans as a language of little practical value. When the authorities responded with force and fired on the schoolchildren, the protests spread across the country and led to the most militant challenge the Nationalist government had faced since 1948.

11. The then-banned party of Nelson Mandela.

formances, would become and continues to be, an important modus operandi in South African theatre.

Black performances in the townships were performed in less than adequate conditions. Empty spaces, all-purpose halls owned by the communities or churches served as the site for most plays. They had neither stages nor other standard theatre facilities. These inadequacies probably helped to contribute to the developing Black South African theatre aesthetic.

Black theatre became increasingly more involved in the struggle against Apartheid in the 1980s. Black theatre groups performed plays on topical issues and called upon audience members to take up action against the particular injustice that was at issue. Often performed under dangerous threats of township violence, some of the plays for this period have been called Theatre of Emergency (Kerr, 1995, p. 232). Audiences of Theater of Emergency tolerated minimal sets, inadequate seating, cast shifts, and actors playing multiple roles when cast members were absent.

One proponent of Theatre of Emergency was playwright, performer, and songwriter Mbongeni Ngema, one of the actors in the two-man South African township-style play "Woza Albert" which played London's West End in the early 1980s.

Ngema's "Asinamali" of 1984, was a play that examined the life of South African political prisoners. Ngema heightened the tension in South Africa by using real township characters in his dramas. Life imitated art when a spy, sent by the police to monitor the play's content, was detected by the audience, pursued, and killed outside the theatre one night. During another evening performance, the police sent thugs in retaliation for the first killing and killed the play's promoter under the mistaken impression the victim was Mbongeni Ngema (Kerr, 1995, p. 233).

The township musicals from this period, especially those involving Mbongeni Ngema, played successfully to overseas audiences. The performances helped to establish the trademarks of Black Resistance, the symbols of the South African struggle. These images included the *toyi toyi* dance (see Chapter 7), the Black Power salute, the freedom song, and the burning tire necklace[12] (Gunner, 1994, p. 30).

But Mbongeni Ngema kept his eye on the international market for theatre. In 1987, Mbongeni produced "Sarafina," a glitzy musical about a young Soweto girl who has been radicalized and who dreams of playing Nelson Mandela in a school play. On February 11, 1990 when Mandela was finally released from prison, the play was still running in South Africa. The play became a symbol of hope of the new South African State.

The success of "Sarafina," partly attributable to its fortunate timing, helped make Mbongeni Ngema, a South African superstar adored by the South African media. His marriage to the star of Sarafina was extensively covered therein. In 1996, he became embroiled in a controversy surrounding the production of

12. Necklacing refers to a form of violence that has been common in South African political manifestations and other conflicts. A victim is surrounded (necklaced) by a stack of gasoline-drenched tires and set alight.

"Sarafina II," a play about the AIDS crisis. AIDS activists criticized Ngema for squandering vast sums of health information money in the production of this second Sarafina (Gibbs, 1999, pp. 120–121). The latter musical, moreover was said to misinform the public about the AIDS crisis and to send the wrong message about HIV prevention. (See Chapter 3).

Theatre and the AIDS Epidemic in South Africa

As noted in Chapter 3, the AIDS epidemic in South Africa has been particularly virulent since the mid-1990s. Theatre and performance have been involved in the struggle to stem the spread of AIDS. The work of DramAide, both as a project in KwaZulu-Natal in the early 1990s and as a partner in the Beyond Awareness Campaigns in the late 1990s, was discussed in Chapter 3. The use of theatre in creating awareness of audiences about issues surrounding HIV/AIDS has created many imitators. Indeed it is not possible to attend an AIDS rally, an edu-Fair, an AIDS mural launching, or an AIDS memorial quilt display (see Chapter 7) without being treated to some form of play.

It is interesting to examine the kinds of plays South African youth create. These plays give us a window on the world of young Black South African school pupils just as they have shown DramAide project organizers in South Africa the enormous problems faced by these young people.

The plays I saw performed in 1999 stress the fact that there is no cure for AIDS and hence prevention is the only sensible option. The plays show desperate victims consulting a series of traditional healers, Western doctors, and finally turning to God. The plays also depict the harsh realities of township life for Black South Africans. They feature young people plagued by sexual advances: young girls the targets of older men; and less frequently young boys, the prey of older women. But many of the plays are deeply misogynistic, showing young girls as willing consorts to these men, "party girls," happy to disobey their parents, go out, and have a good time for the right price. The plays also show other plagues of South African township life: inebriated parents, particularly fathers/uncles who can also be physically and sometimes sexually abusive,[13] gun-toting, *dagga* smoking *tsotsis* (thugs) who attract girls with their flashy clothes, their cell phones,[14] and their fast (if stolen) cars. The performances often show defiant youths that have lost their social moorings in the face of overly authoritarian, grossly inept, or severely irresponsible parents. And quite disturbingly, some of the plays feature boys who are HIV+ and who go around infecting others so that they will not have to die alone.

---

13. See Dalrymple and Preston-Whyte, 1995, p. 123. I commissioned a play from a high school teacher, Cele Lindani, who was running his own drama troupe. Cele presented me with a manuscript whose theme was incest/daughter rape as a cure for the father's HIV+ status.

14. Cell phones appear to be an extremely important status symbol in technology-mad South Africa.

When sexist or "classist" storylines emerge within the context of an AIDS awareness workshop, trained facilitators generally talk through these issues with youth. In these ways, students are enjoined to reflect upon their misconceptions and their prejudices. But other plays produced outside "controlled" project settings certainly are problematic. Some of them certainly reinforce existing class and gender stereotypes. The paradox involved in promoting popular theatre is that very often "the people" themselves are part of the problem (i.e., they have regressive ideas). Certainly, the aim in South Africa must be to give power to those most historically disempowered. That would include Black women and children. But the aim of any theatre project must also be to help repair the fractured communities of South Africa's majority. Theatre is a powerful therapeutic tool, one that unlashes powerful forces, rousing people to action. Like its psychotherapeutic counterpart in the North, theatre seems best used in controlled settings with trained professional facilitators.

Clearly the best AIDS theatre work in South Africa is being done by DramAide and groups like it, operating well within the parameters of participatory methodology heretofore described. Two examples of participatory AIDS theatre from South Africa are provided on the accompanying compact disk. Refer to Drama.

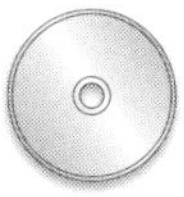

Video 2. School AIDS Play
Scottburgh School Health Promotion Club, Scottburg, South Africa

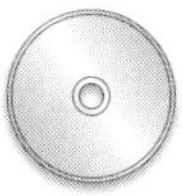

Video 3. AIDS Play
"Live the Message" Drama Troupe, South Africa

As noted in Chapter 3, the DramAide project has evolved along with the AIDS epidemic in South Africa. In many ways, the DramAide project, begun in KwaZulu-Natal has helped to institutionalize participatory methodology. DramAide's theatre projects in junior high schools led to the recognition by South African activists and health officials of the need to teach life skills. DramAide's participatory theatre methodologies have been adopted into a number of projects. And the DramAide project itself has gone on to some new initiatives.

In 1998–1999, DramAide expanded its operation to become a major NGO delivering South Africa's Beyond Awareness 2 AIDS campaign. In this phase of the AIDS struggle, DramAide broadened its operations to include some tertiary (university level) projects. These included the painting of AIDS awareness campus murals and the organization of visits to campuses from the NAPWA, the National Association of People Living With AIDS. The DramAide team also launched the South African AIDS Memorial Quilt project early in 1999. An interview with DramAide mural painters is provided on the accompanying compact disk. Refer to Drama.

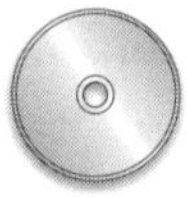

Video 4. AIDS Mural, Dramaide Project
University of Durban-Westville, South Africa

Meanwhile, DramAide facilitators continued to promote life skills development and drama development through the maintenance of health promoting clubs for schools and communities. And they continued to rely on drama workshopping techniques, theatrical warm-up exercises to encourage group participation and group spirit in their AIDS awareness projects. Even when not directly producing plays, DramAide's participatory methodology has continued to inform and to shape the creation of AIDS awareness murals, AIDS memorial quilts or other projects. A demonstration of this methodology is provided in the accompanying compact disk. Refer to Drama.

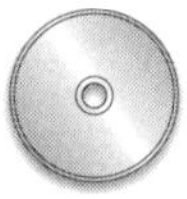

Video 5. Warm-Up Exercise; Sex-Role Reversal Exercise
AIDS Memorial Quilt Project; AIDS Summit for
University Administrators, South Africa

Meanwhile as the new century dawned, the South African AIDS epidemic continued to strike with ferocity. By the end of the 1990s, the ever-evolving AIDS behavioral research pointed at a new causative source of the disease: men. The Panos Institute, among others, reported in 1998, that inordinate male power and skewed gender relations were at the heart of the AIDS epidemic in South Africa, if not the whole continent (Panos Institute 1998). As noted earlier, women are twice as likely to contract HIV from a man than a man is from a woman (Doupe, 2001, p. 7). And women report being far more willing to use condoms, to practice fidelity to one partner, or to abstain from sex altogether. But women are much less able to negotiate the conditions in which sex takes place than are their male partners. And South African girls and women, of all ages and races, married or single, live in fear of the rape that an estimated one in three women undergo. Given unequal pay and conditions of poverty, moreover, women are forced to trade sex for cash or goods in order to assure their own survival and that of their children.

Early in the new century, the current thinking is that the AIDS epidemic in South Africa must now be tackled through a systematic redefinition of gender

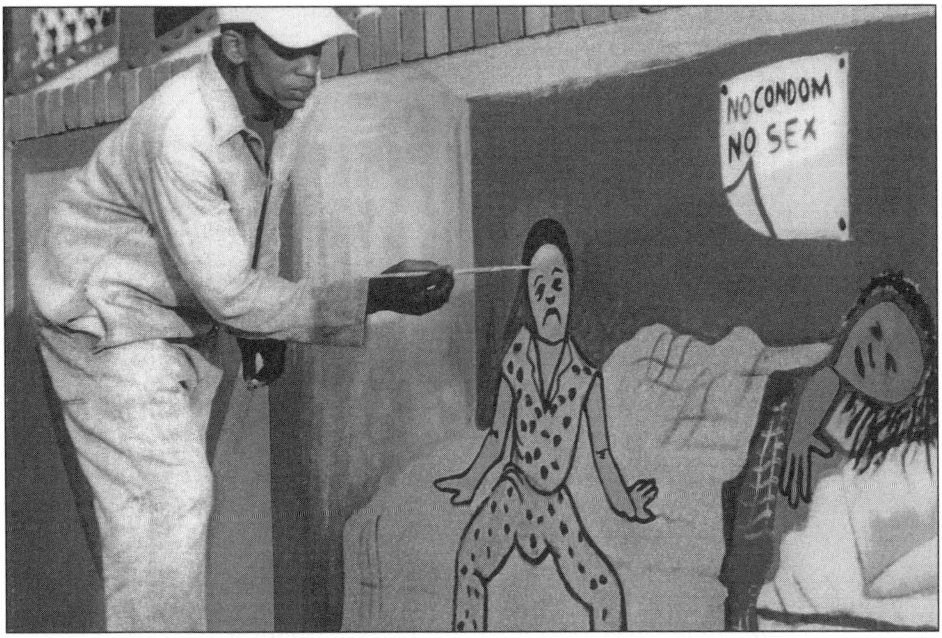

Figure 8-4. Beyond Awareness 2 artists created AIDS awareness murals on several South African university campuses. Photo courtesy the DramaAid Project.

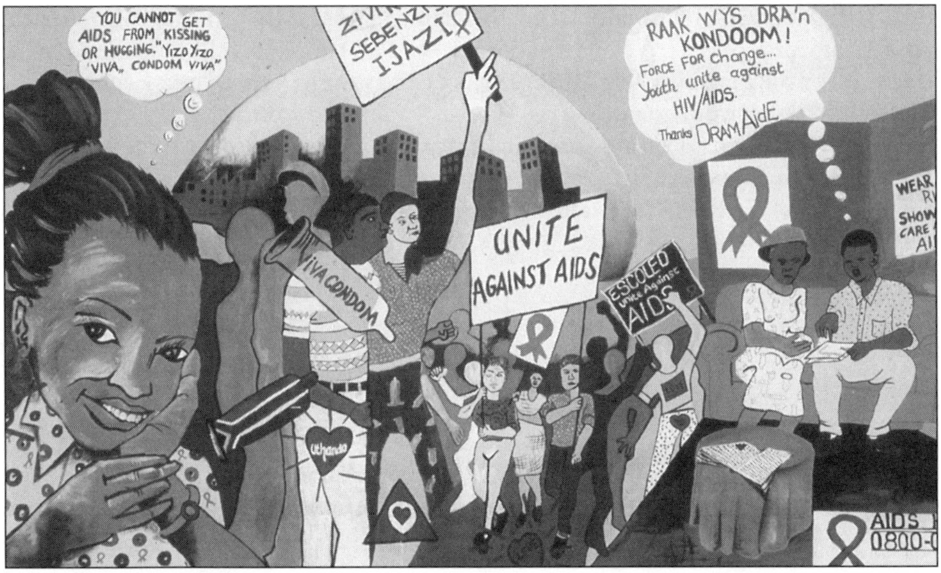

Figure 8-5. Beyond Awareness 2 mural on the campus of Eskhawini College of Education, KwaZulu-Natal, South Africa. Photo courtesy of Neil Cumberlidge.

roles. The DramAide project is well positioned to help. It has already helped to usher in shifts in gender-ascribed behavior. DramAide's project research reports from the mid-1990s found that newly empowered secondary school girls were breaking down gender barriers. On school open days they were surprising their parents with enthusiastic performances of formerly all male dance genres: gumboot, tap, and others (Dalrymple and Preston-Whyte, 1994, p. 126). And in late 1999, DramAide embarked on a new project: workshopping a new (read "kinder," "gentler") South African male. The workshops used participatory techniques to learn from South African young people the essential components of a more caring and attentive male. And the workshops showed how the most sensitive and the least aggressive aspects of these constructs might be reconfigured into new dramas and in other forms of popular culture. In a sense, DramAide is attempting in its way to invent a new South African definition of manhood (DramAide 2000). This project was supported by Johns Hopkins University of Baltimore, Maryland.

South Africa has made great strides in the use of drama to conscientize its citizens about the AIDS epidemic. It has used drama to build AIDS awareness in schools and communities and to begin to institutionalize health promotion and other life affirming behaviors. The DramAide project has been a catalyst in a number of far-reaching AIDS awareness initiatives in South Africa inspiring local groups to come up with plays of their own.

DramAide's involvement in the AIDS crisis has been an ever-evolving, multi sector response the AIDS pandemic. Clearly, DramAide and the participatory drama approaches it has used, have been key instruments in the development of a social movement organized in the fight against AIDS in Southern Africa. And DramAide plays have spawned a number of spin-offs and copies. Some of these groups are inspired by DramAide's effectiveness; others like Eager Artists of Durban is a DramAide off-shoot whose leader and founder Jerry Pooe began his drama career as a DramAide facilitator. A demonstration of an AIDS play performed by Eager Artists is provided in the accompanying compact disk. DramAide's "Walela," an AIDS demonstration play, one used to inspire spin-offs, is subsequently provided on the accompanying compact disk. Refer to Drama.

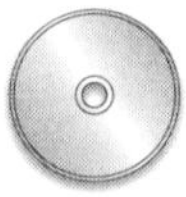

Video 6. AIDS Play, Michigan
Eager Artists of South Africa

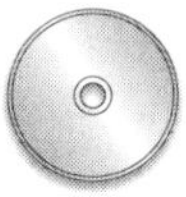

Video 7. Participatory AIDS Play
DramAide Troupe of Durban, South Africa

Soul City Dramatic Television Series

Another remarkable performance product to emerge from the South African AIDS crisis is a television drama series entitled Soul City. Soul City can be viewed as a kind of slick edutainment counterpart to DramAide's homegrown school dramas.

Soul City is a thirteen part serial that is designed to explore health promotion themes wrapped in dramatic storylines. The hour-long dramas are set around characters employed in a government clinic in the fictitious Soul City, a venue that represents a South African Black township. The program is broadcast on South African Broadcasting's TV 1, a channel with the highest Black viewership of the three SABC TV channels. Subtitled in English, the program, much like life itself in South Africa, is multi-lingual.[15] Some of the issues tackled on the series include racism, alcoholism, abuse of women, high blood pressure,[16] child health, smoking, and AIDS.

The program is the inspiration of Dr. Garth Japhet who concluded in the 1980s that South African Broadcasting's enormous pool of talent and its vast resources could be better used in health promotion campaigns. Eventually Japhet created an NGO that was a major participant in the Beyond Awareness Campaigns of the late 1990s.

Soul City uses a multi-media approach to get its messages across. The flagship of the project is the weekly television drama. There is also a 60-segment radio series featuring similar messages but using different characters and different themes. These radio dramas are broadcast in nine African languages on nine regional South African Broadcasting stations. Twelve major South African newspapers cooperate with Soul City by publishing reviews of the upcoming drama. These newspapers also carry glossy magazine inserts distributed by Soul City on given educational topics. These magazines feature photographs and cartoons illustrating major lessons. The magazine insert on AIDS, for example, gives advice that includes visuals about breastfeeding for HIV+ mothers. It also shows how to put on a condom. Through cartoons depicting multiple relationships, the magazine illustrates how and why AIDS is spreading so rapidly. And it demonstrates the importance of care and support for those who are HIV+. It provides advice for healthy

15. Like most urban Africans, Black South Africans live in a world of many languages. Two Black Africans from the same ethnic group may well speak to one another in their native language, Pedi, Zulu, Sotho, or Xhosa, for example. But oftentimes, in multiethnic contexts they will use English that serves as a kind of *lingua franca* in much of the country. They may also use Afrikaans, though for reasons of history, this language is less popular among Blacks. Highly urbanized Blacks, even when speaking to a member of the same ethnic group may use a mixture of languages, according to their individual level of comfort. For reasons of education and because of social mobility, Blacks may be more familiar with technical terms in English than in their native language. In moments of high tension, however, most people resort to their native language for maximum expressiveness.

16. High blood pressure is a major health problem in South Africa, especially among Blacks.

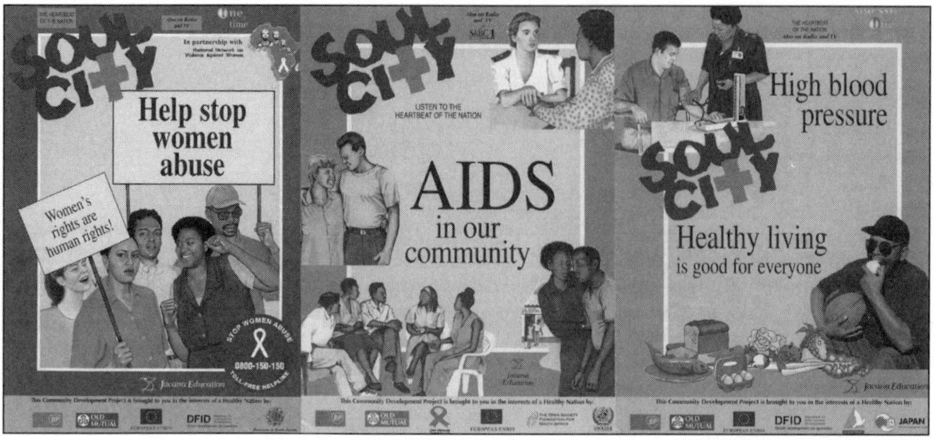

Figure 8-6. Major South African newspapers include glossy inserts expanding on the subject of that evening's Soul City broadcast.

living for those infected with the HIV virus. Finally the magazine supplies lists of national and regional organizations where readers can go for help about AIDS.

Soul City also produces health education packages containing comics, information pages, audio tapes, and workbooks. These are distributed to schools and community centers for use in formal health education classes.

Soul City is based on the sophisticated notion that an entertaining program helps create and sustain a climate favorable to social change. Its creators recognize the importance of personal involvement of audience members, in and with the program. The show presents a range of South African characters representing all races and classes. The producers are cognizant of the need to get audiences talking about the stories, the characters, and the series. To this end, they've developed a number of public relations strategies designed to keep Soul City on the national agenda. They've organized "Search for the Stars" campaigns designed to help find talent for future seasons. They promote coverage of the lives of the Soul City actors in newspapers in magazines. They sponsor games of chance featuring monetary prizes that audiences can win by answering questions that appear in the magazine inserts. They have also created national award competitions such as the "Soul City Health Care Worker of the Year" and a youth award for Community Development.

The creators of Soul City are careful to research all story lines through formative evaluation techniques. And they have done a number of summative evaluations that included ratings; and "before and after" tests of knowledge, attitudes, and behaviors. The results have shown that the program is one of the most popular programs on TV; it imparts knowledge; it stimulates discussion among family and friends; and it can shift attitudes in a direction favored by the series producers. All of these are important precursors to behavior change.

Episode 5 from Series 4 (1999b) of Soul City is an episode whose theme dealt with HIV and AIDS. I am providing the broad lines of the episode to give the reader a flavor of the drama. Readers should note that the series, like much of South African television, makes a concerted effort to present a new non-racist/non-sexist picture of society suitable for the New South Africa.

Two nine-year old boys, Bongani and Luke are nearly hit by a truck while playing soccer in their upscale neighborhood. Bongani's mother Martha who works as a housekeeper for Luke's parents, the Scotts, saves the boys from harm. Martha is injured and goes with the boys to the local clinic for treatment. She calls Katrina, Luke's mother to come to collect her and the boys. When Katrina arrives at the clinic, she begins to tell the woman attending Martha, a Black woman (whom she assumes is a nurse) what to do. To Katy's surprise, the woman assures her she is a doctor and that she has ordered all the needed tests.

Later that evening Katrina discusses the accident with her husband Greg. She decides they should purchase a life insurance policy for Martha, one that would include disability coverage. Katrina informs Martha about the need for medical tests in order to qualify for the insurance. It is clear that Martha and Bongani live in servant's quarters in the Scott's home. Martha agrees that she will get the requisite tests for the insurance when she returns to the clinic for a follow up on her injury.

At the clinic, Martha learns she must undergo an HIV test for insurance purposes. A counselor tells her she may refuse the test or she may decline to be given the results. Martha is surprised to hear this and wonders what all of the concern is about since she is a widow with no sex life. She accepts to be told her results and is shocked to learn she is HIV+. The clinic counselor, Sol explains that she may have gotten AIDS from her husband who may have had other partners. Martha is dismayed to hear this, claiming her husband died of TB, not AIDS.

Sol, the clinic counselor assures Martha she can live a long and productive life even with HIV. Martha retorts that this is easy for him to say because he has not just been told he has HIV. No, he adds, he learned that fact one year ago. Sol assures Martha that they are not alone, that there are 3.5 million other persons in South Africa with the same problem.[17]

Martha comes home and struggles with how to disclose her status to the Scotts. When she does tell Katrina, Katrina is shocked, but she assures the housekeeper she will not lose her job. Later that evening, Katrina discusses the matter with her husband Greg. Mr. Scott, seeing Katy's growing concern, affirms that it is illegal in South Africa to fire someone because of the his or her HIV status. Katy says she knows but her sense of anger, confusion, and fear is palpable.

Soon Katy begins to treat Martha differently. She becomes impatient and short with Martha when the maid gets near any cutting implements. Finally, when Katy comes upon Martha bandaging Luke's cut knee, she explodes. Martha resigns and goes to stay with her sister Mzwayi, the wife of the clinic porter (orderly) in the Soul City clinic.

---

17. This was the HIV+ rate when the show was aired in August 1999.

Bogani comes back to see Luke and the two go off in a mini-bus (public transportation) to Soul City. It is clear that the White child has never seen the ramshackle homes he now sees as he passes through the township. They boys are chased by some bigger street boys and are forced to hide in a shebeen.

When Katrina arrives at home from work, her gardener tells her that Luke and Bongani have gone to Soul City. Alarmed, Katy asks the gardener for help to find the boys. The two of them go off to Martha's sister's in search of the boys. (Martha would not be able to find the home of Mzwayi without help because as a White woman she would not normally go to the township). Katrina calls Mr. Scott on her cell phone to recount the situation. Katrina and Martha go looking for the boys. Soon a vehicle pulls up behind them and Katy is convinced she is about to become a car-jacking victim. Panic-stricken, she remarks disparagingly about the "bloody-township" where she is forced to look for her son. Martha reminds her that many people are also obliged to live every day of their lives in this same "bloody township." Martha adds that the alleged car-jacker behind them is Mr. Scott. Martha and the Scotts find the boys in the shebeen, well taken care of by a matronly owner, who has given the boys soft drinks and chased the big boys off with a broom. Luke is all-aglow with his township adventures. The Scotts are only relieved. As they thank the kind proprietress, it is clear that this experience has helped to dispel for them a myth of the shebeen as a den of iniquity.

The boys go with Greg Scott, and Katrina drives Martha back to Mzwayi's place. Katy apologizes to Martha and asks her if she will come back to work for the family. Martha accepts.

(Synopsis derived from Episode 5, Series 4 in my videotape collection and the Soul City Website, [Soul City 1999b, 1999c]).

A number of AIDS issues are tackled forthrightly in the series. Human Rights of people with AIDS are clearly underlined. People with AIDS in South Africa cannot legally be fired from their jobs. And people must be given the option to learn or not to learn the results of HIV tests. Issues of HIV transmission are clearly mentioned in the program. Monogamy is no protection against AIDS if one has relations with an HIV+ partner. AIDS cannot be transmitted through casual contact with an infected person. Coping strategies for those suffering with HIV are also highlighted. Martha is reminded she is not alone in her struggle. She can come to the clinic or other groups for help at any time.

Equally interesting (for an outsider at least) are the obvious attempts by the program to present a new South Africa. Comfortable White South Africans are encouraged to consider the long-term futures for their domestic servants as this category of employees has never enjoyed worker benefits. Whites are reminded that the crowded, smoky, crime infested townships that they so fear and have so long avoided provide the only housing option available to many of their Black countrymen. Katy is quietly dispelled of her assumption that the Black woman attending to Martha could not possibly be a physician.

Soul City teamed up with a number of important associates to produce this slick multi-media product based in television. UNICEF, one of its partners, con-

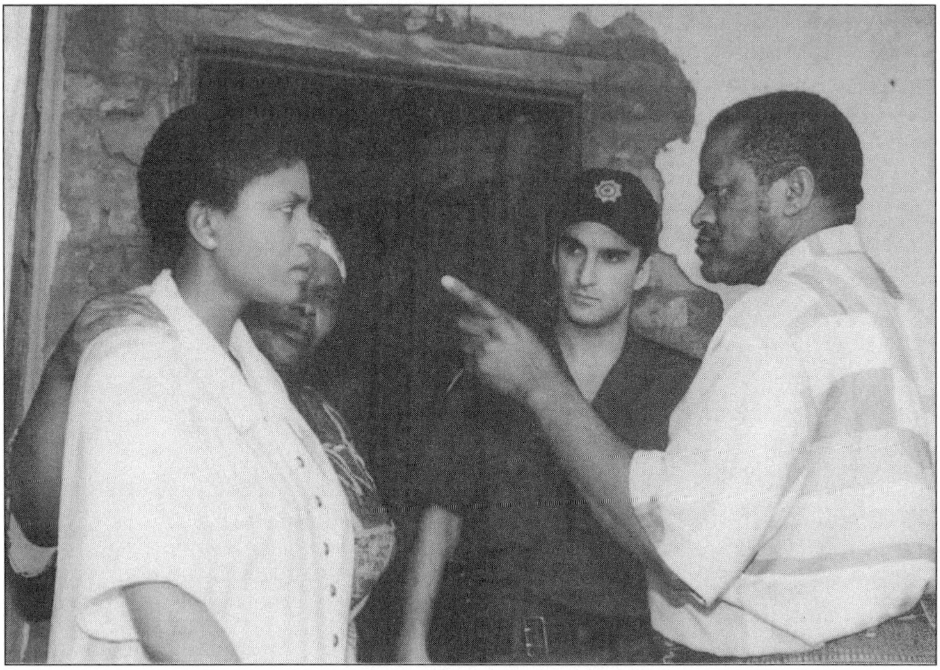

Figure 8-7. A drama on gender violence in Series 4 of Soul City. Photo courtesy of Soul City.

siders the Soul City experience an example of best practice. Indeed Soul City reaches an average of 2.5 million people per episode. Soul City materials have been distributed in neighboring countries in Southern Africa where they have proven very popular (Singhal and Rogers, 1999, p. 217).

Soul City has been the recipient of numerous awards including a Recognition for Excellence Award at the Third World-Enter-Educate Conference in the Netherlands and several South African broadcast production honors. Soul City also received an award from the One World Broadcasting Trust in the United Kingdom in 2001. In 2000 Soul City launched its 5th television series. The themes for the series include rape, disability, small, medium and micro-enterprise, and care and support for people with AIDS.

Theatre and the AIDS Epidemic in Mali

In the West African nation of Mali, drama has been used in a way different from South Africa to promote AIDS awareness. As noted above, Mali has a theatrical tradition called *Kòtèba* that predates the colonial period. Played "in the round," *Kòtèba* used stock characters, stock themes, music, and dance to advance the action. In the 1960s, the newly independent Malian government revived the *Kòtèba* genre under the name of le *Groupe Dramatique Kòtèba du*

Mali. Keen to promote Mali's proud indigenous arts tradition, then President Modibo Keita created the *Théatre Nationale du Mali* (Malian National Theater). Mali's National Theater assembled and supported four groups of actors, musicians, and dancers: the "*Ballets Maliens,* the *Ensemble Instrumentale du Mali*, the *Orchestre Moderne: Le Badéma*, and the *Groupe Dramatique Kòtèba*. Mr. Ousman Sow, a renowned playwright, later became director of the *Groupe Dramatique* in 1980s. His play "Warri" is said by many to have played a key role in the quiet revolution that led to Mali's free elections in 1991.

In 1987, after the United Nations held a conference on AIDS in Bamako, Sow was contacted and asked to produce a play. The conferees had decided that theatre and other genres familiar to the audience would be used to convey the AIDS message. Sow's play, the first to address the AIDS issue in Mali, was done in *Kòtèba* style. It has set the tone for plays that would follow (Sow, November 1999, interview).

Sow's play was called *Weretigi*, which means "cattle market owner." *Weretigi* refers to the eponymous head of the household in this drama, the protagonist. The play used a number of stock characters. There was Djenne, the sexually promiscuous young wife who grants sexual favors to all and sundry save her husband. There was a duplicitous griot, who acts as narrator for the audience, as well as advisor and confidant to the husband while snatching sexual favors from the wife. There was the cuckolded and foolish husband Diallo. Much of the play is farce-like, centering on the trysts of the wife and her efforts to deceive her naïve, but pompous husband.

By the end of the play, the entire cast, minus the cuckolded husband [who has practiced a forced abstinence] is tainted with HIV. The play concludes with the village doctor leading a march of singing school children promoting condoms. The doctor speaks to the audience directly saying that if parents did as much as their children to promote safe sex, there would be far fewer cases of AIDS.

Weretigi uses a typically West African method of gentle humor as a means of social correction. The reader should be sensitive to the strongly patriarchal lines of this drama. It's the protagonist's wife whose errant behavior is focussed upon. It is also the male protagonist who is exonerated. The play uses a griot as a spokesperson because such persons have the power to say things other members of society cannot. Griots are said to have *nyama*, the power of the word, an occult power that can protect against evil forces (Hale, 1998, p. 119–120; see also chapter 5).

Well attuned to the genre, Sow and his collaborators in the Troupe Niogolon, the most well-regarded *Kòtèba* troupe in Bamako,[18] produced a second AIDS play, *Kurusidjala*, a few years later. Aired on Malian television,[19] this drama takes place in the family compound of another cuckolded husband/family head named Ladji. It also draws from stock character types. There is Kadia, a mischievous, lascivious, and greedy young wife who sells home-made Malian yo-

---

18. Ousman Sow works periodically with Niogolon and he trained a number of the troupe's actors who were his students at Bamako's National Institute of the Arts (INA).

19. *Kurusidjala* was designed and conceived primarily as a play. Camera work in the televised version was minimal and generally static so the production when broadcast retains the feel of a performance of *Kòtèba*.

gurt in the marketplace.[20] There is also Kadia's paramour, Djanguine who's also a [disloyal] friend of her husband. There is Madou, the shiftless, drug-taking, oversexed son of Ladji. There is Tosh, Madou's main pal. There is a local unnamed somewhat pompous young physician who is also friends with Madou and Tosh. Then there are Madou's sex-crazy female companions especially Fifi, the daughter of Djanguine. Finally there is the hapless, hayseed of a country cousin, Zantigi and a corrupt policeman. The play takes place in a family compound in Bamako. Most of the action is farcical centering on the sexual escapades of the characters, and the near misses at detection they suffer at the hands of one another. For example, promiscuous Fifi comes to the family compound disguised as an Islamic holy man. Ladji encourages her to instruct Madou in the ways of the Holy Quoran. Out of sight of the old man she removes her disguise and reveals the sexy miniskirt she is wearing for Madou.

Humor is also created through the use of Zantigi, a country relative who comes to stay in the Bamako household. The butt of family jokes, Zantigi puts a damper on Kadia's escapades so she sends him out to fetch rice and to run other errands. Unused to city life, Zantigi now encounters phenomena and situations with which he is unfamiliar. His village values and instincts inevitably get him into trouble. While on his errand for Kadia, he mistakes a house of prostitution for a rice store. So he queues patiently outside it so as to make a purchase. While standing in line, Zantigi recites a lengthy soliloquy on his love of rice and his need for lots of it several times a day. Zantigi's naiveté on matters sexual generates great hilarity for this conservative Islamic audience well used to double entendre. Humor is also created by the fact that many of the female roles, including some of the prostitutes, are played by men. These men in drag also play other roles in the play.[21]

One of the prostitutes overhears Zantigi's monologue and imagines making a fortune from this country customer. She demands money from him, and tells him to wait. Zantigi overhears prostitutes tell customers they only accept business with *manani* (literally "plastic"), the *fougoulan nefamma* (literally indispensable hat) both Bamana euphemisms for condoms. Patting his hatted head, Zantigi shows his displeasure at being forced to wait to be served despite of his proper attire. When another customer gets his turn before the country bumpkin the latter loses his temper. Zantigi assaults the customer for apparently "cutting in line" (jumping the queue) for what he still thinks is a sack of rice rather than a time in the proverbial sack.

Zantigi's misadventures multiply as a policeman appears at the brothel and demands and receives free service after Zantigi has paid and received no service/rice. The policeman tries to arrest Zantigi who flees and is stuck and injured by a moving vehicle. Zantigi is taken to the hospital whereupon he is said to be in need of a blood transfusion. The entire family comes to the hospital, their

20. Urban women's commercial activities are viewed with considerable ambivalence by the religious leaders and by the patriarchy because these activities help women to elude male supervision. The activities are particularly suspect when they take place in disreputable locations such as long distance taxi (motor) parks or train stations.

21. As noted, traditionally women did not appear in the *Kòtèba*. It is still considered less than respectable for women, especially married women, to act in dramas.

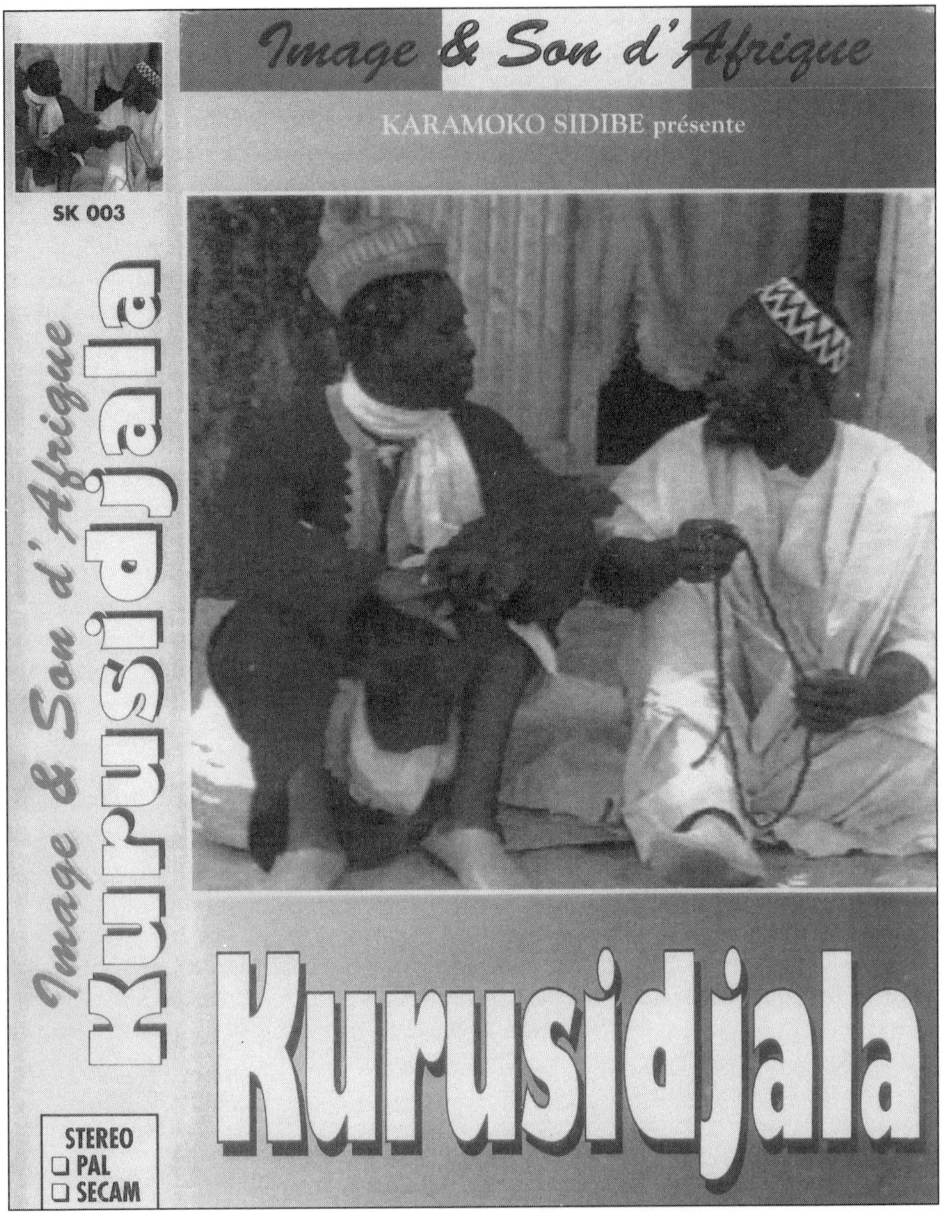

Figure 8-8. A scene from "*Kurusidjala*," a Malian AIDS awareness play performed in the *Kòtèba* tradition. This video is available for rent or purchase in Mali.

blood is tested, and they are all diagnosed as HIV+. The doctor who himself has done the testing comes to Ladgi's compound to announce the results and is surprised to see his girlfriend Fifi there among the HIV+. The scene ends with the whole group, including the doctor, crying over their HIV+ status.

Besides supplying interest and adding humor, some of the conversations held at the brothel are instructive. Stock characters like Zantigi (derived from *Kòtèba* tradition) make it possible to convey messages that normally would be unacceptable in polite society or mixed company. Zantigi is an oaf and is recognized as such through a genre that reserves this place for him. Stylistically and socially he can be used much like a jester to say things others cannot say.

It is noteworthy that indigenous forms of communication, namely griot song have long been used on Mali Radio to convey lessons in morality and social conduct as well as lessons in development (Bourgault, 1995, p. 87). Mali's decision to use indigenous drama in AIDS education can be viewed as part of a trend established since the 1970s to use grass roots theatrical forms in development (Mlama, 1993, p. 96). Sow's plays represent the best of the genre, a modernized *Kòtèba* that is widely appreciated in Mali. True to its roots in the patriarchy, the genre pokes gentle fun at those in power, especially older heads of households. It laughs at them for their pomposity and for their arrogance. These are men who conduct themselves as mature heads of families, serious Muslims, role models for the community. Yet their young wives take their husband's friends and confidants as lovers. And their unmarried children tryst comfortably at home with companions of the opposite sex.[22] The plays are valuable because they present life as it is lived, at least in rapidly urbanizing Bamako where social change has increased pre-marital and extra-marital sex in recent years (see Brand 2001). These farces are useful in that they attract audiences and through humor are able to keep audience attention long enough for the viewing public to hear the message. Indeed, research in Mali estimates that 77% of Malian women and 96% of Malian men had heard of AIDS and knew something about it (*Plan Stratégique*, 1999, p. 11).

Sow is an effective promoter of Theatre for Development and is regularly called upon by NGOs to write or produce plays, including recorded audio plays[23] on their behalf. In touch with the people, Sow leans nevertheless toward political satire and the creation of a rather singular artistic vision. But development work is more steady than plays about national politics and AIDS plays are in demand. So like many an artist, he has become a producer of AIDS performances.[24] Trained in Croatia, Sow is more of a playwright than a playmaker. He leans more in the direction of literary drama than does the Niogolon Troupe of actors with whom he often works.

Theatre Niogolon is said to be the best private theatre group in Mali. Founded by Philippe Dauchez, an expatriate drama professor, formerly on the staff at INA (*Institut National des Arts*), the troupe was the first Malian theatre group to produce Theatre for Development. The Niogolon Theatre troupe claims to have two

22. In Bamanan households or compounds, the head of the household has own hut or room. Each of his wives has her hut or room that she shares with her young children. Older sons living in their father's compound will have their own room or hut, located at some distance from the elders making it possible to receive guests of the opposite sex without easily being seen.

23. The audio serials are used by primary health care workers in village settings. They are used for *causeries,* discussions on the subjects of HIV/AIDS.

24. There is no question that creativity with an AIDS message sells (to NGOs and aid agencies) at this juncture in the history of the AIDS pandemic in Africa. The subject of AIDS as a "patron of the arts" is a worthy one, one that the reader is invited to consider.

different missions in Mali. The first aims to preserve Mali's traditional indigenous culture through the production and enactment of traditional folklore. The second strives to work in the area of development with Non-Governmental Organizations on AIDS awareness, health education, and other issues. Given the nature of funding in Mali, Niogolon's preoccupation leans toward the development work. Niogolon actors-directors Malick Drame and Teneman Sanogo work quite closely with audiences. They try out different storylines and different ways of rendering a scene, checking to be certain audiences are both pleased and informed with their work on development. Open to improvisation, they are eager to try some of the Boalian Forum Theater techniques they learned about in drama school, techniques that have been displayed in Ouagadougou, at the bi-annual African film festival (Drame and Sanogo, 8 December 1999, interview).[25]

In many ways, the work of Ousman Sow and the troupe Niogolon have set a standard against which others in Mali's performance sector measure themselves, and try to imitate. There is no shortage of theatre groups in Mali. Again, as in the pre-colonial period there are troupes of young people producing drama on an amateur basis throughout the country. Those located in Bamako make use of space available at the French Cultural Center for rehearsals. The presence of NGOs using indigenous drama in development projects helps to support budding theatre professionals and the development of theatre in the country. And much like South Africa, new groups continue to proliferate.

There is general consensus among NGOs and theatre people that issues surrounding HIV/AIDS in Mali should be handled in forms that can be considered edutainment. Dramas and griot singing seem to be the most common. And as noted in Chapter 3, some local groups producing dramas are making use intermittently of participatory methodology. But lack of overall coordination seems to keep the results of research by one organization out of the hands of the next, despite the clear need to share information as widely as possible. Unfortunately, Mali is plagued with a tendency toward administrative inflexibility, a top-down, centralized, and hierarchical style of management inherited from French colonial administration. Even though the 1990s have seen considerable progress toward decentralization and "user-friendliness," old habits sometimes die hard. The system sometimes values protocol over action. Administrative inflexibility in Mali is underlined by a tendency among some managers to jealously guard information that could be best shared among members of the AIDS campaigns communities. Generally speaking, the non-governmental sector is far more effective and accessible than those in government. Given the ever-changing contours of the epidemic, it is imperative that all players be fully up-to date on the latest findings. Reports of best practice appear in relatively short supply. And the application of Action Research methodology is warranted.

If critical reflection of AIDS dramas is needed, then two major issues raised by Malian AIDS dramas warrant further discussion. First there is the question of humor in many of the productions. Those who know Mali argue quite convincingly that Malians, especially the least educated, expect humor in theatre, particularly theatre genres in indigenous languages (for example, Dauchez n.d.). Many argue that the masses would lose interest in a drama that contained no laughs. But this

25. FESPACO, the West African film festival held every second year in Ouagadougou, Burkina Faso, added a section on Theater for Development in the mid-1990s.

matter has not been thoroughly researched. An interesting and flexible genre, *Kòtèba* has been adapted to modern political satire, TV commercials, and AIDS awareness campaigns. But it's use in commercials has sometimes proven problematic (Traoré 2000). Though humor may attract and hold the attention of audiences, it is unclear whether these melodramatic comic farces are the best delivery vehicle for the dissemination of such serious messages. Does the laughter they engender serve to weaken the apparent threat of the disease? Does humor make AIDS that much more acceptable? If so, is this functional or dysfunctional to the spread of the virus? Can humor take Malians 'beyond awareness'? And if laughter is effective, it would be useful to learn how it is working, so that it might be applied to other situations.

Second, there is the issue of sex role stereotyping embedded in an ancient theatrical genre. Planners need to consider to what extent stereotypical and highly gendered dramas in fact contribute to the AIDS problem rather than to the solution. Creators need to take seriously the role of unfaithful men (both officially monogamous and polygamous) in the spread of the virus. And rather than recreating the patriarchal past, they need to begin to spotlight as counterproductive the sexual double standard. Women's relative powerlessness in the face of the AIDS epidemic certainly cannot be aided by plays which help reinforce the myth that women are responsible for the AIDS epidemic. Action research and other participatory methodologies could begin to present the keys to unpacking some of these dangerous stereotypes. The Niogolon actors, Teneman Sanogo and Malick Drame say they are ready to use Boalian techniques. They are simply waiting to be commissioned to do so (Drame and Sanogo, 8 December, 1999, interview).

One project that presents new theatrical trends is the project *Danaya So*, a Malian NGO that has enjoyed support from the Swiss charity Caritas and the Canadian government through its regional SIDA2 project. The project uses troupes of former and actual prostitutes who produce plays in bars, in motor parks, and in the street, instructing potential clients and others about condom use and warning against the dangers of HIV/AIDS. *Danaya So's* plays tell women's stories. A synopsis of one of the AIDS play of the Yassa troupe of *Danaya So*, Bamako, is provided here.

> An urban family consisting of three, a mother, an adult daughter, and a young girl must survive. The young daughter Miriam is enrolled in school and needs money for tuition, school supplies, and clothing. The family depends for survival on the earnings brought in by Fifi, the older daughter. Fifi, a prostitute, is under pressure to bring more money home in order to satisfy the family's needs. The mother is old, but she's savvy about condoms, and gives a lesson on their use to Fifi (and the audience) before the latter goes off to work. Fifi is offered a high price, 50,000 CFA (about U.S. $73.00) by a client for sex without a condom.[26] At first Fifi refuses, but her prostitute friends convince her she should accept the offer. But soon after the unprotected sexual encounter, Fifi falls

26. Prices for sex in Bamako in 2000 were running as low as 500 CFA francs (about 73 US cents) to about 10,000 CFA francs (about US $14.00), the price suggested in the play.

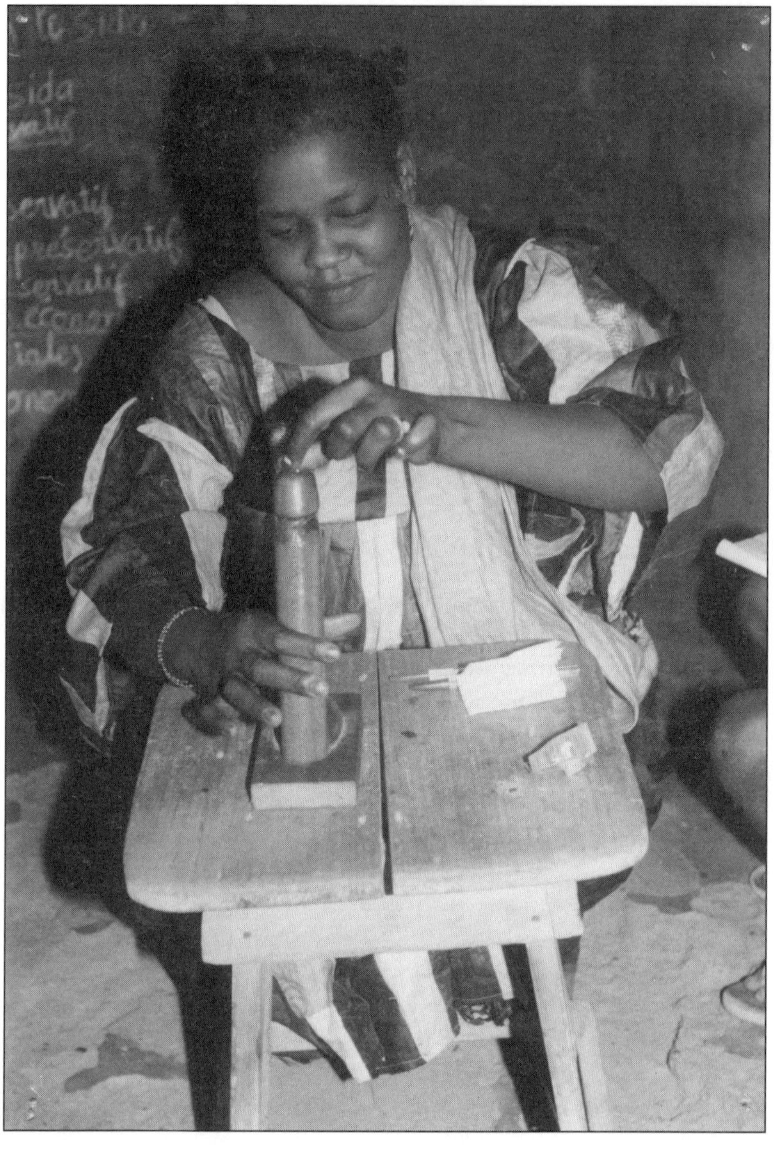

Figure 8-9. A member of Danaya So demonstrates how to put on a condom. Such demonstrations typically follow *Danaya So* street theatre performances and constitute part of Danaya So's social marketing efforts. Photo courtesy of SIDA 3.

ill. Her mother tries to treat her for malaria, and failing that, the mother takes Fifi to a traditional healer who gives a false diagnosis and charges high fees. Meanwhile, at school, young Mariam is mistreated for being the sister of a young woman with AIDS. Fifi eventually dies, and when the performance ends, Mother is trying to determine how to survive without encouraging Miriam to turn to prostitution.

Danaya So's dramas are followed by questions from the audiences and group discussions. The storyline and the point of view of *Danaya So* provide audiences with a rare public glimpse of a women's perspective on the AIDS epidemic. The women dress in trousers and baseball caps, and parody through gesture and stance, male sexual bravado. Their attitude makes it clear they reject the notion that females are the cause of the global pandemic! The fact that women in Mali do not normally appear in stage plays makes these plays even more extraordinary. These female actors appear to have the potential to hold up a mirror on a social group in Mali long protected from critical scrutiny: men, especially older men. The plays of *Danaya So* appear to offer up the potential of chipping away at a patriarchal system that has helped to fuel the AIDS epidemic. The discussion of AIDS and gender will continue in Chapter 9.

Review Questions

1. What is the importance of ritual in society? How is theatre related to ritual on the Africa continent?
2. What new forms of theatre and performance did Europeans introduce to Africa? How did Africans adapt European performance genres and traditions to their own needs, tastes, and purposes?
3. What is DramAide? In which ways does DramAide draw upon Black South African performance traditions in its approach to playmaking?
4. What is Soul City? In which ways does Soul City illustrate the principles underlying edutainment as a catalyst for behavioral and social change?
5. What is *Kòtèba*? How has *Kòtèba* been adapted for use in Mali's struggle against HIV/AIDS?
6. What is *Danaya So*? How does *Danaya So* attempt to address important AIDS-related issues ignored by some other groups in Mali. What are the limitations of *Danaya So*'s work in the areas of Information, Education, and Communication?

Chapter 9

AIDS and Performance for the 21st Century: Toward a Theory of Ritual and Performance

Origins of Performance; Theories of Performance

In Chapter 4, I noted that many African performance traditions date from ancient times. I also showed that many scholars believe that the earliest performances were based in religious ritual, and that such performances aided ancient peoples in communicating with their gods and ancestors. These theories tend to imply, without actually so claiming, that early humankind was preoccupied largely with supernatural matters. Some scholars question this notion arguing that some performance, at least some dance and music, must have come about as a way for a group to pass time during idle moments, after harvests for example. These latter theorists argue that performance has also long been about play and about socializing. In any case, both camps recognize that ritual and performance have been close partners in human activity down through the ages and that both have had tremendous transformative power.

As I noted earlier, the study of performance is still in its infancy at this time early in the third millennium. One of the goals of a study of this kind has been to examine performance in Africa more carefully and to consider its use in the struggle against the scourge of AIDS. Such an examination could uncover commonalties across groups. These deliberations, it is hoped, will lead to the refinement of a theory of performance and social change.

Performance theory draws its inspiration from a variety of disciplines. Here I will take up a brief discussion of the different threads important in the development of performance theory. Two scholars whose work is particularly important to us in this context are anthropologist Victor Turner and performance scholar Richard Schechner.

Anthropologist Victor Turner argued (as did Suzanne Langer) that performance descends from sacred rituals. He expounded upon this topic in one of the last essays he wrote shortly before his death in 1984. The reader should be sensitive to the sweeping breadth of Turner's definition of performance.

> Theatre is one of the many inheritors of that multifaceted system of preindustrial ritual which embraces ideas and images of cosmos and chaos, interdigitates clowns and their foolery with gods and their solemnity, and uses all the sensory codes to produce symphonies in more than music: the inter-twining of dance, body languages of many kinds, song, chant, architectural forms (temples, amphi-theatres), incense, burnt offerings, ritualized feasting and drinking, painting, body painting, body markings of many kinds, including circumcision and scarification, the application of lotions and drinking of potions, the enacting of mythic and heroic plots drawn from oral traditions. And so much more (1990, p. 12). (Reprinted with the permission of Cambridge University Press).

But Turner also averred that performance, sacred and otherwise, originated in social drama of the kind envisioned by Goffman.

> The social drama, then I regard as the experimental matrix from which the many genres of cultural performance, beginning with redressive ritual and juridical procedures, and eventually including oral and literary narrative, have been generated (Turner, 1982, p. 78). (Reprinted with permission of Performing Arts Journal Publications, 1982).

And he argued that social drama was universal.

> My observations convince me that it [social drama] is a spontaneous unit of social process, and a fact of everyone's experience in every human society (Turner 1982, p. 68). (Reprinted with permission of Performing Arts Journal Publications, 1982).

Turner also believed like Goffman, that performance in everyday life in Africa was an unending series of dramatic engagements for which he felt African rural life was particularly attuned.

> In the simpler pre-industrial societies acting a role and employing a status was so much a part of everyday life that the ritual playing of a role even if it was different from that played in mundane life, was the same kind as the one played as son, daughter, headman, shaman, mother, chief, or queen sister (1982, p. 115). (Reprinted with the permission of Performing Arts Journal Publications, 1982).

Performance scholar Richard Schechner, who collaborated closely with Victor Turner, has also argued for example that both theatre and ritual must have come from cave dances of our Paleolithic ancestors (1985, p. 22). But Schechner also notes that some of this activity may have had non-sacred intent.

> The "origin" of the aesthetic genres—theatre, dance, music—could as well be themselves, these activities being co-existent with the human species, or if one demands a functional origin, they could be rooted in healing, in fun-making or teaching (as story-telling and imitations) (1990, p. 24). (Reprinted with the permission of Cambridge University Press).

And Schechner points out that Turner's formulations (about the original sacredness of performance) can neither be proved nor disproved. He allows that some aesthetic forms may have generated spontaneously in pre-history.

The work of these two scholars establishes the close ties, probably evolutionary, between ritual and performance. These ties clearly developed in conditions of human sociability. And some of them evidently emerged in human awe-filled contemplation of the sacred.

Theories of Ritual and Social Change

Anthropologist Victor Turner's lifelong work on ritual recognized two different kinds of ritual distinguished due to purpose: rites of passage and redressive ritual. Turner's discussion of the former drew straight from van Gennep's writings. Social theorist Arnold van Gannep was the first to identify the function of ritual as an aid in helping humankind to cope with life's awesome dramas. These rituals or "rites of passage," as he called them, help people to negotiate their way socially through birth, puberty, pair bonding, parenthood, old age, and death (1908). Anthropologist Victor Turner elaborated on the way participation in these rites of passage helped bring about the transformation of a person from one stage of the individual's life to the next.

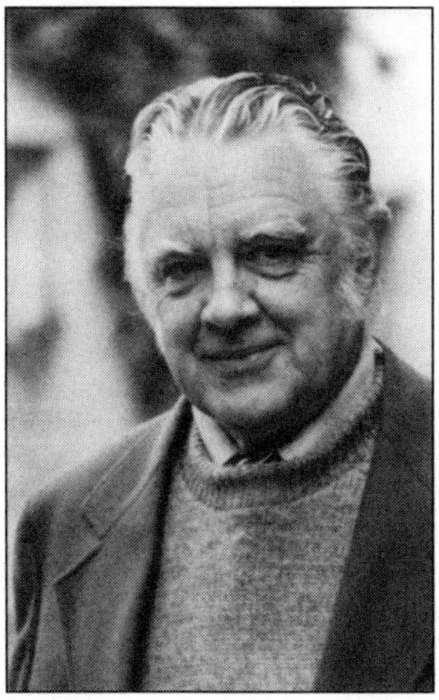

Figure 9-1. Victor Turner's (1920–1983) work showed how ritual can function in the process of social change. Photo courtesy of Edie Turner.

Turner showed that redressive ritual, rituals of compensation or healing, grew out of the need to solve conflicts. He argued that these conflicts derived from social drama, i.e., disputes between one or more members—spats, marital conflicts, wars, sickness, etc. Redressive ritual, he noted, worked to restore community or individual balance. These included mock warfare, judicial processes and legal punishments, healing rites, community sacrifices to angry gods, and so on.

Turner argued that rites of passage described by van Gennep took the same ***form*** of redressive ritual. This is because individuals undergoing them had

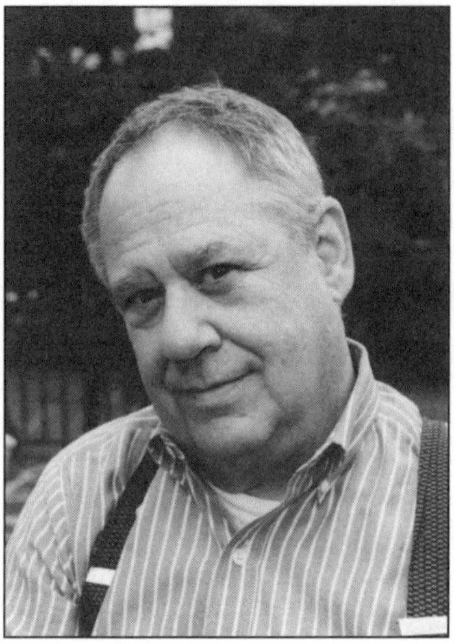

Figure 9-2. Richard Schechner's work introduced the concept of "flow" in performance, and argued that "flow" is the portion of the performance where personal and social transformations take place. Photo courtesy of Richard Schechner.

reached a crisis point in their lives, a crisis whose contradictions could only be mediated by a rite of passage.

Turner's ritual theories introduced the world to the concepts of ***liminality*** and ***communitas***. *Liminality* refers to a condition of being outside of normal everyday life, of being marginal to the society. *Communitas* refers to a feeling of solidarity experienced by persons who undergo a group experience together outside normal life experience. Understanding these concepts is key to an appreciation of the role of ritual in people's lives and the mechanisms by which it operates.

The concepts of *liminality* and *communitas* may easily be applied to the processes college students undergo should they choose to become members of a fraternity.[1] When a brother is "pledged" by a fraternity, he could be said to be in a "***limin***al" phase of social membership. He is neither a fully-fledged member of the fraternity, nor truly a member of the "non-Greek" campus community, but rather he is somewhere "betwixt and between." Fraternity hazing (despite its growing unpopularity among university administrators) is designed partly to engender ***communitas*** among pledge groups. The logic here is that people who suffer together under unusual circumstances bond together. The bonding provides the strength needed to undertake important tasks needed in society. It also provides a common worldview, a common way of seeing life among all members.

1. Fraternity hazing rituals derive their origins from rites of passage in traditional societies wherein boys learned to be and "became" men.

Structure of Ritual

Turner argued that the basic structure of a ritual was tripartite, i.e., it contains three events or phases: the pre-liminal; the liminal; and the post-liminal. The pre-liminal involves the dramatic separation of the individual or the group from his or her peers. The liminal involves an intense period of activity during which the initiate or ritual subject undergoes a series of activities or transformations all leading the initiate to his changed state. The liminal period culminates with a peak or dramatic ceremony (ritual within a ritual) that is the heart of the ritual. It is at this moment that the actual transformation takes place. The third phase of ritual enactment is the post-liminal. Here the new initiate is welcomed back into the community in a new and transformed state.

Until sometime well into the mid-twentieth century the process by which couples in the United States were wed followed the ritual structure laid out by Turner. A dating couple could be said to be in a pre-liminal phase of marriage. When a dating couple decided to marry, it was customary to announce their engagement to the community. Typically, the future groom symbolized his intentions by the giving of a ring to his future bride. And the couple's families held parties or celebrations to mark their engagement. The engagement announcement/celebration marked the beginning of the liminal phase of the marriage ritual, a phase of mini rituals leading up to the central ritual. The engagement also served notice to the community that the future bride and groom were leaving their single peers, their colleagues still looking for mates. The young man and young woman were socially liminal (marginal) because they were neither "really single" (available) nor "really married." The liminal period (the engagement phase) consisted of a series of steps or activities (mini rituals) designed to prepare both partners for their new roles in society. In some churches, engaged couples were expected to undergo marriage instructions in preparation for the life change. These instructions were often shared with other betrothed couples so a kind of *communitas* could be built up among similarly jittery couples. Other activities involved the material life. The woman was usually expected to begin gathering her trousseau. Bridal showers were organized to help her accomplish this task. The groom was supposed to prepare himself for his new role as a family head. He was charged with assuring a dwelling place for his new bride. In some communities this meant actually building a home, in others, placing a down payment on a mortgage or paying the first month's rent. Bridal showers and the traditional bachelor party also helped integrate the couple into the social worlds of married women and married men in the community while retaining their ties with their single cohorts. As the wedding date loomed closer, the drama of the coming event intensified with the final marriage preparations.

The **liminal** phase of the marriage ritual culminated in the actual wedding ceremony (the core ritual within the ritual), the most dramatic part of the process and the point where the most important transformations took place. The ritual of the wedding ceremony was highly processual. The bride and groom each entered the church separately; the bride and her father marched down the aisle to music as they preparing to meet the groom already standing before the congregation. When the father and the bride arrived at the altar; the father would hand over his daughter to her awaiting future husband. During the ceremony, the couple would be joined before God and society by a recognized figure of the community. At the end the couple would march triumphantly out of the service transformed from individuals into a married couple, i.e., as husband and wife.

The **post-liminal** phase of the marriage ritual involved a social portion, the wedding banquet where the new couple was reintegrated into the community, and a private phase, the honeymoon, where the new couple adjusted to living with one another as man and wife.

Victor Turner alerted readers to the importance of the processual form of a ritual, to the fact that it is a ***patterned enactment.*** The ritual, according to Turner is like a road map marking the way to the accomplishment of certain goals. The map shows how to move from childhood to puberty; how to proceed from being single to being married; how to turn the condition of barrenness to one of fertility; or how, for example, to send a member of the living off to the land of the spirits. In Turner's formulations, the steps in a ritual are irreversible. The bride does not get unmarried by walking out of the church backward.[2] ***Indeed a ritual is transformative because it is sequenced.***

For many years, anthropologists known as structural-functionalists had focussed their research on showing how social phenomena including ritual and other performance activities supported the social system, i.e., how they cemented the status quo. Turner and other anthropologists he inspired were more concerned with the ***role of ritual in change.*** Turner observed that all rituals contained "invariant passages" which kept rituals intact from generation to generation, and thus maintained the social stability over time. But he noted that rituals contained "variable passages, which both at the verbal and non-verbal levels, improvisation [was] not merely permitted, but required" (Turner, 1982, p. 81). These variable passages in Turner's view "contain[s] the potential for cultural innovation, as well as the means of effecting structural transformations within a relatively stable socio-cultural system" (Turner, 1982, 85). To proceed with the current example of a wedding ritual, many American couples in the 21st century script their own wedding vows or edit the existing ones so as to de-emphasize time-honored but passé notions such as spousal obedience by the wife. The fact that these couples retain the core promises to "Love, honor, and cherish," the partner and the fact that they still undergo the "typical church wedding ceremony" provides stability for the community and continuity across the generations. But the fact that the couple can alter the ritual helps the couple and the wedding guests to socially process the changing relationships between men and women. The notion of ***variation in performance*** is then key to an appreciation of the role of ritual or ritual-like experiences in social change including development.

Theories of Performance and Social Change

For anthropologist Margaret Drewal, the processes of transformation are embedded in African performance traditions. Performances are re-represented, or repeated, but they are never done the same way twice. Each re-enactment has the

2. If the marriage falters, a redressive ritual, a legal divorce must be undertaken to disengage these two individuals.

power (inherent in the variable parts observed by Victor Turner) to bring new elements of social life to the surface. In a given ritual or performance in a given year or at a given moment, performers may decide to bring "frontstage"—to make public/to tell a story about—realities which had formerly been kept "backstage."[3] Drewal, like Turner, is well aware that rituals and other performances may be presenting or communicating ideas that the performer has not consciously processed (Drewel, 1991, pp. 1–64). This makes their dialogic or ritual approach to communication far more inclusive and powerful than those of the earlier dramatistic communication theorists (Mead, Burke, and Goffman) whose theories implied consciousness on the part of communicators. Both Turner and Drewal, but especially Drewal, would fall into the post-modernist camp, while Burke, Mead, and Goffman were considered modernists as explained in Chapter 4.

Turner recognized the close relationship between ritual and other types of performance including theatre. And Turner argued that all performance arose in social drama or social conflict. Because all societies are rife with social conflict he argued, humans have invented ritual and performance to help people overcome their differences.

Liminal and Liminoid Genres

It should be recalled that in Turner's ritual formulation, social transformations take place during liminal (separation/out of society) phases of ritual, during that portion of the ritual when participants are symbolically cut off from the rest of society. Turner, in fact, regarded ritual as a liminal performance genre, ***(i.e., as a genre of performance that exists on the margins of normal life).*** And Turner, moreover, also contended that Western performance entertainment genres descended from ritual. But he argued that industrialization and division of labor had over the centuries replaced ritual with a set of "entertainment genres flourishing in the leisure time of society" (1990, p. 12). Some of Turner's academic work involved exploring differences between ancient ritual and modern performance genres. He termed the former ***liminal*** and the latter ***liminoid*** genres. He showed that differences in the social uses of the two kinds of performances led to differences in their ability to transform participants/audience members.

Turner noted that liminal genres used a common set of symbols, the meanings of which are shared by the entire group while liminoid genres represented one person or one group's view, i.e., a particularistic view of the whole. He argued that while liminal genres of ritual were compulsory and involved the entire community, modern performance genre participation is optional and involves only fringes of the social group. He showed that where traditional ritual (liminal) incorporated both work and play, modern entertainment forms (liminoid) involve only genres of play. He pointed out that the purpose of ritual forms was deadly serious but that entertainment forms are about diversion and play.

Turner argued that liminal genres peaked historically in the tribal and early agrarian societies; and that liminoid genres began to develop with the city-states,

---

3. The notions of "frontstage" and "backstage" were first raised by Goffman in 1974.

Ancient Ritual-Liminal	Modern Performance-Liminoid
Origin in Social Drama	Origin in Social Drama
Historical peak: Tribal and early agrarian societies	Age of Enlightenment/Baroqe
Involement: Entire Community	Segment of Society: Fringes
Audience: participant	Differentiated & passive
Social Function: Integration of whole	Social Criticism of one social segment by another
Mode of consciouness: Group	Individual
Combines work and play	Play Only
Participation Required	Participation optional
Involves much flow	Involves little flow
Is deadly serious	Is entertainment/Diversion
Transformation is permanent	Transformation is temporary/ a transportation

(Bourgault 1991, pp. 56–60, used with permisssion, *Journal of Development Communication.*)

Figure 9-3. Ancient ritual versus modern performance.

and peaked during the Western Age of Enlightenment of the 17th and 18th centuries. Turner noted that ritual performances functioned to integrate the whole community while modern performance genres tend to serve up criticism of one segment of society by a different one (the playwright's/the actor's/the theatre company's) segment. He observed the importance of performance genres in preindustrial times as compared to the marginality of performance genres in modern life. And he commented on the religious and cosmic significance and the awe-inspiring nature of liminal genres in ancient times as compared to the secularity and relative triviality of today's performances. He argued that the liminal (ritual) genres were "no longer in a central driving place." And that "the pronounced numinous supernatural character of archaic ritual has been greatly attenuated" (1990, p. 12).

Turner noted that *liminal* phenomena mute individuality, merging the identities of the actors with the action of the ritual, and hence the cosmos and society's belief about it. In so doing, they achieve ***flow***, a kind of "self-propelled" take off, which results in a transformation (Turner, 1982, p. 53). But he found that *liminoid* genres tended to heighten the sense of particularity of spectators by distancing audiences from actors and the stories depicted on stage. For this reason, flow for spectators was difficult to achieve.

Anthropologist Victor Turner and performance artist and scholar Richard Schechner did much collaborative work on performance. And some of Schechner's findings will be discussed below. Elsewhere (Bourgault 1991) I have laid out in table form a Turner/Schechner model of the differences between ancient ritual and modern performance genres. It is reproduced here in this volume in Figure 9-3.

It is worth highlighting that the Western world has certainly under emphasized and perhaps misunderstood theatre in many parts of the world because our own theater is of the liminoid variety, the entertainment variety. We in the Western world have long overlooked the relationship between ritual and theatre. We have long underestimated the power of performance because we have tended to consider it mere entertainment, unconnected with cosmic matters. Not content to merely establish the links between ritual and theatre, Schechner's work explores the nature of the relationship between the two. Indeed Schechner argues that this relationship is braided, that ritual can turn into theater and that theater can turn into ritual (1988, pp. 106–152). His discussion implies that a performance that starts out as play can become supremely significant. People, especially people playing their own selves, in an experimental performance workshop, in a political demonstration, in an encounter group, in popular theater, under the right circumstances can "click" into liminal modes of consciousness and undergo permanent transformations.

Concept of Flow

The concept of ***flow*** is important to the discussion of social change and merits further discussion.[4] Much of the collaborative and experimental work of Turner and Schechner was devoted to the study of flow and the attempt at its creation in performers. This is because, as noted above, it is during the process of ***flow*** that social transformations occur. And both scholars were deeply interested in social change or social transformation.

According to Schechner, flow represents a phase in the performance genres where the ego of the actor is lost through a merging with experience. This can occur because the consciousness of the individual has been narrowed so that his/her complete focus is on the action of the enactment. Here the actor has complete control over the work/play of the performance. He/she has mastered the lines; he/she knows the moves. He/she "goes with the flow." Turner adds that flow is coherent because the demands of the action are non-contradictory. The rules of engagement are clear. This control is also "autotelic," i.e., it seems to need no rewards outside itself (1982, p. 58).

Both Turner and Schechner have recognized that modern Western performances do not engender much flow for audience members. They say this is because modern audiences are differentiated and passive. These theorists would argue that transformations occurring during plays and within audience members are temporary, and not permanent. They are ***transportations,*** not transformations. And neither Turner nor Schechner would think that the actors in these modern plays undergo significant transformations.

Schechner (1985) notes that flow often occurs during trance-like states induced "through repetition and accumulation." In his work with theatrical and ritual forms, he has devised all night dances to demonstrate the pattern of flow. He describes the experience.

4. See Turner 1982, for a more detailed discussion of the differences between liminal and liminoid genres. See also Bourgault 1991, for the application of Turner and Schechner's theories to a village-based radio drama project conducted in Liberia in 1989.

> Each time I've participated in this kind of dance I've had, and others too have had, a trance-like experience...where for varying periods the sense of me as an individual, the amount of time passing, the awareness of the environment I was in (outdoors in a field and inside a gymnasium to name two) were abolished. What was left were vaguely recollectable sense of moving in a circle and the feel of other persons, the other bodies, to either side of me (1985, p. 11). (From *Between Theatre and Anthropology* by Richard Schechner. Copyright© 1985. Univeristy of Pennsylvania Press).

In a later work Schechner describes physical aspects of ritual performances.

> Individual and collective anxieties are relieved by rituals whose qualities of repetition, rhythmicity, exaggeration, condensation, and simplification stimulate the brain into releasing endorphins directly into the bloodstream yielding relief from pain and a surfeit of pleasure (1995, p. 233).

For Schechner, the flow is the portion of the performance where the transformations occur in those participating. Schechner finds that flow, however absent in modern Western performances, occurs during the enactment of tradition-based Asian dance performance genres. And it certainly occurs as well in African ritual contexts. Indeed Turner wrote of the power of flow unleashed in Zambian performance of "thin, ill-nourished old ladies, with only occasional naps, [to] dance, sing, and perform ritual activities for two or three days and nights together" (1990, p. 13). Certainly trance and possession is common in African ritual.[5]

Schechner argues that conventional Western theatre fails to transform its audiences because they have no role to play in a performance other than spectator. Western audiences never achieve true flow during a conventional performance. What they achieve at best, is some form of "private sentimental empathy." In order to be transformed through performance flow a person must actively take part in the experience (1985, p. 145).

For a permanent change to occur through a performance, a performer must be restored to ordinary life (life after the ritual or the performance), in a changed state. The performer must return transformed. Schechner regards Western theatrical performances as ***transportations*** rather than transformations because professional actors do not emerge from a performance with a change in status or a change in consciousness.

> During the performance the performers are 'taken somewhere,' but at the end, often assisted by others, as they are 'cooled down' and reenter ordinary life just about where they went in (1985, p. 125). (From *Between Theatre and Anthropology* by Richard Schechner. Copyright© 1985. Univeristy of Pennsylvania Press).

5. See for example Rosenthal 1998, on trance and possession among the Ewe; see also Hackett 1996, on trance and possession among the Yoruba, the San, and many other groups. See Amankulor 1997, who offers a discussion of the experimental theatre of Jerzy Grotowski who also collaborated with Turner and Schechner.

Less absolutist, Turner argues that flow, though rare in modern life, ***can*** happen with liminoid forms. Artists become immersed in the creative activity, and make "art for art's sake," giving themselves over completely to the rules of the genre. Some of the transformation that derived in "the flow" then "sticks" with the artist, even after he or she has recovered from the work. And Turner further argues that artists, actors, and spectators alike reincorporate aspects of the theatrical genre in a piecemeal fashion into their everyday lives. This he feels is a partial transformation, one that stands in sharp contrast with complete transformations engendered by traditional ritual—transformations incorporated wholesale into the lives of society members.

Richard Schechner has studied in a comparative perspective the transformative power of various performance genres. These have included conventional Western theatre, ancient Greek drama, Japanese *Noh* dancing, and quasi-religious enactments of Hindu mythology. Schechner's work contrasts levels of involvement of audience members in the various genres. In Japanese *Noh* and in the Indian mytho-religious enactments, the spectators actively participate. And in the ancient Greek Drama, the chorus, who represented worshippers of the god Dionysus, actively commented on the events in the play and thereby served as a bridge between the spectators and the actors. All of these forms were participatory, he maintains, and all were transformative. Again, in order to be transformed through performance ***flow***, a person must ***actively take part*** in the experience. Indeed, Schechner believes that flow occurs among performers in many of the religious performances of the classical oriental tradition. This has led Schechner to the further study of Eastern performance practice.

Schechner's more recent research work has brought him to explore questions surrounding human performance consciousness and the role of consciousness in performance technique. Schechner draws upon the work of Paul Ekman who has studied the relationship between facial displays of emotion and the autonomic nervous system (ANS). As noted above, Ekman is also known for his cross-cultural work identifying human universals in the facial display of emotion across cultures. Ekman has shown that actors who relive an emotion in order to display it on stage [the Stanislavski method] experience the same autonomic nervous response (ANS) responses as those who consciously create the facial expressions mechanically "as they looked at themselves in the mirror" (Schechner, 1990, p. 30). Schechner notes that the second, the mechanistic method of acting is the kind despised by most American performers. It is similar in technique, however, to that used in classical Asian dance. In these systems, the *kutiyattam* and the *kathakali* of India, and the Balinese and Javanese classical dances of Indonesia, dancers learn to display stylized emotion by practicing extensive muscular manipulations of the face and body.

Schechner draws from the training for *Natyasastra*, centuries old and no longer performed sacred Sanskrit theatre texts, to develop his arguments. *Natyasastra* is a system for acting that describes eight basic emotions or *rasas*. Schechner notes that *Natyasastra* not only teaches how to convey these feelings to an audience, but how to achieve feelings themselves through the appropriate performance of gesture. Like yoga training, *Natyasastra* uses external body manipulation to affect and change the internal spirit. *Natyasastra* training then clearly involves the use of biofeedback techniques to alter the emotional stages of the actor.

Schechner shows that six of the eight classical *rasas* correspond to Ekman's six basic emotions. He comments on the significance of this finding for ritual theory.

> The *Natyasastra*—and the arts based on it—insist on what Ekman's experiments show: there are links between "mechanical acting" and feelings! The causal chain can go in both directions: feelings can lead to stage action while the practice of specific stage exercises can arouse feelings in actors (1990, p. 35). "Magnitudes of Performance," reprinted with permission of Cambridge University Press. First printed as "Magnitudes of Performance," in *Performance Theory* @Routledge, 1988.

Schechner has argued that the techniques used by performers to transform themselves for performance are the same processes that occur in the 'ritual process' first described by van Gennep and later explained by Turner.

Schechner makes a very important point about the role of performance in communication. The sensitive reader should hear the echo of Suzanne Langer in these words.

> Human communication systems are not reducible to the static model of "sender—channel—receiver," or any variation thereof—that assumes the existence of discrete parts. The human system is an extremely subtle multiplex—feedback, [sic.], one in which the originator of feelings is also affected by the emotions s/he is expressing—even if these emotions are a lie. That is what Ekman's experiment, and good acting are saying: the doing of the action of a feeling is enough to arouse the feeling both in the doer and in the receiver (1990, p. 41).
>
> "Magnitudes of Performance," reprinted with permission of Cambridge University Press. First printed as "Magnitudes of Performance," in *Performance Theory* @Routledge, 1988.

Schechner cautions scholars against relying too heavily on language or on artistic conventions as tools for analyzing what goes on in a performance. He notes there are no language universals. But he highlights the fact that there are non-verbal signals which "come close to conveying the same feelings everywhere." Moreover, these feelings he points out, "constitute the very heart of human performing art and ritual as well as individual human experience." His conclusion of this discussion is central to the work of this volume.

> Performance of theatre, dance, music, ritual by the very nature of their existence as behavior—as things done—give us our best examples for the intercultural study of human communication (1990, p. 42). "Magnitudes of Performance," reprinted with permission of Cambridge University Press. First printed as "Magnitudes of Performance," in *Performance Theory* @Routledge, 1988.

Schechner has argued that performance, like ritual with which it is closely related, has enormous transformative power. He has argued further that the study of performance promises to make great strides in the field of human communication.

It seems equally obvious from Schechner's comments that the performance process offers both a supportive channel for the adoption of new ideas in a given society and a comfortable venue for sharing ideas across cultural divides.

Transformative Power of Participatory Methodology and Edutainment

We have already defined edutainment as it is practiced today as educative media that are also entertaining. We have noted that some of today's edutainment consists of small media, such as posters or audio cassettes, and that other edutainment consists of large media. National TV broadcasts such as Soul City in South Africa are excellent examples of edutainment. We have noted that good edutainment strives to engender para-social communication, i.e., it tries to get audience members involved with the broadcast. Audiences may engage with the program entity itself by joining its contests, by following the lives of its stars, or by discussing its story lines and program content.

The role of the para-social communication is to foster interaction, the doing of, or acts of participation. The social participation reinforces the message of the broadcast or of the edutainment. The weakness of much edutainment is that it is often large scale and generally impersonal. The recipients of the message have generally not engaged in its construction though some (or more often others like them) may have participated in formative research during the design phase of the media product in question. To use the author's Schechner/Turner schema provided above, edutainment products would be liminoid genres.

Chapter 2 discussed the nature of participatory methodology in relation to AIDS awareness campaigns in Africa. It noted that participatory methodology, though related to edutainment, implies a broader role for the audience. Here the targets of the message have participated in its creation. Such audiences obviously have a great deal of ownership over the messages they design, and these are clearly relevant to their social circle. Performances created through participatory methodology would fit many of the criteria of a liminal genre. They involve entire communities (or sub-communities—a school, a youth group, etc.); they involve audiences; they work to integrate a whole group; they foster and operate from group consciousness; and ***they offer opportunities to perform that are less than optional.*** In other words, the experience of creating a performance or a media product through participatory methodology tends to be a liminal one, one approximating (if not actually replicating) the experience of ritual. And the degree of flow that develops in the creation of a media product through participatory methodology will normally be quite high. Of course, the levels of secularization and industrialization of the group involved will certainly affect the experience. According to theory, the less industrialized and less secularized the society, the easier it is for performers to slip into a liminal state during performance. Indeed the Turner/Schechner model identifies tribal and early agrarian societies as the historical peak of ritual.

Certainly, in some rural parts of Africa, the associations of theater with ritual seem intuitive.[6] Nobel Prize-winning Nigerian author Wole Soyinka expounded on these relationships in *Myth, Literature, and the African World* (1976). Soyinka noted herein that "the supposed dividing line between ritual and theatre

6. See Bourgault 1991 that describes an experiment in village-based drama for development in Liberia. The author argues that in the creation of the performance, a ritual-like event occurred.

should not concern [his readers] much in Africa, [because] the line...[was] largely drawn by the European analyst" (1976, p. 7). Soyinka is known to ask forgiveness from the Yoruba gods before bringing them out on stage. Soyinka claims he needs the presence of the gods to demonstrate power to audiences (Doho, personal communication, July, 2001).

Cameroonian playwright and popular theatre producer Dr. Gilbert Doho tells of the power of a participatory theatre piece "*L'Illuminée du bois sacré*" ("The Enlightened One of the Sacred Forest") which he helped to facilitate. The play, created by and about local women, centers on a group of rural Cameroonian women who confront their chief for selling off tracts of their village's sacred rainforest, sections of which were theretofore reserved for ritual purposes.

After Doho's group created the dramatic piece, the women invited the chief to see their performance during his next visit to their village. As they performed their play, they drew strength from one another, presenting the reality of their own community to this errant chief. And the exercise worked! Embarrassed by the power of this theatrical display and its public sanction of his behavior, the chief relinquished the logging permits he had dispensed to local lumber companies.

Clearly, something communal had "clicked" among these performing women and connected with their audience. Flow had indeed been achieved. The exercise (or as Turner would have it, the ritual) left the women forever changed. They had been empowered by their creative performance activity, an exercise in power they'd heretofore thought impossible. Playing themselves, they had stood up to their chief and reclaimed the village's sacred forest. Henceforth, they would not go back to being powerless. Even today, the women of the particular village in question are no longer content to leave decision-making to men. They demand a voice in village governance! (Doho, personal communication, July 2001).

In another theater for social change workshop, the people in the village of Mayoka, Cameroon, created a play about a mayor who embezzled money from the village. The mother of the mayor played the judge in a fictitious impeachment trial of the mayor. After hearing all arguments in the putative case, the mother pronounced in favor of impeachment. So shamed was the mayor/son by his mother's public condemnation, that he stepped down and left the village. While Doho does not exactly aver that the event had ritual-like quality, he posits that it was more powerful than the mere liminoid experience of entertainment (Doho, personal communication, July 2001).

Schechner points out that the narrative aspect of performance works together with its motor aspects.

> ...the narrative cognitive stimulus works from the cerebral cortex down while the movement-sonic stimulus works from the lower brain up. Performing a ritual, or a ritualized theatre piece or exercise, is both narrative and affective. These work together to form the experience of ritualizing (1995, pp. 239–240).

The reader may wonder if ritual-like transformations can occur in modern secularized industrialized societies like South Africa. One has only to hear accounts of apartheid era marches to know the power of performance. Young

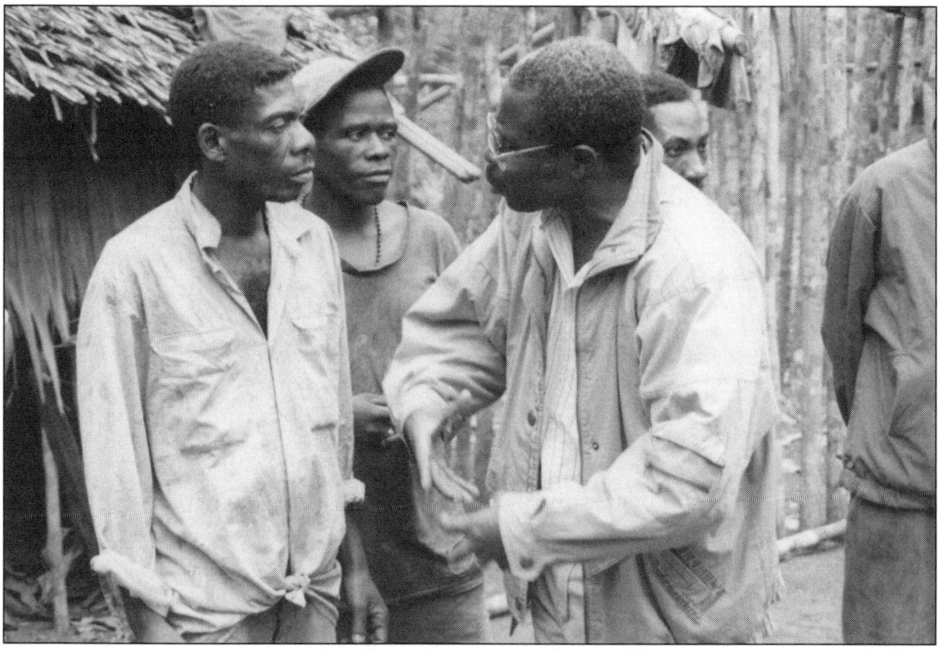

Figure 9-4. Dramatist Gilbert Doho provides direction for "Alien in my Land," a Theatre for Social Change production of a rainforest pygmy (Mekon) band in Cameroon. Photo Courtesy of Gilbert Doho.

South African protestors would *toyi-toyi* for hours in illegal gatherings facing police armed with tear-gas, bullets, dogs, and automatic weapons. The *toyi-toyiing* never failed to unnerve police.

Dalrymple reports that school Open Days in South Africa feature girls wearing men's suits and declaring defiantly that "We are in charge of our bodies." Elsewhere she reports that girls who were about to be sexually harassed on the school grounds responded in a burst of feminine solidarity by singing AIDS songs they had learned through DramAide (Seidel, 1995, 157). Performance is clearly a powerful weapon in Africa. It draws from forces both within individuals, builds solidarity between them, and binds them together with spiritual forces beyond them. This is why colonial governments tried to repress African performance, and why many post-colonial African governments have also tried to contain certain aspects of it.

Issue of Gender

This brings us to the next point in our discussion: that of gender and the AIDS epidemic. This volume has repeatedly argued that gender relations must shift if the HIV infection rate on the African continent is to slow down. It is worth repeating that sub-Saharan Africa is the region with the highest percentage of female infections. And it is the only continent where heterosexual sexual contact alone is significant as a means of HIV transmission. It is also noteworthy

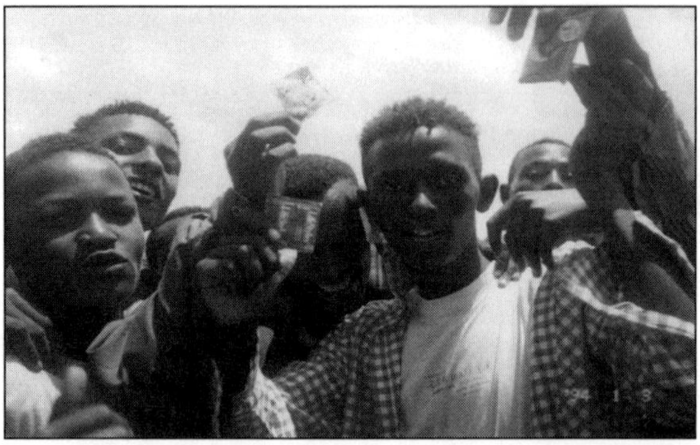

Figure 9-5. Young men must develop sexual responsibility. Photo courtesy of David Schein, Awassa Children's Project.

that the spread of HIV occurs more frequently from men to women than from women to men, as I have already observed. Throughout the AIDS epidemic women have been unfairly victimized and they have suffered a double burden. For years campaigns that focussed on prevention erred by making the tacit twin assumptions that sex was always consensual and that more information about risks would lead to safer behaviors. Both of these notions have been disavowed. By the time of the new millennium, AIDS prevention projects were seeking ways to influence men specifically. And the United Nations took the lead in 2000 and 2001 with their AIDS campaign theme: "Men Can Make a Difference." This seems to be an important step in the right direction. Half way into the first decade of the new millennium we may be in a better position to see how these projects have fared. Even before the results of these special efforts have been assessed, I glimpse ever cautious at the possibility of a paper-thin silver lining in the AIDS epidemic for Africa. The silver lining is that gender relations are finally being critically appraised and tackled within the context of, and as a result of, the AIDS pandemic. And performance clearly figures into this agency. Efforts to change the status of African women have emerged at a number of levels.

On a social level, many projects have recognized the importance of women in AIDS prevention activities, and as a result, have targeted projects to them. African women, well organized into NGOs since the 1980s, have been in a position to cooperate with INGOs. They have proven responsive to AIDS projects of all kinds, so their networks have been strengthened. As noted earlier, projects have recognized the positive role of performance. And they have stressed the need for women's inclusion. As a consequence, more women are performing than ever before. Projects like Mali's *Danaya So* are tackling women's issues head on, encouraging women to perform theatre in public, something that Malian tradition and Islamic popular practice had made taboo. And if, as in South Africa, women are victims, they are at least taking their victimage out onto the public stage, where they share their stories and build up solidarity rather than suffer in an isolated silence. In so doing, they cannot but expose and undermine the excesses of the patriarchy. The stories of women and girls will be repeated and discussed through participatory methodologies. Many African countries, like South Africa, have a host of AIDS and gender awareness projects. They have taken

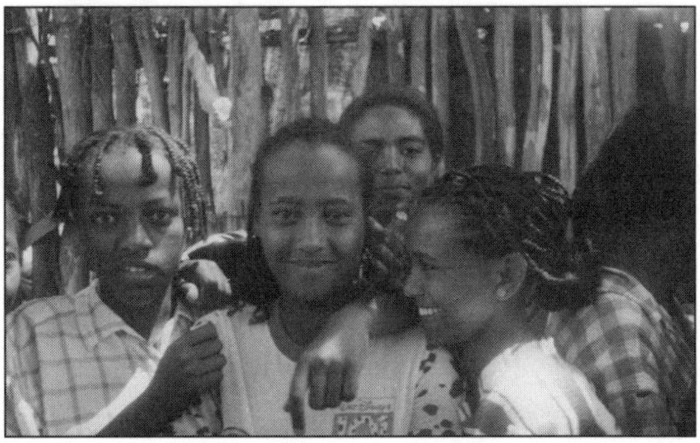

Figure 9-6. African's future depends on better gender relations. Photo courtesy of David Schein, Awassa Children's Project.

their cues both from the UN's third millennium's agenda, and from the evolution of their own AIDS campaigns.

The epidemiological context of the AIDS epidemic has brought a number of related women's issues to the forefront. These include family planning, pre-natal care, women's education, women's access to health care, and female genital cutting or mutilation (FGC/FGM). Now that these issues are in the forefront they too are being tackled.

On a symbolic level, it also seems women are gaining ground through the AIDS epidemic. Discussion of the AIDS issue is leading to the demystification of sex, and a demystification of the male penis. Demonstrations of the male phallus, bring "frontstage" what was once hidden and adulated backstage. Male power is finally being "outed" in this epidemic and being shown to be both in need of, and in receipt of, a dose of control. The once mighty phallus is being tamed in public by females in performance. They respond to the penis by wrapping it in rubber! Effigies of the phallus, once hidden from women and uninitiated males in sacred houses along with masks and other venerable objects, are now in public display. Male power is being demystified, and through the self-same process reduced.

On an economic level, AIDS projects wishing to help the HIV+ are giving more attention to women. This is because women are the main care givers in society. Micro-finance projects are aimed at HIV+ women caring for themselves (for such women are likely to have been abandoned by spouses) and for those people dependent upon them.

Issue of Globalization

This volume has repeatedly pointed out that AIDS is a problem of poverty. The volume has noted, and it is worth repeating, that negative economic growth rates, continued degradation of the natural environment, increased pollution, decreased spending on health, decreased protein intake, and so on, all continue to erode the general health of Africans and to weaken their immune systems.

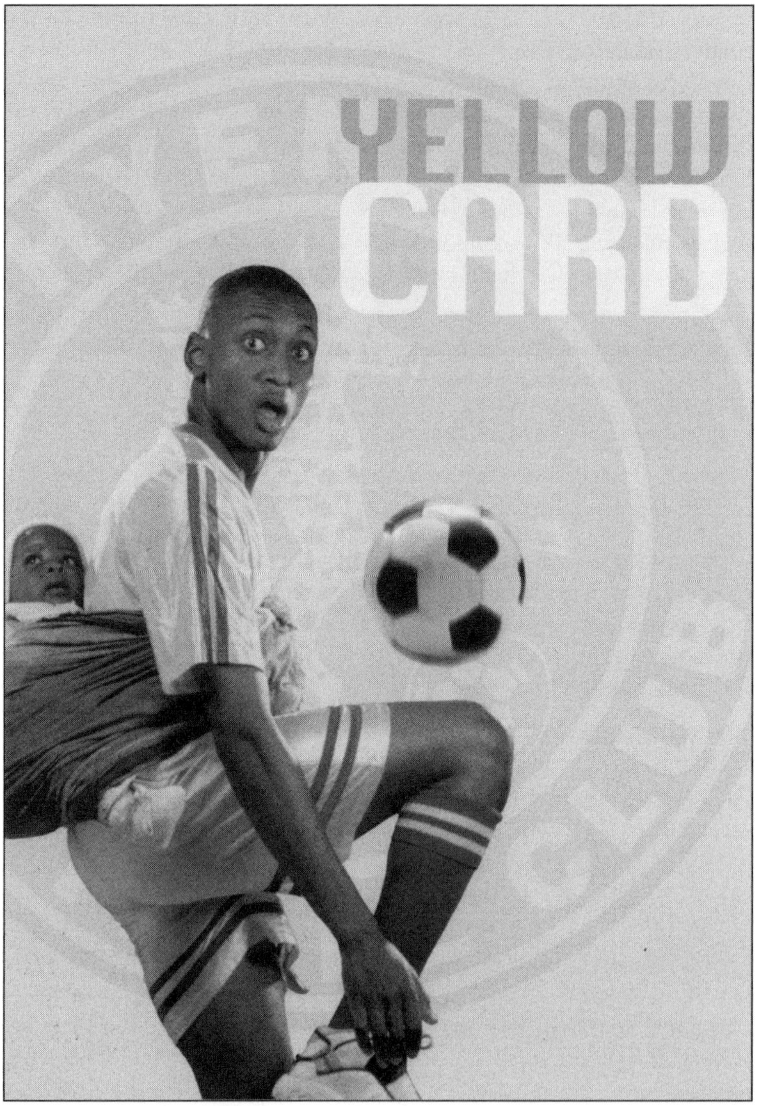

Figure 9-7. "Yellow Card," a feature film produced by John and Louise Riber of Media for Development Trust (Harare, Zimbabwe) that promotes male sexual responsibility. Photo courtesy of Media for Development Trust.

Salih Booker and William Minter from Africa Action argue that Africa's inordinate share of the AIDS case-load is largely a consequence of the economic policies of the Western world, policies based on economic rather than human considerations. They note that access to life-saving drugs and access to care for people with HIV is largely a matter of race, class, gender, and geography (Booker and Minter, 2001, p. 11). They further maintain that globalization, based on the ideology of free trade and the magic of the price mechanism, is a device for minority rule of the world's resources. It fosters a double standard that guarantees human rights including the right to health, only to a privileged few and denies them to the rest of the world's "Others." They argue that the developing world and especially Africa operates in a system of global apartheid. Indeed, forty-four of the fifty-two countries in the world with life expectancies of less than fifty years are in Africa. Those who consider Africa Action's position extreme should note that the US continues to refuse to ratify a UN Declaration on Human Rights recognizing that "access to medication in the context of pandemics such as HIV/AIDS is one fundamental element...of the right...to health." The US, a major proponent of globalization has stood alone in its position against the unanimous vote at the UN (Booker and Minter, 2001, p. 12).

UN Secretary General Kofi Annan has taken the lead on the world's stage in organizing the fight against HIV/AIDS. In 2002 he launched an independent Global AIDS fund, one whose initial goal was to amass 7–10 billion dollars to tackle AIDS and other tropical diseases. He has asked the rich countries, the members of the G7[7] nations and multi-national corporations to supply most of the cash. The purpose of the fund is to provide treatment and build a health infrastructure to support the primary international response to the greatest health pandemic since the Black Death. As of summer 2001, the Bush administration had pledged $200 million dollars to the Global AIDS Fund.[8] The Bill Gates Foundation had pledged $100 million dollars. Coca-Cola announced it would use its massive distribution network in Africa to assist the UN with AIDS prevention programs (Lindsay 2001).

Activists of all stripes argue that the US contribution of $200 million is a paltry sum in view of the fact that the US received $200 million dollars ***per week*** in debt repayment from the developing world. The Washington Post estimates this amount represents $4.90 per year for every person with HIV/AIDS, and an expenditure of $.73 per year per American (Washington Post 2000). The U.S. pledge is also paltry in view of the $50 billion + targeted for homeland security in the wake of the September 11, 2001 attacks. In 2002, despite considerable fanfare on the part of the Bush administration to increase support for the Global Fund, the U.S. government's pledge was again for only $200 million (Physicians for Human Rights 2002). Nevertheless, the U.S. government has pledged to increase funding to $500 million by 2004. This amount falls far short of the $2.5 billion activists say represents the U. S. proportionate share of fighting the epidemic(Physicians for Human Rights 2002).

Kofi Annan's initiative is a brave and ambitious one designed to give high visibility to this epidemic. What is interesting and noteworthy about the Global Fund is that it has helped to focus and combine the energies of AIDS activists with forces fighting globalization. This is because both types of groups have realized they were working on a common and related problem—African poverty. Indeed, Jubilee 2000 Activists argue that cancellation of debt should be linked to programs that will help purchase anti-retroviral drugs and other services needed in the AIDS epidemic.

The group Act Up, famous for its "AIDS theatrics," has now formed itself into an international anti-globalization alliance that concentrates on access to

7. The G7 nations include the world's major capitalist democracies: the U.S., the United Kingdom of Great Britain, France, Germany, Canada, Italy, and Japan. Russia became a member of the body in 1989 and the group became known as the G8.

8. If maintained at this level for 10 years, it will represent less than 0.2% of the 2001 Bush tax cut!

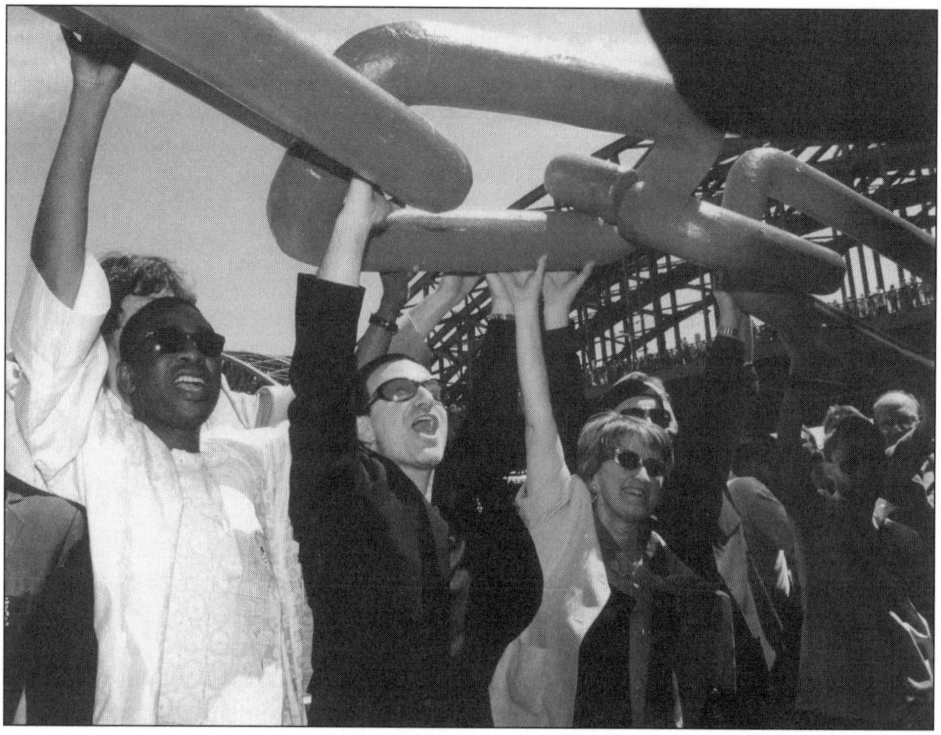

Figure 9-8. Pop Star Bono of U2 was active in anti-globalization campaigns in 2002 and in efforts to convince the George W. Bush administration to drop Third World Debt. Photo courtesy of Jubilee 2000.

healthcare. Act-Up's two most important branches are those of Philadelphia and of New York. They have joined a broader Health Gap Coalition, "a network of AIDS and trade activists formed in 1999 when its members realized that no organization existed within the United States focusing exclusively on the global AIDS epidemic" (Kim, 2001, p. 17).

Act-Up, the AIDS Coalition to Unleash Power, it should be recalled, is a grassroots organization that gained public attention in the 1980s and early 1990s for its use of guerilla theater tactics. The group achieved a level of notoriety when it shut down the New York Stock Exchange and later when it interrupted a mass at St. Patrick's Cathedral in New York in order to protest Roman Catholic teachings on condom use.

More recently Act Up used public political performance to call attention to AIDS treatment issues. They disrupted the Gore presidential campaign kickoff in Carthage, Tennessee, in protest of Gore's support for sanctions against South Africa for the import of generic AIDS drugs. Gore shifted his policy as a result of their actions (Act Up n.d.).

In Summer 2000, after the World AIDS conference in Durban, South Africa, Health Gap teamed up with South Africa's Treatment Access Campaign to form the GTAC (Global Treatment Action Campaign), an international collective of AIDS activists. GTAC was the group in the forefront of the fight against Big Pharmaceuticals, the group that succeeded in getting "Big Pharma" to drop their suit against the South African government (see Chapter 2). And in 2002, they were forcing the South African government to provide anti-retroviral treatment in government clinics to pregnant women (Africa Action, 2002, March 25).

On June 23, 2001 the Global Health Coalition, Jubilee 2000 activists and others organized a rally at the UN Special Session on HIV and AIDS. They carried signs driving home their message, "Trillions for tax cuts, death for people with AIDS." "Death by patent drugs for Africa." And "Bush AIDS policy: Coffins for kids." Many in the coalition argue that debt relief should be given in exchange for AIDS support and care (Lindsay 2001).

These groups promise to attend future meetings of economic leaders of the world's wealthy nations. They will continue to press their message of increased care and support for the HIV+ and for the related issue of debt forgiveness. Emboldened by the victory against "Big Pharma" activists are increasingly focussing on demands for AIDS treatment for the world's developing nations.[9] In 2002, pundits were saying that noisy anti-global activism was beginning to pay off by making such INGO lobbies as Jubilee 2000, Oxfam, and *Médecins Sans Frontières* (Doctors Without Borders) appear reasonable to international lending institutions (Denny, 2002, p. 10). And in mid 2002, there were clear signs that the Bush administration was also beginning to get the message. Despite disappointing funding levels in 2002 for the Global AIDS Fund, the Bush Administration did pledge to increase foreign aid by 50% between 2003 and 2005 (USAID 2002). World poverty, it seemed, had finally gotten the attention of the Bush administration. It seems the U.S. government has come to see the twin problems of AIDS and world poverty as security threats. Besides the attacks of September 11, pundits credit high profile *performers* with focusing the US federal government's attention on the issues of global health. These *players* on the global stage include such individuals as U2's Bono, Microsoft's Bill Gates, Pope John Paul II, and several transnational coalitions: the Global AIDS Alliance, Drop the Debt, Jubilee 2000, the Health Action AIDS Campaign and many more (Brainard 2002).

African Performance and the Struggle against AIDS

It is clear that the issues of globalization, Third World Debt and the AIDS crisis will be on the world agenda for the foreseeable future. The transnational

9. The argument for treatment is in their view, both moral and pragmatic. Activists say it is immoral to allow 35 million+ people to die without treatment because they come from countries too poor to purchase life-extending drugs for AIDS patients. Activists also argue that treatment options will normalize and de-stigmatize the disease. This will result in less denial, encourage more suspected HIV+ persons to come forward for testing, and help them to live responsibly. All this will lead to an ultimate decrease in the rate of infection.

activist groups, the INGOs, the Global Fund for AIDS, Malaria, and TB will keep the issue on the world agenda. Still many fear that the preoccupation of the Western world, particularly that of the U.S. with homeland security, will distract the attention of the rich. The wealthy nations need to focus on this epidemic that is killing not 3,000 in a one time attack, but more than 6,000 every day in sub-Saharan Africa, an epidemic that has already claimed 20 million lives (UNAIDS, 2002, July, Report).

In the upcoming struggles there is a clear role for Africans to play. Africans must organize their capacity for creating mesmerizing spectacles and put these to use in the struggle against AIDS. This volume proposes the idea of creating a master performance, perhaps a musical epic, performed (like many African rituals and African epics) over several days. The epic performance would express the multiple issues that surround the AIDS epidemic. This master ritual-spectacle would incorporate a wide range of African performance genres, both modern and traditional, both sacred and secular, both liminal and liminoid. The full epic would include sacred dances and secular pop stars, together with hymns and hype.[10]

Sacred portions of the proposed event would necessarily include a cadre of religious leaders representing the major world religions and African traditional religion. Prominent figures such as Archbishop Desmond Tutu and other well-respected Mainline church leaders would surely be asked to participate; as would Vimbeni Shembe, the current leader of the Nazarites (Shembe) of Southern Africa. So would the Dalai Lama. African traditional healers would figure prominently in the ritual. Among the sacred portions of the ritual/epic would be a ceremony honoring the world's millions who have died of AIDS. Miles of AIDS memorial quilt panels would be displayed. Those who have not participated in the quilt project could be enjoined to add their own commemoratives for their dead. Photographs of some the worlds famous who have succumbed to AIDS would be prominently hung in the performance space: Arthur Ashe, Freddie Mercury, Rock Hudson, Philly Lutaaya, Fela Kuti, Liberace, Ryan White, Nkosi Johnson, and so on. Those currently suffering from AIDS would also be asked to participate. Both the unwell in the later stages of the disease and the fit (like Magic Johnson) would be asked to be involved.

Major politicians would be also be invited. This would be a good opportunity for ex-presidents to become active once again on a world stage. The political cohort would be led by an African leader of stature: Nelson Mandela and Gracia Machel immediately come to mind.

To guarantee the interest of spectators unfamiliar with African performance and to make it suitable for a global age, the epic must include a sampling of Western and other world media celebrities. Such individuals would be invited to donate their time and talents for this endeavor.

The spectacle must necessarily also contain a number of variable passages where audiences would be enjoined to participate. With appropriate media fan-

10. Inspired by the success of the Live Aid concert of the 1980s, Red Hot AIDS charity has pledged to organize star-studded fund raisers for Aids work to be held at the Millennium Stadium in Cardiff, United Kingdom every two years. Such efforts represent the sort of spectacle/entertainment aspect of what is being proposed herein. They are a good beginning.

fare, the epic performers must converge upon a major international public meeting and perform the spectacle. They might choose the opening of the next World Cup Soccer tournament or the opening of the next Olympic games.

The spectacle, The African AIDS Epic, like other epics, must give ample opportunity for Africans to present themselves to the world through the media. Throughout the course of the years to come, abbreviated performances, parts of the African AIDS Epic, could be repeated at different venues such as AIDS international meetings, G7/G8 and World Trade Organization meetings, and forums organized by the United Nations. Sacred portions could be performed in churches, temples, and mosques and scared shrines around the world. Informative portions of the AIDS Epic could be repeated in schools for children. And some parts of the narrative could be designed for lawmakers and journalists. Other AIDS Epic components could be targeted at industry, featured at labor rallies, company picnics, and stockholder meetings. There would even be portions of the African AIDS Epic directed at major pharmaceutical corporations and lending agencies.

Who will create the master narrative, the African AIDS epic opera of the millennium? Perhaps a playwright such as Wole Soyinka could be enjoined to help out providing he agrees to invite the Yoruba gods to descend upon the performance space. Important healers from the continent would be asked to join the effort. Perhaps Stephen Spielberg would care to create the definitive AIDS spectacle that could expiate the North's collective guilt for its treatment of Black humankind. And surely creative Black women writers—Maya Angelou, Tony Morrison, Buchi Emecheta, and Tsitsi Dangaremba must help create the master spectacle. African pop stars, Youssouf N'Dour, Salif Keita, Oumou Sangaré, Oliver Mtukudzi and the like would share in the creative process. New talents, representative of Africa's youth must also be enjoined to participate in the proposed African AIDS Epic. Perhaps some of the young AIDS performance activists featured in this volume will take up the challenge. Thabo Mbeki's dream of an African Renaissance could surely be embodied in this production. And no doubt Mali's artists could contribute their impressive performance skills to such an endeavor. In this juncture, in this post-modern age, I prefer to leave open the authorship of the future master AIDS performance. But it's clear that if Africans can perform the plight of their AIDS epidemic on the world stage and get the North to participate, they can change hearts and minds.

In the 1950s, African peoples introduced text-bound Americans to political action through the performative process. The Civil Rights agenda became a movement through the demonstration of passive resistance and through active marching. The term "movement" came into use during that era, symbolizing political processes that were being unleashed through the power of people's bodies performing. And the Civil Rights Movement led to many shifts in the social landscape as several movements emerged in its wake: the anti-war movement, the women's movement, the Indian rights movement, the environmental movement, and so on. Ultimately the Civil Rights movement led to a change in the way people in the U.S. perceive reality. It led to post-modernism in the humanities and the social sciences, a digression from text-bound Eurocentric perspectives.

Today, African peoples are engaged in a new struggle. As we have seen, they have a formidable array of performance tools. Africans must find a way to create an African AIDS Epic and to perform it, not once but several times, for a planetary audience. This volume challenges creative African peoples everywhere to come together to Play for Life. When they do, the ancestors will surely join them on the world stage and usher in a transformation.

Performance troupe Eager Artists represents some of South Africa's finest new post-apartheid theatrical talent. The group was founded in 1993 by Jerry Pooe, a playwright, librettist, choreographer, and producer-director. Born in Soweto, Pooe was moved to rural KwaZulu-Natal at 16 by his mother who wished to deliver him from township violence so that he could develop his writing. By the age of 17 he had written his first play.

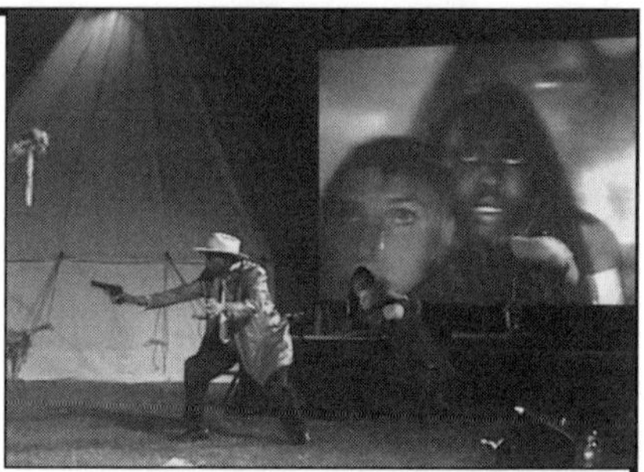

Since 1993, Eager Artists have performed more than 12 different original plays. They have performed throughout South Africa as well as in Canada and the United States. The troupe's leader, Jerry Pooe, said he founded the group in order to bring a new kind of theatre to the South African stage. If apartheid theatre was created to move people to activism, post-apartheid is about a new kind of consciousness. "In protest, we agitated the audience, now we need to calm them down," insists Pooe. Done in the style of the Black township musical, Pooe's plays have addressed such issues as South African history, township violence, health, and AIDS. Very committed to social change, Eager Artists conduct playmaking workshops and sensitivity groups on a number of social issues. These include human rights, gender violence, electoral fairness, and the HIV/AIDS pandemic. In 2002, Eager Artists teamed up with *Het Waterhuis* of Rotterdam, Netherlands. Within this partnership, the two groups produced "Free Birds," a performance that uses multi-media techniques to spread messages surrounding the issues of HIV/AIDS, especially sexism, high risk lifestyles, and the need for tolerance for those infected with HIV. The performance has been described as a hymn to life, love, and mourning. The photographs featured here are scenes from "Free Birds," performed at the Curries Fountain Stadium, Durban, South Africa in July 2002. "Free Birds" was also featured in the 2002 Grahamstown Theatre Festival in South Africa's Eastern Cape Province. In 2003, Eager Artists and Het Waterhuis are scheduled to tour the Netherlands and Germany presenting their co-production, "Free Birds."

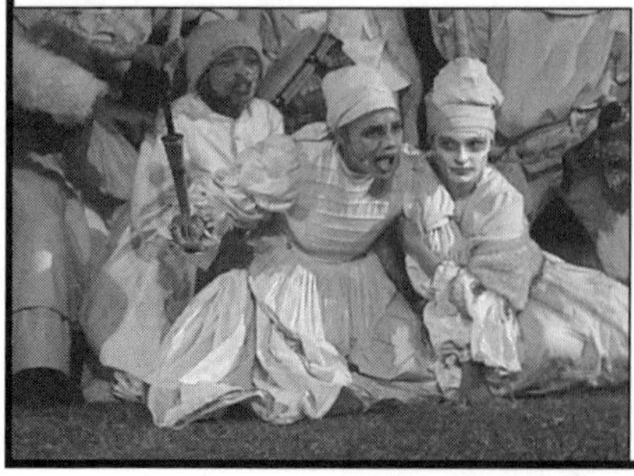

Figure 9-9. Scenes from 'Free Birds,' a bi-national theatrical extravaganza addressing the AIDS issue.

Review Questions

1. How do Turner and Schechner's discussions of liminal genres aid us in understanding the role of ritual in social change? In which ways and under which conditions can performances in Africa be considered liminal genres?
2. What is participatory methodology? How does it function to bring about social change?
3. What is the nature of the proposed African AIDS Epic? How should it be designed and organized to work for global awareness of the AIDS pandemic and ultimately a decrease in the world's number of cases of HIV/AIDS?

Glossary

Abron: A West African ethnic group inhabiting areas of Cote d'Ivoire, Ghana, and Burkina Faso that are part of the Akan ethnic groups.

Action Research: A style of evaluative research wherein the evaluator is engaged in an ongoing dialog with the recipients of communication interventions, i.e., one in which the evaluator critically inserts him/herself into a social process of change rather than standing dispassionately outside to evaluate given media products.

Age graders: A social grouping comprising a fellowship of peers of the same age and gender who have undergone initiation rituals together.

Age of Enlightenment: (Also called the Age of Reason), a period of history initiated at the end of the seventeenth century by a group of intellectuals who attempted to popularize the ideas of the Scientific Revolution by applying theories from the natural sciences to human behavior.

Agonistic: Of or relating to aggressive behavior; a defensive social interaction (such as fighting, fleeing, or submitting) between individuals.

AIDS: Acquired Immunodeficiency Syndrome, a set of symptoms that indicate that a person has become infected by a retrovirus called HIV that seriously damages the body's immune system. The retrovirus attacks the body's T-cells (lymphocytes). A key symptom is the development of one or more of a range of 'opportunistic' infections that attack when the immune system has been weakened. HIV is introduced into the body through the exchange of bodily fluids or blood products.

Apartheid: The official doctrine that formally institutionalized a rigid social and political system that segregated and discriminated South African people on the basis of race, and enforced a program of separate development. In South Africa, this system was the official policy of the White minority government from 1948-1994.

Ashanti: One of Ghana's largest ethnic groups concentrated in south-central Ghana. The Ashanti are part of the Akan ethnic group; their language is known as Asante or Twi.

Ashanti/Asante: A pre-colonial West African empire located in present-day Ghana. The Ashanti Empire was influential over other peoples in the region and was heavily involved in the 18th century slave trade. As the Ashanti expanded they engaged in persistent clashes with the British colonial powers until the Ashanti were finally annexed by the British into the Gold Coast in 1902.

Aurature: See orature

Bard: A poet-singer skilled in composing, reciting, and singing verses on heroes and their deeds.

Bikutsi: Fast and furious dance/music from southeast Cameroon. From "*biku*," (to thump) and "*tsi*," (the ground). The lyrics of *bikutsi* music always incorporate political controversy, social debate, and sex and have a reputation for being pornographic.

Bi-lateral Aid: Aid agreements made between two countries, one the recipient and the other, a donor country.

Boer (Dutch for farmer): An early White settler of South Africa who made a living as a semi-nomadic farmer and rancher. May also be called an Afrikaner. Can also refer to the descendents of these settlers.

Clientism: A social system characterized by unequal relations in which the superior, or patron, provides benefits in the form of financial resources or physical security to the inferior, or client, who is in return expected to offer respect and obedience to the patron. The relationship is also referred to as a "patron-client" relationship. The system is also called a system of "patronage."

Cold War: The conflict over ideological differences between the United States and the Soviet Union that existed between 1945 to 1989 and that divided much of the rest of the world into two camps aligned with either side. The conflict was carried on by methods short of sustained overt military action usually while continuing to maintain diplomatic relations.

Colonialism: The policy of officially occupying and governing a territory by a foreign power through a combination of invasion, partition, and conquest.

Communitas: A profound experience of social solidarity, equality, and community that arises in participants of ritual as they undergo a group experience that is outside the boundaries of everyday life.

Counter-Reformation: The reform movement in the Roman Catholic Church in seventeenth century Europe resulting from and responding to the Protestant Reformation's ascetic style. The Counter-Reformation in Europe emphasized the importance of flamboyant dramatic style in music, art, and architecture, all in order to restore mystery to the church experience. The collection of styles from the Counter-Reformation period are known as Baroque.

Coup d'etat: The sudden and forceful overthrow of a government by way of force by a small unrepresentative group.

Cult: A small circle of persons united by devotion or allegiance to a particular religious figure, spirit, totem, artistic tradition, or intellectual movement.

Dahomey Kingdom: A precolonial West African kingdom located in present-day Benin, West Africa. The Dahomey Kingdom became powerful through its involvement with the 18th and 19th century Atlantic slave trade.

Diaspora (African): The scattering of the peoples of African origin into other parts of the world. The African diaspora resulted largely from the slave trade and more recently from economic migration and the "brain drain."

Divination: The art or practice that seeks to foresee or foretell the future; to discover hidden knowledge; to offer explanations of misfortune; and to identify of preventative measures to be taken against conflict, misery, and illness usually by the interpretation of omens or by the aid of supernatural power and unusual insight.

Diviner: A person with instinctive foresight who assumes the role of mediating communication between other-worldly spirits and earthly clients

Djeli (See Griot): A Mande bard or griot of West Africa whose present-day role is to maintain family histories and traditions. Historically, the griots served the kings of the great empires by acting as praise-singers, advisers, and spokespeople.

Dagoma (Dagomba): The largest ethnic group in the northern region of Ghana occupying the east-central territory and parts of Togo. The Dagoma speak Dagbani and trace their heritage back to the Mossi-Dagamba kingdoms of the medieval period in West Africa.

Drama: Literary work that tells a story and can be performed through the use of dialogue and actions.

Edutainment (Entertainment-Education): A media product or message resulting from an attempt to combine education and entertainment in order to increase audience awareness of a social issue, to influence attitudes, and to change behaviors.

Efe: A masquerade performance of the Yoruba people of West Africa that consists of buffoonery, joking, or play, even though it may also have a serious purpose. Efe is performed primarily at night

ELISA: (Enzyme-Linked Immunosorbent Assay). A blood test that indicates the presence of antibodies in response to a specific antigen. Various ELISA tests are used to detect a variety of infections. The ELISA test for HIV indicates only that a viral infection has occurred.

Epic: A long poetic tale, usually centered upon a legendary or historical hero, that covers a great deal of time, and a multitude of events and achievements, and is narrated in an elevated style.

Epidemiology: The branch of medicine that studies the prevalence, distribution, and control of epidemic disease in large populations.

Ethnography: The description and interpretation of human social groupings, accomplished through a variety of data collection methods, the most important of which is participant observation.

Explanatory tale: A narrative that serves to explain and account for the origin of events and experiences in a culture.

Fable: A fictitious story used to teach moral lessons or to enforce a useful truth, usually in which animals speak and act like human beings.

FGC (Female Genital Cutting): The collective name given to the practices that involve partial or total cutting away of the female external genitalia for non-therapeutic reasons. Also referred to as "Female Circumcision," Female Genital Excision, or "Female Genital Mutilation," the last being a more inclusive term. The procedure involves at least three clinically distinct kinds of surgery. The *sunna* alters the prepuce of the clitoris; *excision* removes the clitoris and parts of the labia minora; and *infibulation* excises the clitoris and the labia minora, and then sutures together the remaining labia majora.

FGM: (Female Genital Mutilation). A collection of practices that involve partial or total cutting away of the female external genitalia for non-therapeutic reasons and or practices that involve the introduction of foreign substances into the vaginal cavity purportedly to alter the vaginal mucosa for non-therapeutic reasons. See FGC.

Flow: Self-induced transformation that occurs within the course of performance whereby the performer fully merges with the experience.

Forum Theatre: A collection of theatrical techniques designed to conscientize oppressed people concerning their social, political, and economic situation and then to empower them through performance so as to alter their life situation. This approach was first implemented by playwright Augusto Boal in Latin America as a means of educating peasant farmers.

Formative Evaluation/Formative Research: Research or evaluation conducted as an ongoing part of an information campaign aimed at ensuring that messages are appropriately constructed to meet changing audience needs, understandings, and interpretations.

Fulani: Pastoral people living in communities throughout West Africa occupying parts of Senegal, Gambia, Guinea, Mali, Burkina Faso, Niger, Nigeria, and Cameroon. The Fulani are the only cattle-raising people of West Africa. Also known as Pulaar, Peulh or Fula.

Ghana Empire: An early kingdom (700 –1200 A.D.) of the western Sudan including present day Mali and southeastern Mauritania. Trade in gold and slaves with the Arabs to the north in exchange for salt led to the apex of the empire's power, as well as its decline from competition by the end of the 11th century A.D.

Globalization: The process of denationalization of a country's markets, labor, political and legal systems, and the rise of the global economy, greatly facilitated by supranational trade organizations and treaties such as the North American Free Trade Agreement (NAFTA), the European Union (EU), and the World Trade Organization (WTO). In the humanities, globalization refers to the process whereby individual lives and communities are affected by economic and cultural forces that operate world-wide.

GDP (Gross Domestic Product): Annual value of all goods and services produced in an economy, plus income earned by residents outside the country, minus incomes accruing to foreign residents of the country.

GNP (Gross National Product): The total monetary value of all goods and services produced in a country in one year.

Grand Narrative: The notion of a universal truth or totality, which has been derived from scientific principles, and which can be applied to whole populations.

Great Trek: A massive northern and eastern exodus in ox-drawn covered wagons of thousands of Afrikaners (Boers) that took place in South Africa in the 1830s. The *voortrekkers* moved out from the Cape Colony of South Africa in response to the British annexation of the colony and to the abolition of slavery.

Griot: (Djeli): A West African, caste-based professional hereditary musician-oral historian. Probably a frenchification of a local African term. Male griot, female griotte.

Hausa: An ethnic group of northern Nigeria and southern Niger with a reputation for astute trading. The Hausa are well known for their political organization derived from ancient Hausa city states of 1000 to 1800 A.D.

HIV (Human Immunodefficiency Virus): A variable retrovirus that invades and impairs the body's T-cells of the immune system and is the cause of AIDS.

Homeland: A region created and designated by the government for a particular race or ethnic group. In Apartheid South Africa, a homeland referred to one of 10 ethnic territories set aside for the exclusive use of Black Africans. Four homelands became "independent" between 1976 and 1981. All homelands were reabsorbed into South Africa under the constitution of 1994.

Horon: A social grouping in the Mande society of West Africa made up of nobles who engage in farming, governance, and military activities

HDI (Human Development Index): A multidimensional scale developed by the United Nations Development Program to distinguish between levels of development, as defined by the variety and value of options available to people for shaping their own destinies.

Ideophone: An idea in sound, i.e., a word whose sound, in the context of an oral performance, conveys the event, object, or being to which the word refers.

Igbo: One of the three major ethnic groups of Nigeria who inhabit the southeastern part of the country. Historically known for having mastered the arts of metalwork, weaving, and woodcarving. The Igbo have a non-centralized political and social organization in which age-grade associations, elders, and title-holders play important political functions.

Imbongi: A Zulu poet who composes and recites court praises.

IMF (International Monetary Fund): An international agency originally founded in 1944, that oversees the "credit worthiness" of nations and determines terms for loans. In this capacity, it has forced most African countries to accept Structural Adjustment Programs. (See below).

INGO (International Non-Governmental Organization): An organization founded to address a single or a related group of issues broadly concerned with human development and welfare on a global scale. The organization is comprised of a body of volunteers together with some paid staff who function according to the organizations own constitution. INGOs typically form linkages with local and national NGOs in the countries where they operate.

Inyanga: A traditional Zulu naturopath, herbalist, or pharmacist who treats illness and misfortune using naturally occurring substances, mostly plant-based.

Isangoma: A traditional Zulu diviner, part psychologist, part healer, who through the use of herbs, roots, barks, snakeskin, dried animal parts, and so on, is able to communicate with the spirit world in order to diagnose illness, find lost objects, ferret out unsociable individuals, and ward off evil for the community or on behalf of a client.

Isicathamiya: A creative twentieth century South African a capella call and response singing style accompanied by a dance form that fuses Western dance elements with Zulu men's team dance styles. The style became recognized worldwide after the release of Paul Simon's Graceland album with its acclaimed *isicathamiya* group Ladysmith Black Mambazo.

Izimbongo: Zulu court praises recited by a court poet known as an *imbongi*. The genre has been adopted to serve many popular struggles, notably the AIDS crisis.

Jùjú music: A 20th century form of popular music that originated as street music in Yorubaland in southwestern Nigeria and uses electrified guitar/banjo, tambourine, and traditional instruments such as *dùndún* (talking drum) and *sèkèrè* (a netted bottle-gourd rattle). Jùjú is rooted in the tradition of singing about social and cultural issues through the use of parables and proverbs.

Kamba: A Bantu-speaking ethnic group of Kenya and Tanzania. The Kamba maintain agricultural plots, keep livestock, and trade their crafts for subsistence.

Khoi Khoi: An ethnic cluster of Khoisan-speaking pastoral groups of Southern Africa who base their livelihood on herding cattle and foraging in Southern Africa. Khoi Khoi may also be referred to as Khoe Khoe, Khoi, or by the derogatory name Hottentot.

Khoisan: A linguistic term referring to the family of languages spoken primarily in Southern Africa that make use of click consonants. The languages are spoken by the San foragers and the Khoi Khoi pastoralists.

Kòtèba: An unmasked theatrical form of entertainment popular among the Bamanan people of central Mali originally performed by a young all male cast who used humor and irony to mock societal quirks and social transgressions.

Kwaito: A genre of South African pop music deriving from township jive that integrates performance aspects of rap and hip hop with techno instrumentation and beat. Kwaito is thought to be reflective of life in the crowded Black townships of South Africa.

Legend: A story, or set of related stories, passed down from earlier times, often by word of mouth, associated with admirable people or events believed to be true although not historically verifiable.

Levirate marriage: The custom of marriage between a man and his brother's widow required under certain circumstances in certain African societies.

Liminal: Existing in an ambiguous social position.

Lingua franca: A language that serves as a means of communication among speakers whose native tongues differ. Swahili, Hausa, and Pidgin English are widely used in Africa as lingua franca.

Mali Empire: A West African kingdom that was located along the upper Niger River. The Mali Empire flourished between the thirteenth and sixteenth centuries by trading gold and produce and probably rose to prominence in the wake of the collapse of the Ghana Empire.

Mande: A West African linguistic group belonging to the larger Niger-Congo language family. The Mande dialects are found throughout the region of the upper Niger River and the Atlantic coast of West Africa. The term Mande is also a cultural term used to describe a number of related groups who absorbed the culture and values of the Mali Empire.

Masai: An ethnic group of Kenya and Tanzania who live as semi-nomadic pastoralists. Masai men have a reputation for being fierce warriors who effectively defend their stock and may even raid the stock of others.

Masquerade: A form of dramatic ritual enactment or entertainment used in conjunction with dance and mime whereby spirits are called up and/or characters and atmosphere are created through the use of fantastic costumes, masks, and disguises.

Mfecane ("the crushing"): The early-nineteenth-century period of warfare and forced migration throughout Southern Africa resulting from the rise of the Zulu King Shaka's campaign for conquest and expansion together with European colonial settlement and capitalism.

Middle Ages: An era of European history between ancient and modern times, around 500 A.D. to 1400 A.D.

Migrancy: A form of labor mobility in which workers and their families are dependent on both wage earnings and subsistence production to make ends meet. Migrancy typically involves the separation of family members, often husband and wife, one of whom leaves the farm in search of paid employment, the other who remains behind to tend the crops.

Misogynistic: Of, or relating to, a hatred and distrust of women.

Modern Western Period: An historical period dating roughly from 1500-2000 A.D. which based its notions of reality on written, text-based, and scientifically codified knowledge. The Modern Period was socially and intellectually estranged from the spirit world, folk art, folk wisdom, and common law.

Multilateral Aid: Aid channeled through international agencies (usually agencies of the United Nations) rather than from a single donor country.

Neo-Pentecostalism: A broad-based Christian religious movement of the middle and late 20th century whose focus, like that of early 20th century US Pentecostalism, is on salvation and on the receipt of charismatic gifts, but whose emphasis includes modernistic prosperity theology, and positive thinking. Neo-Pentecostalism is interested in world-wide expansion, and uses mass media widely in the dissemination of its messages.

NGO (Non-Governmental Organization): An organization founded to address a single or a related group of issues broadly concerned with human development and welfare on a national or local scale. An NGO is comprised of a body of volunteers together with some paid staff who function according to the organization's own constitution. An NGO in a given country often provides on-the-ground assistance to a sister international organization, an INGO with similar philosophy, objectives, and modes of operation.

Ngoni: A plucked lute instrument used in most parts of West Africa. The number of strings and size varies.

Nguni: A subdivision of the Niger-Congo language family. This term is commonly used to refer to ethnic groups, such as Zulu, Xhosa, and Swazi, who speak related Bantu languages and inhabit Southern Africa.

Nyamakala: A social grouping in the Mande society of West Africa made up of hereditary specialized artisans and griots who worked with spiritually charged materials including metal, especially iron, leather, music, and words.

Onomatopoeia: The naming of a thing or action by a vocal imitation of the sound associated with it such as "boom" or "buzz."

Orality: The quality or state of living in a world in which one's cultural heritage and human experience is passed down to succeeding generations by word of mouth, rather than by the written word.

Orature/Aurature: The process of orally transmitting cultural heritage, human experience, insights, and customs to successive generations. Orature is a practice that stores knowledge and information in the individual and collective memories of members of a society, as opposed to storing them in written texts housed in a library. Also, the collective body of orally transmitted cultural heritage.

Paradigm Shift: A sweeping change in patterns of thinking or ways of seeing the world.

Parastatals: Companies or agencies established by governments and allowed to operate semi-autonomously in a designated commercial or service field. Examples might include a state telecommunication company, a state power company, and a state airline.

Parallelism: A speaking or writing technique that structurally arranges and coordinates sentences, paragraphs, ideas, and images so as to balance them in terms of meaning and rhythm.

Participatory Methodologies: Methodologies used for the purpose of engaging an audience in the creation of a message. Communication strategies in which the consumers of a message are also the producers of that message and therefore assume ownership of it.

Patriarchy: A system of social organization in which descent, succession, and family rule are traced through the male line.

Performance: The intentional use of the human body by a human actor in a series of structured actions designed to create meaning for a community of participants or spectators.

Pentecostalism: Of or relating to Christian religious bodies that emphasize revivalistic worship, salvation, charmismatic gifts of the Holy Spirit, especially glossalia, and premillennial teaching. Early 20th century US Pentecostalism also preached a strict code of moral and ethical behavior that required sect-like avoidance of the wider secular world.

Polygamy: Marriage in which a spouse of either sex may have more than one mate at a time.

Polygyny: The state or practice of a man having more than one wife or female mate at a time.

Post-Modernism: A movement in art or literature that is a reaction against modern theory's emphasis on rationality and a unitary world-view. Post-modernism denies that there is one over-arching reality or a single truth. Rather, post-modernism favors a focus on fragments of human experience and bits of reality, including apparently 'non-rational elements of human life, such as emotion and play.

Pronatal (Pro-natalist): In favor of reproduction and birth. Likely to adopt policies aimed at maintaining high birth rates or increasing fertility.

Protestant Reformation: A reform movement of sixteenth century Europe that aimed to cleanse the Roman Catholic Church of its then-perceived artistic and ritual excesses. The movement resulted in the rejection or modification of many Roman Catholic practices and the establishment of Protestant Churches.

Redressive: Compensatory or avenging action for wrongdoing; making or exacting reparation or healing.

Retrovirus: Viruses that contain RNA and use an enzyme known as reverse transcriptase to produce a DNA analog of their RNA.

Rites of Passage: Rituals associated with major changes in one's social status, condition, or age.

Ritual: A socially established and symbolically significant procedure observed and performed with regularity and in a set manner.

Ritual View of Communication: A view of communication that sees communication in terms of sharing information, of social participation, of fellowship, and of possession of a common faith, culture, or set of values.

San: A term encompassing several Southern African Khoisan-speaking societies who traditionally lived primarily by hunting and gathering. May also be referred to as Bushmen, although this term is considered to be derogatory and sexist.

Schistosomiasis (bilharzia): A disease caused by the blood fluke (Schistosome) whose larvae enter through the skin of persons standing or swimming in an infected pond or stream. The young flukes travel in the bloodstream to the liver where they mature, causing anemia and problems of the urinary tract.

Scientific Revolution: A period of history established by a small group of scholars during the seventeenth century who created a new scientific view of the universe and laid the foundation for the modern sciences. It was not until the Enlightenment period that the ideas of the Scientific Revolution were popularized and widely spread.

Sect: A dissenting or schismatic religious body, especially one regarded as extreme or heretical; a group, usually religious, adhering to a distinctive doctrine or to a distinctive leader.

Seropositivity: Showing a significant level of serum antibodies indicating previous exposure to the infectious agent being tested.

Shaka: A nineteenth Southern African warrior chief of the Zulu kingdom who introduced new fighting tactics and campaigns of expansion and conquest against neighboring Black African groups and Europeans, notably the British, who were infiltrating their lands in eastern South Africa.

Shona: An ethno-linguistic group located in southeastern Africa in the present-day countries of Zimbabwe and Mozambique.

Simian Immunodeficiency Virus (SIV): A virus that is closely related to the HIV retrovirus that infects African apes and monkeys.

Sororate Marriage: The custom of marriage with a wife's sister, following the wife's death.

Soweto (South-western townships): A collection of famous South African townships near Johannesburg and one of the largest urban areas in Southern Africa. Historically known as the center for the massive uprisings opposing Apartheid. Today, it is one of the largest urban areas in Southern Africa.

Stone Age: The earliest period of prehistoric human culture characterized by the use of stone tools dating back in Africa some two million years.

Structural Adjustment Programs (SAP): A package of reforms, designed by the IMF and World Bank to remedy the perceived structural flaws in the economies of developing nations and to restore their economic health through reforms that devalue currency, reduce public sector expenditure, and strengthen market forces.

Summative Research: A final evaluation of a media or communication project, one which addresses the successes and failures of a project and which usually makes recommendations for further or alternative communication interventions.

Sundiata Keita: Founder and ruler of the Mande Empire, (also known as the Mali Empire) in West Africa. After defeating the Susu group of the Soninke clan, Sundiata rose to power and established a centralized monarchy enabling him to control the region's trade routes and gold fields

Talking Drum: A West African hourglass-shaped drum used to imitate the tones of spoken language.

Tonal: Of or relating to the importance of tone in the determination of meaning of specific morphemes or units in language.

Toyi-toyi: A creative South African dance historically used for protest during the liberation struggle against Apartheid.

Trekboers: Adventurous European pioneers who moved away from the Cape colony from the beginning of the 18th century and who settled the interior of South Africa, competing with the Khoisan and Nguni-speaking peoples for farming and grazing land

Transportation View of Communication: A view or theory of communication that uses a metaphor of geography, defining communication as the sending or transmission of signals or messages across space and time, often for the implied purpose of control.

Tribe: A loose collection of people united by ties of language and culture and descent from a perceived common ancestor. Closely associated with the colonial era, the notion of tribe is today perceived to have reified differences among colonized peoples. Those who oppose the term charge that colonial powers exaggerated the importance of ethnicity among African people and sometimes falsely or incorrectly assigned groups to specific geographical territories. For these reasons, the term tribe is out of favor among African scholars who consider it to be politically incorrect and culturally misleading.

Trickle Down: The assumed gradual spread of development from large national urban centers, particularly capital or port cities, to the agricultural hinterlands, and from relatively economically well off people to the less fortunate in the developing world, including Africa. Trickle down has been a major theory underlying capitalism in the Western world and the development aid given by the West to the developing world and Africa from 1960 until the mid 1980s.

United States Agency for International Development (USAID): An agency of the federal government of the United States that provides economic, development, and humanitarian assistance around the world in support of the foreign policy goals of the U.S.

UNAIDS (United Nations Joint Programme on HIV/AIDS): A joint program of the United Nations created in 1996 to help meet the challenge of the HIV/AIDS pandemic. In 1996 UNAIDS consisted of UNICEF (United Nations Children's Fund); the UNDP (United Nations Development Programme); UNFPA (United Nations Fund for Population Activities); the UNESCO (United Nations Educational, Scientific, and Cultural Organization); the WHO (World Health Organization); and the World Bank. The joint programme was joined in 1999 by the UNDCP (United Nations Drug Control Program) and in 2000 by the ILO (the International Labor Organization).

Voortrekker: Afrikaner pioneers who migrated from the Cape colony at the tip of South Africa north and east in search of new land and in flight from British rule at the time of the Great Trek.

Widow cleansing: A Southern African custom among some ethnic groups wherein a widow must engage in sexual intercourse with a designated person in the community, sometimes a member of the husband's family, so as to expunge the spirit of the deceased from the wife or to ward off evil.

World Bank: Established in 1944 at the same time as the IMF, the World Bank, (originally the International Bank for Reconstruction and Development) aims to assist member states in their development efforts with the provision of loans and technical assistance.

Xhosa: An ethnic group of South Africa who depend on farming and migrant labor as their livelihood. The majority of Xhosa inhabit the Eastern Cape Province of South Africa.

Yaka: A Bantu-speaking ethnic group of west Central Africa inhabiting parts of Democratic Republic of the Congo and Angola.

Zhem: An important and sacred drum dance that is performed by drummers of the Dagoma people of northeastern Ghana to signify very significant occasions such as the induction or a funeral of a Chief. *Zehm* uses a secret drum language and can only be played after drummers have performed appropriate rituals.

Zulu: The largest ethnic group in South Africa, concentrated in the Province of KwaZulu-Natal. Traditionally, the Zulu people cultivated grains and kept cattle, which became an important symbol of wealth.

References

"Abuse of Women Escalates HIV Infections in Africa." n.d. Retrieved June 10, 2001, from http://www.afrol.com/Categories/Women/backgr_abuse_aids.htm.

Act Up. n.d. Retrieved July 2001, from http://tensegrity.critpath.org/actup/index.html

AFP. 2000. 14 September. "Mbeki told to come clean on AIDS policy." Retrieved September 6, 2001, from http://www/mg.co.za/mg/za/arhive/2000sep/14sep-news.html.

"Africa Action," Africa Policy Electronic Distribution List: An Information Service Provided by Africa Action, incorporating the Africa Policy Information Center, the Africa Fund, and the American Committee on Africa, 2002, 25 March. Retrieved March 25, 2002, from http://www.africaaction.org.

"Africa Action," Africa Policy Electronic Distribution List: An Information Service Provided by Africa Action, incorporating the Africa Policy Information Center, the Africa Fund, and the American Committee on Africa. 2002, 27 March. Retrieved March 27, 2002, from http://www.africaaction.org.

"Africa Action," Africa Policy Electronic Distribution List: An Information Service Provided by Africa Action, incorporating the Africa Policy Information Center, the Africa Fund, and the American Committee on Africa. 2002, 6 July. Retrieved July 7, 2002, from http://www.africaaction.org.

Africa in Figures. 1998. Retrieved June 1, 2001, from http://www.un.org/Depts/eca/newweb/html/africa-in-figures.htm.

Africa-Dance Rhythms from Algeria to Zimbabwe. 2001. Compact Disk. London: World Music Network with Oxfam and New Internationalist.

African National Congress. 1994. *The Reconstruction and Development Programme*. Johannesburg, South Africa: Umanyano Publications.

Africa Policy Information Center. 1998. "Africa's Debt." Background Paper 12 (December). Washington, D.C.: Africa Policy Information Center.

Ahlberg, Beth Maina. 1993. "Is There a Distinct African Sexuality?" Department of International Health Research (IHCAR). Stockholm, Sweden: Karolinska Institute and Uppsala University.

AIDS Analysis Africa. 2000. 10, 6 (Apr./May): 9.

AIDS Analysis Africa. 2001a. "Open Secret: People Facing Up to HIV and AIDS in Uganda." *Aids Analysis Africa* 11, 5 (Feb./Mar.): 2.

AIDS Analysis Africa. 2001b. "Drug Availability in Botswana and the HIV prevalence increases." *Aids Analysis Africa* 11, 6 (Apr./May): 9.

AIDS Analysis Africa. 2001c. "2000 South Africa Sero Prevalence Results." *Aids Analysis Africa* 11, 6 (Apr./May): 3.

AIDS Analysis Africa. 2001d. "The Port of Durban and its Role in the Spread of HIV in KwaZulu-Natal." 2001. *Aids Analysis Africa* 11, 6 (Apr./May): 6–7.

"AIDS at 20: Timeline of Events." 2001. *Newsday*, 29 May. Retrieved May 30, 2001, from http://www.newsday.com/coverage/current/news/Tuesday/nd3124.htm.

"AIDS Control/AIDS in Mali-Djeli Daouda, the Highway Troubadour." 2000, 4 Sept. Retrieved May 31, 2001, from http://www.acdi-cida.gc.ca/cida_ind.nsf/vLUall.

Alland, Jr., Alexander. 1990. *When the Spider Danced: Notes from an African Village*. Prospect Heights, Ill.: Waveland Press.

Ajayi, Omofolabo S. 1998. *Yoruba Dance: The Semiotics of Movement and Body Attitude in a Nigerian Culture*. Trenton, N.J.: Africa World Press.

Alder, M; S. Foster; H. Grosskurth; J. Richens; H. Slavin. 1998. *Sexual health and health Care*: Sexually *Transmitted Infections: Guidelines for Prevention and Treatment*. 2nd ed. London: International Family Health & Department for International Development.

Amankulor, J. Ndukaku. 1993. "English Language Drama and Theater." In *A History of Twentieth-Century African Literatures*, ed. Oyekan Owomoyela, 138–172. Lincoln and London: University of Nebraska Press.

Amankulor, J. Ndukaku. 1997. "Jerzy Grotowski's Divination Consultation." In *The Grotowski Sourcebook*, ed. Richard Schechner and Lisa Wolford, 356–364. London & New York: Routledge.

Amin, Samir. 1990. *Maldevelopment*. London: Zed Press.

Amon, Jospeh. 2001. Plan International Mali STD/AIDS Project Final Evaluation Report. Bamako, Mali. Unpublished Report.

Apter, Andrew. 1993. "Attinga Revisited: Yoruba Witchcraft and the Cocoa Economy." In *Modernity and its Malcontents: Ritual and Power in Postcolonial Africa*, ed. Jean Comaroff and John Comaroff, 111–128. Chicago and London: University of Chicago Press.

Arens, W. and Ivan Karp, eds. 1989. *Creativity of Power: Cosmology and Action in African Societies*. Washington, D.C.: Smithsonian Institution Press.

Bascon, William. 1972. "African Dilemma Tales: An Introduction." In *African Folklore*, ed. Richard Dorson, 143–155. Garden City, New York: Anchor Books.

Bebey, Francis. 1969. *African Music: A People's Art*. Trans. Josephine Bennett. Westport, Conn.: Lawrence Hill and Co.

van Beek, Walter and Thomas Blakely. 1994. "Introduction." In *Religion in Africa: Experience and Expression*, ed. Walter van Beek and Thomas Blakely, 1–20. Portsmouth, N.H.: Heineman; London: James Currey.

Begho, Felix. 1996. "Traditonal African Dance in Context." In *African Dance: An Artistic, Historical and Philosophical Inquiry*, ed. Kariamu Welsh Asante, 163–182. Trenton, N.J: African World Press.

Bellman, Beryl. 1984. *The Language of Secrecy: Symbols and Metaphors in Poro Ritual*. New Brunswick, N. J.: Rutgers University Press.

Bilodeau, Dennis, Coordinator, Information and Communication, USAID, Bamako, Mali. 2000 & 2001. Personal Communication.

Bird, Charles. 1972. "Heroic Songs of the Mande Hunters." In *African Folklore*, ed. Richard Dorson, 275–295. Garden City, New York: Anchor Books.

Boal, Augusto. 1979. *Theater of the Oppressed*. Trans. Charles and Maria-Odilia Lead McBride. New York: Urizen Books.

Booker Salih and William Minter. 2001. "Global Apartheid." *The Nation*, 273 (2): 11–12; 14–16.

Bourgault, Louise M. 1989. Unpublished Field Notes from a Gola-Kpelle Village in Liberia.

Bourgault, Louise. 1991. "Village Based Drama for Development in Africa." *Journal of Development Communication* 2, 2 (December): 49–73.

Bourgault, Louise M. 1995. *Mass Media in Sub-Saharan Africa*. Bloomington: Indiana University Press.

Bourgault, Louise M. 1996. "Television Drama in Hausaland: the Search for a New Ethic and a New Aesthetic." *Critical Arts* 10 (1): 61–84.

Bourgault, Louise M. 1998. *Manuel de Radio Rurale*. Bamako, Mali: USAID/US Peace Corps. Risographed.

Brainard, Lael. 2002, June 26. "With Help from the Famous, Foreign Aid Resurges." Retrieved August 2, 2002, from http://www/brook.edu/view/oped/brainard/20020626.htm.

Brand, Saskia. 2001. *Mediating Means and Fate: A Socio-Political Analysis of Fertility and Demographic Change in Bamako, Mali.* Leiden, Netherlands: Brill.

Braun, Kwame. 2000. "Picture This: Video Artists as Researchers in Ghana." Video presentation and talk presented at the 43rd Annual Meeting of the African Studies Association. Nashville, Tessessee. November.

Bread for the World Institute. 1994. Hunger 1995: Causes of Hunger, 5th Annual Report on the State of World Hunger. Silver Springs, Md. Bread for the World Institute.

British Broadcasting Corporation. 2001. World Service. 21 July. Radio News Broadcast.

Brooke, Pamela. 1989. "Adapting Village Drama to Radio." A Report presented to the Institute for International Research. Monrovia, Liberia. Unpublished paper.

Brown, Duncan. 1998. *Voicing the Text: South African Oral Poetry and Performance.* Cape Town, South Africa: Oxford University Press.

Brümmer, Stefaans and Sam Sole. 2002. "The ANC's Virodene Backers." *Mail and Guardian* (Johannesburg) 5–11 July, 2–3.

Burke, James. 1991. "Communication in the Middle Ages." In *Communication in History: Technology, Culture, Society*, ed. David Crowley and Paul Heyer, 67–77. New York: Longman.

Byabarumwanzi, F. 2001. "*Point de vue d'un homme.*" *SAFCO, Aids in West and Central Africa* (Abidjan, Côte d'Ivoire), 1 (Jan.–Mar.): 7.

Cameron, Joan and Karen Rawlings Anderson. 1998. "Circumcision, Culture, and Health-care Provision in Tower Hamlets, London." In *Gender and Development: Violence Against Women*, 48–54. Oxford, U.K.: Oxford University Press.

Campbell, Catherine. 1997. Migrancy, Masculine Identities and AIDS: The Psychological Context of HIV Transmission on the South African Gold Mines. Social *Science and Medicine* 45, (2): 273–281.

Campbell, Catherine and B. Williams. 1995. Mineworkers Perceptions of Health and Illness: A Pilot Study. In *Epidemiology Research Unit Report Series*, 32. Johannesburg, South Africa: Epidemiology Research Unit.

Campbell, Susan. 1998. *Called to Heal.* Epping, Ill.: Zebra Press.

Carey, James. 1975. Review of *The Interpretation of Cultures*: Selected Essays by Clifford Geertz. *Communication Research* 2 (April): 129–137.

"Catastrophic impact could be substantially reduced with relatively modest contribution from the developed nations." 2000–2001. *Aids Analysis Africa* 11, 4 (Dec. 2000–Jan. 2001): 16.

Cele, W. Lindani. n.d. *Mqothi Wembokido Nesisekelo (*"Annihilator"). (Musa Ndlovu, Trans. 2000, Jan.), Durban, South Africa. Unpublished Poetry.

Cele, W. Lindani. n.d. *Mthakathi Ndini Uyascleka* ("You Scary Sorcerer!"). (Musa Ndlovu, Trans. 2000, Jan.). Durban, South Africa. Unpublished Poetry.

Charry, Eric. 2000. *Mande Music.* London and Chicago. University of Chicago Press.

Chernoff, John Miller. 1979. *African Rhythm and Sensibility.* London & Chicago: University of Chicago Press.

Chisvo, M. and L. Munro. 1995. A Review of Social dimensions of Adjustment in Zimbabwe, 1990–1994. Harare, Zimbabwe: UNICEF.

Comaroff, Jean and John Comaroff. 1993. "Introduction." In *Modernity and its* Malcontents: *Ritual and Power in Postcolonial Africa*, eds. Jean and John Comaroff, xi–xxxvii. Chicago and London: University of Chicago Press.

Connaissances, Attitudes et Comportements des Jeunes (15–25 *ans*) *vis à vis de la Santé de la Reproduction.* 1999. Bamako, Mali: Ministère de la Santé et de la Personne; Direction Nationale de l'Action Sociale; Centre National d'Information, d' Education, et de Communication pour La Santé (CNIECS).

Cope, Trevor, ed. 1968. *Izibongo: Zulu Praise-poems.* Oxford, U.K.: Clarendon Press.

Crewe, Mary. 2000. "How Do We make Sense of President Mbeki?" *AIDS Analysis Africa* 11, 1 (June/July): 10–11.

Crowley, David and Paul Heyer, eds. 1991. *Communication in History: Technology, Culture, Society*. New York: Longman.

Daba, Habib Ahmed. 1981. "The Case of Dan Maraya Jos: A Hausa Poet." In *Oral Poetry in Nigeria*, ed. Uchegbulam N. Abalogu; Garba Ashiwaju; and Regina Amadi-Tshiwala, 209–229. Lagos: Nigeria Magazine.

Dagron, Alfonso Gumucio. 2001. *Making Waves: Stories of Participatory Communication for Social Change*. New York: Rockefeller Foundation.

Dalrymple, Lynn and Eleanor Preston-Whyte. 1994. "Participation and Action: reflections on community-based AIDS Intervention in South Africa." In *Is DramAide Making a Difference? Evaluations of* the *DramAide Programme*, ed. Lynn Dalrymple and Eleanor Preston-Whyte, 111–128. Durban, South Africa: the DramAide Project.

Dalrymple, Lynn. 1997. DramAide Funding Proposal. Durban, South Africa. Risographed.

Dalrymple, Lynn. 1999. Founder, The DramAide Project, University of Zululand, KwaZulu-Natal, South Africa. 1999. Interview by author, August, Durban and Port Shepstone, South Africa. Audio cassette and unpublished notes.

Dalrymple, Lynn. 2001. Founder, The DramAide Project, University of Zululand, KwaZulu-Natal, South Africa. Personal Communication. July.

Dauchez, Philippe. n.d. "Useful Theatre in Mali." Retrieved May 27, 2002, from http://www.iias.nl/host/ccrss/cp/cp2_Useful.html.

Dembele, Daouda, and Hawa Dembele. 1999. "Yiriba." Tale with music recorded on cassette. 1999. Produced by *Projet Appui à la Lutte Contre le SIDA en Afrique de l'ouest*, coordinated by the Centre de Coopération Internationale en Santé et Développement (CCISD Inc.). Financed by ACDI, Agence Canadienne pour le Développement International. Translated from Bambara to French by Moutaga Ly and from French to English by author. Bamako, Mali. November 1999.

Dembele, Teme. n.d. "SIDA." AIDS Song [private videotape recording]. Transcribed and translated from Bambara to French by Moutaga Ly and from French to English by author. Bamako, Mali. November 1999.

Denny, Charlotte. 2002. "School doors finally being pushed open." *Guardian Weekly* (Manchester, U.K.), April 25–May 1, 10.

Department of State. 2001. Background Note: South Africa. Retrieved June 24, 2001, from http://www.state.gov/r/pa/bgn/index.cfm?docid=2829.

Desai, Gurav. 1991. "Research Resources on Popular Theater and Development in Africa." *Research in African Literatures* 22, (3): 91–132.

Devisch, René. 1991. "Mediumistic Divination Among the Northern Yaka of Zaire." In *African Divination Systems: Ways of Knowing*, ed. Phillip Peek, 112–132. Bloomington and Indianapolis: Indiana University Press.

D'Haem, Jeanne. 1997. *The Last Camel: True Stories of Somalia*. Lawrenceville, N.J.: The Red Sea Press.

Diabaté, Naïni. n.d. "SIDA." [Audio cassette]. Produced by Wanda Records, Bamako, Mali. Translated from Bambara to French by Jacques Keita, Bamako, Mali. Feb. 2001. Translated from French to English by author.

Diarra, Tieman and Abdoulaye Diarra. 1996. *Etude CAP sur* les *MST/SIDA en direction des jeunes des milieux urbain, semi-urbain et rural au Mali*. Bamako, Mali: Plan International. Unpublished Report.

Dinozzi, Robert (Producer) and Jhally, Sut (Director). 1994. *Killing Screens: Media and the Culture of Violence*. [Videotape]. (Available through Media Education Foundation, Amherst, Mass.).

Diop, Waly. 2000. "Lessons from the Field: From Government Policy to Community-Based Communication Strategies in Africa: Lessons from Senegal and Uganda," *Journal of Health Communication* 5 (Supplement): 113–117.

Doho, Gilbert. 1989. "*Les Funérailles bamiléké: Eléments de théàtralité.*" *Notre Librarie* (Paris): 99 (octobre–décembre): 78–82.

Doho, Gilbert. 1997. "Petit Piment." Yaoundé, Cameroon: Editions Clé.

Doho, Gilbert. 2000. "*Theatre populaire ou reappropriation du pouvoir par les masses au Cameroun.*" Paper presented at the 43rd annual meeting of the African Studies Association. Nashville, Tenn. November. Unpublished paper.

Doho, Gilbert. Playwright, Associate Professor, Université de Yaounde, Cameroon. 2001. Personal Communication. July.

Doho, Gilbert. n.d. "Secret Societies and Good Governance in the Grassfields of Cameroon." Unpublished paper.

Doho, Gilbert and Eileen Julien. In press. *Théatre populaire: Essai de réarmement des masses au Cameroon.* Bloomington: Indiana University Press.

Doupe, A. 2001. "Why Focus on Men?" *SAFCO: Aids in West and Central Africa* (Abidjan, Côte d'Ivoire), 1 (Jan.–Mar.): 6–7.

DramAide. 2000. "See You at Seven." [Educational Videotape and Users' Manual]. Tape produced by Wireless Additive of Johannesburg, South Africa. Users' manual compiled by Dr. Lynn Dalrymple and Paul Botha. KwaZulu-Natal, South Africa: DramAide Project.

Drame, Malick & Teneman Sanogo. Actors, Troupe Niologon, Bamako, Mali. 1999. Interview, December, Bamako, Mali. Cassette and unpublished field notes.

Drewal, Margaret Thompson. 1991. "The State of Research on Performance in Africa." *African Studies Review* 34 (3): 1–64.

Drisdelle, Rhéal. 1997. *Mali: A Prospect for Peace.* London: Oxfam.

"Dramatic Increases in AIDS Orphans." Retrieved August 8, 2001, from http:www.afrol.com/Categories/Health/health009_aids_orphans.htm.

Dubuch, C. 1985. "*Langage de pouvoir, pouvoir de langage.*" *Politique Africaine* (Bordeaux) 20: 44–55.

Durkheim, Emile. 1961. *The Elementary Forms of Religious Life.* Trans. John Ward Swain. New York: Collier.

Ekman, Paul, Wallace Friesen, and Phoebe Ellsworth. 1972. *Emotion in the Human Face.* New York: Pergamon Press.

Ekman, Paul and Wallace Friesen. 1975. *Unmasking the Face.* Englewood Cliffs, N.J.: Prentice-Hall, Inc.

Economic Commission for Africa. 1989. *African Alternative Framework to Structural Adjustment Programs.* Addis Ababa, Ethiopia, 1989.

Ericcson, Susan and Sanjay Taireja (Producers); Jhaly, Sut (Director). 1999. *Tough Guise: Violence Media and the Crisis in Masculinity.* [Videotape]. (Available from Media Education Foundation, Amherst, Mass.).

Eyoh, Hansel. 1984. "Trends in African Theatre: The Popular Theatre Approach." Paper presented at the International African Literature Conferences. Budapest. Unpublished paper.

Eyoh, Hansel. 1986. Hammocks to Bridges. Yaounde, Cameroon: Bet & Co.

Eyoh, Hansel. 1994. "Popular Theatre Re-Visited. With an Additional Bibliography on Popular Theatre and Theatre for Development." *Matatu: Journal for African Culture and Society* (Amsterdam & Atlanta): 20: 95–134.

Fage J. D. 1969. *A History of West Africa, 4th ed.* Cambridge, UK. Cambridge University Press.

Family Health International. *1998. Mali and HIV/AIDS: Key Talking Points.* Washington, D.C. and Bamako, Mali: United States Agency for International Development. Unpublished Paper.

Family Health International. 2002. Corridors of Hope in Southern Africa: HIV Prevention Needs and Opportunities in Four Border Towns. Washington, D.C.: Family Health International. Monograph.

Filter, H. 1986. *Paulina Dlamini: Servant of two kings*, ed. S. Bourquin. Pietermaritzburg, South Africa: University of Natal Press.

Forgey, H.; T. Dimant; T. Mophuthing; J. Spratt; D. Pienaar; and N. Peter, 2001. *South Africa Survey 2000/1*. Johannesburg: Institute of Race Relations.

Freire, Paolo. 1974. *Pedagogy of the Oppressed*. Trans. Myra Berman Ramos. New York: Seabury.

Gausset, Quentin and Hanne O. Mogensen. 1996. "Sida et pollutions sexuelles chez les Tonga de Zambie." Paris: *Cahiers d'études Africaines* XXXVI (3): 143; 455–476.

Geertz, Clifford. 1973. *The Interpretation of Cultures*. New York: Basic Books.

Geertz, Clifford. 1983. *Local Knowledge: Further Essays in Interpretive Anthropology*. New York: Basic Books.

Gibbs, James. 1999. "Noticeboard." In *African Theatre in Development,* ed. Martin Banham, James Gibbs, and Femi Osofisan, 117–126. Oxford, U.K.: James Curry; Bloomington & Indianapolis: Indiana University Press.

Goffman, Irving. 1974. *Frame Analysis: An Essay on the Organization of Experience*. Cambridge, Mass: Harvard University Press.

Gould, P. 1993. *The Slow Plague: A Geography of the AIDS Pandemic*. Oxford, U.K.: Blackwell.

Graham-White, Anthony. 1974. *The Drama of Black Africa*. New York: Samuel French, Inc.

Griesgraber, Mary Jo. 1997. "Forgive Us Our Debts: The Third World's Financial Crisis." In *Developing World 99/00,* ed. Robert J. Griffiths, 55–60. 9th ed. Guilford, Conn.: McGraw-Hill/Dushkin.

Grove, A.T. 1989. *The Changing Geography of Africa*. Oxford, England. Oxford University Press.

Grosskurth, H.; F. Mosha; J.Todd; K. Senkoro; J. Newell; A. Klokke *et al.* 1995. "A Community trial of the impact of improved sexually transmitted disease treatment on the HIV epidemic in rural Tanzania: 2. Baseline survey results." *AIDS* 9 (8): 927–934.

Gumisai, Mutume. 2001. "Experts Assail Condom-Obsessed AIDS prevention." Interpress Service, 12 May. Retrieved June 10, 2001, from http:www.afrol.com/categories/health/health057_aids_condom.htm.

Gunderson, Frank. 2000. "Witchcraft, Witchcraft and Musical Warfare: The Rise of the Bagiika-Bagaalu Music Competitions in Sukumaland, Tanzania." In *Mashindano!: Competitive Music Performance in East Africa*, ed. Frank Gunderson and Gregory Barz, 407–419. Dar es Salaam, Tanzania: Mkuki na Nyota Publishers.

Gunderson, Frank. 2000. "Kifungua Kinywa, or 'Opening the Contest with Chai'." In *Mashindano! Competitive Music Performance in East Africa*, ed. Frank Gunderson and Gregory Barz, 7–20. Dar es Salaam, Tanzania: Mkuki na Nyota Publishers.

Gunner, Liz. 1994. "Introduction: The Struggle for Space." In *Politics and Performance: Theatre, Poetry, and Song in Southern Africa*, ed. Liz Gunner, 1–34. Johannesburg, S. A.: Witwatersrand University Press.

Hackett, Rosalind. 1996. *Art and Religion in Africa*. London: Cassell.

Hale, Thomas. 1998. *Griots and Griottes*. Bloomington and Indianapolis: Indiana University Press.

Hambridge, Martha. 1995. "Report of a Case Study on the impact of DramAide on STD levels among High School scholars." In *Is DramAide Making a Difference?* ed. Lynn Dalrymple, 63–110. KwaZulu-Natal, South Africa: The DramAide Project.

Hanna, Judith Lynne. 1987. *To Dance is Human: A Theory of Nonverbal Communication*. Chicago and London: University of Chicago Press.

Hansen, H. 1972/73. Clitoridectomy, Female Circumcision in Egypt. *Folk*, 14/15, 25–6.

Haring, Lee. 1972. "A Characteristic African Folktale Pattern." In *African Folklore*, ed. Richard Dorson, 165–179. Garden City, New York: Anchor Books.

Harvey, Brian, James Stuart, and Tony Swan. 1993–94. "Comparative Intervention Trial of the DramAide Programme in KwaZulu High Schools." In *Is DramAide Making a Difference?* ed. Lynn Dalrymple, 33–56. KwaZulu-Natal, South Africa: The DramAide Project.

Heywood, Mark. 2002. "Pretoria High Court hands down precedent-setting judgment: 'A countrywide MTCT programme is an ineluctable obligation of the state'." *AIDS Analysis Africa* 12, 6 (Apr./May): 12–13.

Hickey, Alison. 2002. "What Budget 2002 means for SA government's response to HIV/AIDS." *AIDS Analysis Africa* 12, 6 (Apr./May): 1–3; 7.

Hinzen, Heribert, Frederick B. James, Jim M. Sorie, and Sheikh Ahmed Tamu (eds.). 1987. *Fishing in* Rivers *of Sierra* Leone *Oral Literature*. Freetown: Peoples Educational Association of Sierra Leone.

"HIV/AIDS: Drowning by Numbers." 2002. *New Internationalist* (Market Harborough, U.K.), 346 (June): 18–19.

Hornik, Robert. 1988. *Development Communication: Information, Agriculture, and Nutrition in the Third World*. White Plains, N.Y.: Longman.

Human Rights Watch/Africa. 1995. *Violence Against Women in South Africa: State Response to Domestic Violence and Rape*. New York: Human Rights Watch.

Hunter, Susan and John Williamson. 2000. *Children on the Brink: Strategies to Support Children Isolated by HIV/AIDS*. Washington, D. C.: United States Agency for International Development (USAID).

International Encyclopedia of Dance, ed. 1998. "Sub-Saharan Africa." In *International Encyclopedia of Dance*, Vol. 6, 12–26. Oxford, U.K.: Oxford University Press.

Janzen, John. 1994. "Drums of Affliction: Real Phenomenon or Scholarly Chimera?" In *Religion in Africa: Experience and Expression*, ed. Thomas Blakely, Walter E.A.van Beek, and Dennis L. Thompson, 160–182. London & Portsmouth, N.H.: James Currey.

Jhally, Sut. (Producer, Writer, and Director). 1995. *Dreamworlds II: Desire, Sex, and Power in Music Video*. [Videotape]. (Available through Media Education Foundation, Amherst, Mass.).

Kaleeba, Noerine, Joyce Kadowe, Daniel Kalinki and Glen Williams. 2000. *Open Secret: People Facing Up to* HIV *and AIDS* in *Uganda*, *Strategies for Hope*, No. 15. London: ACTIONAID.

Kalipeni, Ezekiel. 2000. "Health and Disease in Southern Africa: A comparative and vulnerability perspective." *Social Science and Medicine* 50: 963–983.

Kamuzora, C. Lwechungura. 2001. "HIV/AIDS bitter-sweet future: the demographic impact of the epidemic in Africa." *AIDS Analysis Africa* 11, 4 (Dec. 2000/Jan. 2001): 7–8, 14.

von Kapff, Uli. 1997. *Zulu: People of Heaven*. Umhlanga Rocks, South Africa: Holiday Africa Publications.

Keim, Curtis. 1995. "Africa and Europe before 1900." In *Africa*, ed. Phyllis M. Martin and Patrick O'Meara, 115–134. 5th ed. Bloomington & Indianapolis: Indiana University Press.

Kelly, Kevin. Professor of Psychology, Rhodes University & Evaluation Specialist, Grahamstown, South Africa. 1999. Interview, September, Grahamstown, South Africa. Cassette tape & unpublished field notes.

Kerr, David. 1995. *African Popular Theatre*. London: James Curry, Ltd. & Portsmouth, N. H.: Heinemann.

Kidd, Ross. 1979. "Liberation or Domestication: Popular Theatre and non-formal education in Africa." *Educational Broadcasting International* 12 (1): 3–9.

Kidd, Ross. 1983. "Popular theatre and popular struggle in Kenya: the story of Kamiriithu." *Race and Class* 24 (3): 287–304.

Kidd, Ross and Martin Byram. 1981. "A Fresh Look at Popular Theater in Botswana: Demystifying Pseudo-Freirian Non-Formal Education." *Rural Development Participation Review* 3 (1): 19–24.

Kim, Richard. 2001. "Act-Up Goes Global." *The Nation* 273 (2): 17–18.

Kimama, Lawrence. 2001. "The Maiden." Unpublished Kenyan Folk Tale. Emailed.

Kloph, Donald W. 1991. *Intercultural Encounters: The Fundamentals of Intercultural Communication.* Englewood, Col.: Morton Publishing Company.

Knappert, Jan. 1995. *African Mythology: An Encyclopedia of Myth and Legend.* London: Diamond Books.

Kofoworola, Ziky O. 1981. "The Hausa Example". In *Oral Poetry in Nigeria*, ed. U. Abalogu, G. Ashiwaju, and R. Amadi-Tshiwala, 290–308. Lagos, Nigeria: *Nigeria Magazine.*

Komba-Malekela, Betty and Rita Liljeström. 1994. "Looking for Men." In *Chelewa, Chelewa: The Dilemma of Teenage Girls*, ed. Zubeida Tumbo-Masabo and Rita Liljeström, 133–149. Tryckeribolaget, Östersund, Sweden: Nordiska Afrikainstitutet.

Konaré, Adame Ba. 1998. *Ces Mots Que Je Partage: Discours d'une Première Dame d'Afrique.* Bamako, Mali: Editions Jamana.

Langer, Suzanne. 1976. *Philosophy in a New Key: A Study in the Symbolism of Reason, Rite*, and *Art*, 3rd ed. Cambridge, Mass.: Harvard University Press.

Lightfoot-Klein, Hanny. 1989. *Prisoners of Ritual: An Odyssey into Female Genital Circumcision in Africa.* New York: Harrington Park Press.

Lindsay, Daryl. 2001, 25 June. "Aids Activists Change Their Act, Parts 1 and 2." Salon. Com. Retrieved July 22, 2001, from http://www.salon.com/news/feature/2001/06/25/aids/index.html.

Lutaaya, Philly Bongoley. n.d. "Alone." [Cassette Tape]. Stockholm, Sweden: Swedish Red Cross, Producer.

Maart, Brenton. n.d. *Community, Radio, and AIDS Action.* Pretoria, South Africa: Beyond Awareness 2 Campaign.

Machipisa, Lewis. 2000, 19 Jan. "Health-Zimbabwe: Government Urged to Stop Deducting AIDS Levy." Inter Press Service. Retrieved June 9, 2001, from http://www.aegis.com/news/ips/2000/op000106.html.

Malinowski, Bronislav. 1948. "Magic, Science, and Religion," in *Magic, Science, Religion and other Essays by Bronislav Malinowski*, text. ed. Selected and with a Foreword by Robert Redfield, 1–64, Glencoe, Ill.: Free Press.

Maloka, Tshidiso. 1997. "The Struggle for Sunday: All-male Christianity in the Gold Mine compounds." In *Christianity in South Africa: A Political, Social, and Cultural History,* ed. Richard Elphick and Rodney Davenport, 242–252. Berkeley and Los Angeles: University of California Press.

Mann, J., D. Tarantola, and T. Netter (eds). 1992. *AIDS in the World: A Global Report.* Boston: Harvard University Press.

Mashinini, Dudsile Phindile. 2000. "Why there are differences between Black People and White People." Unpublished South African Folk Tale. Emailed.

Mbarga, Prince Nico & Rocafil Jazz. 1976. "Sweet Mother," [Cassette]. Nigeria: Rogers All Stars Ltd.; 1991. Cambridge, Mass.: Rounder Records.

Mbembe, Achille. 1992. "The Banality of Power and the Aesthetics of Vulgarity in the Postcolony." Trans. Janet Roitman. *Public Culture* 4, 2 (Spring): 1–30.

McPake, B. 1993. "User Charges for Health Services in Developing Countries: A Review of the Economic Literature." *Social Science and Medicine* 36 (11): 25–30.

McGeary, Joanna. 2001. "Death Stalks a Continent." In *Africa*, ed. F. Jefress Ramsay, 206–213. 9th ed. Guilford, Conn.: Dushkin/ McGraw-Hill.

Mda, Zakes. 1993. *When People Play People: Development Communication through Theatre.* Johannesburg: Witswatersrand University Press; London: Zed Books.

Mead, Geroge Herbert. 1934. *Mind, Self, and Society.* Chicago: University of Chicago Press.

Médecins sans Frontières. 2001. "Treating HIV/AIDS." 6, 2 (Summer), Special Issue.

Mlama, Penina H. 1991. *Culture and Development: The Popular Theatre Approach in Africa*. Uppsala, Sweden: Nordiska Afrikainstitutet.

Morlet, A.; J.J. Guinan; I. Diefenthaler; and J. Gold. 1988. "The Impact of the Grim Reaper National AIDS educational campaign on the Albion Street (AIDS) Centre and the AIDS Hotline." *Medical Journal* Australia. 148 (6): 282–286. Abstract retrieved June 17, 2001, from aidsline: National Library of Medicine at http://ww1.aegos.org/publ/aidline/1988/jun/m8860305.

Morrison, Joy. 1991. "Forum Theater in West Africa: An Alternative Medium for Information Exchange." *Research in African Literatures*, 22 (Fall): 29–40.

Mtukudsi, Oliver. 1988. "Stay With One Woman." [Record]. Harare, Zimbabwe: Development Through Self-Reliance (DSR). (Available through Media for Development International [MFDI], Colorado Springs, Co.)

Mwikisa, Peter. 2002. "Constructions of Masculinity in Traditional African Culture and in Western Popular Culture: Self-Imagination of the African Male and the Fight Against AIDS." Paper presented at the Conference on Language, Literature, and the Discourse of HIV/AIDS in Africa. Gaberone, Botswana. June.

Nafo, F. Traoré. 2001. "World AIDS Campaign: Men Make A Difference." *Safco, AIDS in West and Central Africa* (Abidjan, Côte d'Ivoire), 2 (Apr.–June): 6–7.

Niane, Djibril Tasmir. 1960. "*Soundjata, ou l'épopée mandingue*." (Paris) *Présence Africaine*. In English as "Sundiata, An Epic of Old Mali." Trans. G.D. Pickett. London: Longman, 1965.

Nicoll, Angus. 1998. "Control of Sexually Transmitted Diseases (STDs) and the reduction of Heterosexual HIV transmission in countries where STDs are highly prevalent." London: PHLS Communicable Disease Surveillance Centre. Retrieved June 20, 2001, from http://www.euroserv.org/1998/980723.html#std.

Nketia, J. Kwabene. 1966. "Music in African Cultures: A Review of the Meaning and Significance of Traditional African Music." Legon, Accra, Ghana: Institute of African Studies, University of Ghana. Mimeographed.

Nwoga, Donatus I. 1981. "The Igbo Poet and Satire." In *Oral Poetry in Nigeria*, ed. U. Abalogu, G. Ashiwaju, and R. Amadi-Tshiwala, 230–243. Lagos: *Nigeria Magazine*.

Nyoni, Frowin Paul. 2000. "The Social Significance of Mganda-wa-Kinkachi Dance Contests Among the Matengo." In *Mashindano!: Competitive Music Performance in East Africa*, ed. Frank Gunderson and Gregory Barz, 233–254. Dar es Salaam, Tanzania: Mkuki na Nyota Publishers.

Nxumalo, Henry. 1989. "The Birth of a *Tsotsi*." In *The Drum Decade: Stories from the 1950s*, ed. Michael Chapman, 18–23. Pietermaritzburg, South Africa: University of Natal Press.

Nyangoro, Julian E. and Timothy Shaw, eds. 1991. *Beyond Structural Adjustment: The Political Economy of Sustainable Democratic Development*. Westport, Conn.: Praeger.

Obbo, Christine. 1987. "The Old and the New in East African Elite Marriages." In *Transformations of African Marriage*, ed. David Parkin and David Nyamwaya, 263–280. Manchester, U.K.: Manchester University Press.

Ojaide, Tanure. 1996. *Poetic Imagination in Black Africa*. Durham: Carolina Academic Press.

Okpewho, Isidore. 1992. *African Oral Literature: Backgrounds, Character, and Continuity*. Bloomington and Indianapolis: Indiana University Press.

Okumu, Charles. 1994. "The Place of Oral Poetry in Contemporary Ugandan Society. The Oral Artist as Historian and Commentator." In *Oral Tradition and its Transmission: The Many Forms of Message*, ed. E. Sienaert, M. Cowper-Lewis and N. Bell, 329–345. Durban, South Africa: The Campbell Collections and the Centre for Oral Studies University of Natal.

Olabimtam, Afolabi. 1981. "The Èfè/Gèlèdé Poet of Ègbádo Kétu Yorùbà." In *Oral Poetry in Nigeria*, ed. Uchegbulam N. Abalogu; Garba Ashiwaju; and Regina Amadi-Tshiwala, 157–167. Lagos: *Nigeria Magazine*.

Omond, Roger. 1986. *The Apartheid Handbook*, 2nd ed. Middlesex, Eng.: Penguin Books.

Ong, Walter. 1982. *Orality and Literacy: The Technologizing of the Word*. London: Methuen.

Opland, Jeff. 1983. Xhosa Oral Poetry: Aspects of Black South African Tradition. Johannesburg, South Africa: Ravan Press.

Osofisan, Femi. 1998. "'The Revolution as Muse': Drama as Surreptitious Insurrection in a Post-colonial military state." In *Theatre Matters*, ed. Richard Boon and Jane Plastow, 11–36. Cambridge: Cambridge University Press.

O'Sullivan, Tim, John Hartley, Danny Saunders, Martin Montgomery, and John Fiske. 1994. *Key Concepts in Communication and Cultural Studies*, 2nd ed. London and New York: Routledge.

Panos Institute. 1998. AIDS and Men: Old Problem, New Angle. Panos HIV/AIDS Briefing No. 6. London: Panos Institute, December.

Parker, Warren. 1994. The Development of Community-based Media for AIDS Education and Prevention in South Africa: Towards an Action-based Participatory Research Model. MA Thesis. Centre for Cultural and Media Studies, University of Natal, Durban, South Africa. Unpublished.

Parker, Warren, Lynn Dalrymple, and Emma Durden. 1998. *Communicating Beyond AIDS Awareness: A Manual for South Africa*. Pretoria, South Africa: Department of Health.

Pegrum, Mark. 1997. "Warnings and Fear." *Mots Pluriels*, 1 (3). Retrieved June 17, 2001, from http:www.arts.uwa.edu.au/MotsPluriels/MP397/mpeg2.html.

Perani, Judith and Fred Smith. 1998. *The Visual Arts of Africa: Gender, Power, and Life Cycle Rituals*. Upper Saddle River, N. J.: Prentice-Hall.

Peterson, Bhekizize. 1994. "Apartheid and the Political Imagination in South African Theatre." In *Politics and Performance: Theatre, Poetry, and Song in Southern Africa*, ed. Liz Gunner, 35–54. Johannesburg: Witwatersrand University Press.

Physicians for Human Rights. 2002, 7 June. "Medical Groups Decry Senate Failure on Appropriations for fighting Global HIV/AIDS." Retrieved August 4, 2002, from http://www.phrusa.org/campaigns/aids/release060902.html.

Plan Stratégique National De Lutte Contre le VIH/SIDA 2000–2004. 1999. Bamako, Mali: Ministère de la Santé des Personnes Agées et de la Solidatité; Programme National de Lutte Contre de SIDA. Photocopied.

Pratt, James. 1989. Monthly Report to the Chief of Party of the LRCN Project. Gbarnga and Monrovia, Liberia. February. Unpublished.

Ramsay, F. Jefress. 2001. "Africa: The Struggle for Development." In *Africa*, ed. F. Jefress Ramsay, 2–9, 9th ed. Guilford, Conn.: Dushkin/ McGraw-Hill.

Ranger, Terrence. 1975. *Dance and Society in Eastern Africa 1890–1970: The Beni Ngoma*. Berkeley, Cal.: University of California Press.

Rosenthal. July. 1998. *Possession, Ecstasy, & Law in Ewe Voodoo*. Charlottsville & London: University of Virginia Press.

Sakho, M. L. 2001. "Mobility, Migration Patterns and HIV/AIDS Go Together." *Safco: AIDS in West and Central Africa (*Abidjan, Côte d'Ivoire*)*, 1 (Jan.–Mar.): 11.

Schechner, Richard. 1985. *Between Theater and Anthropology*. Philadelphia: University of Pennsylvania Press.

Schechner, Richard. 1988. *Performance Theory*. London and New York: Routledge.

Schechner, Richard. 1990. "Magnitudes of Performance." In *By Means of Performance*, ed. Richard Schechner and Willa Appel, 19–49. Cambridge, U.K.: Cambridge University Press.

Schechner, Richard. 1995. *The Future of Ritual.* London & New York: Routledge.

Schwab, George. 1947. *The Tribes of the Liberian Hinterland.* Cambridge, Mass: Peabody Museum.

Seidel, Gill. 1995. "DramAide-Towards a Critical Overview." In *Is DramAide Making a Difference?* ed. Lynn Dalrymple and Eleanor Preston-Whyte, 129–173. KwaZulu-Natal, South Africa: The DramAide Project.

Setel, Philip W. 1999. *A Plague of Paradoxes*: AIDS, *Culture, and Demography in Northern Tanzania.* Chicago and London: University of Chicago Press.

Singhal, Arvind and Everett M. Rogers. 1999. *Edutainment-Education*: A *Communication Strategy for Social Change.* Mahwah, New Jersey: Lawrence Erlbaum Associates.

Sithole, Jabulani. 2002. "Cultural Factors in the Spread and Management of HIV/AIDS." Paper presented at the Conference on Language, Literature and the Discourse of HIV/AIDS in Africa. Gaberone, Botswana. June.

Sissoko, Sada. 1995. *Le Kotéba et l'évolution du théatre moderne au Mali.* Bamako, Mali: Editions Jamana.

Smart, Rose. 2000. "Orphans and vulnerable children—'the collateral casualties'." *Aids Analysis Africa*, 11, 2 (Aug./Sept.): 8–9.

Smith, Barry. 1997. "South African Christian Music." In *Christianity in South Africa: A Political, Social, and Cultural History*, ed. Richard Elphick and Rodney Davenport, 316–326. Berkeley and Los Angeles: University of California Press.

Smith, Gordon and Jason Napier. 2001. "Can We Cope with another 'Lost Generation'? A bottom-up risk approach to HIV/AIDS in South Africa." *AIDS Analysis Africa*, 11, 5 (Feb./Mar.): 7–8.

Soul City Institute. 1999a. Violence Against Women in South Africa: A Resource for Journalists. South Africa: Soul City Institute.

Soul City. 1999b. http://www.soulcity.org.za/episode 5.htm.

Soul City. 1999c. Episode 5, Series 4. Videotape.

Sow, Usman. 1999. Playwright and Theatrical Producer. 1999. Interview, November, Bamako, Mali. Cassette and unpublished notes.

Soyinka, Wole. 1976. *Myth, Literature, and the African World.* Cambridge, U.K.: Cambridge University Press.

Spirit of Africa. 2001. Compact Disk. London: Real World Records, Ltd. Distributed by EMI Music, Randburg, South Africa.

Staudt, Kathleen. 1991. *Managing Development: State, Society, and International Contexts.* Newbury Park, Cal.: Sage.

Steps. 2002. Tracks from the Steps documentaries and music inspired by the films. Compact Disk. Johannesburg, South Africa: Distributed by Ghetto Ruff

Stevenson, Robert. 1988. *Communication, Development, and the Third World.* White Plains, New York: Longman.

Stillwaggon, Eileen. 2001. "Aids and Poverty in Africa: Prevention and Treatment Require a Focus on Overall Health and Development." *The Nation*, 21 May, 22. Retrieved June 1, 2001, from http://www.comminit.com/TheDrumRole/sld-1992.html.

Stine, Gerald. J. *AIDS Update 2002.* Upper Saddle River, N.J.: Prentice Hall.

Stock, Robert. 1995. *Africa South of the Sahara.* New York: The Guilford Press.

Stone, Ruth. 1994. "Bringing the Extraordinary into the Ordinary. Music Performance among the Kpelle of Liberia." In *Religion in Africa, Experience and Expression*, ed. Thomas Blakely, Warren van Beek and Dennis Thompson, 388–397. Portsmouth, N.H: Heinemann; London: James Currey.

Stone, Ruth. 1995. "African Music Performed." In *Africa*, ed. Phyllis M. Martin and Patrick O'Meara, 257–272. 3rd ed. Bloomington and Indianapolis: Indiana University Press; London: James Currey, Ltd.

Stride, G.T. and C. Ifeka. 1971. *Peoples and Empires of West Africa: West Africa in History 1000–1800.* New York: Africana.

Stryker, Richard and Stephen Ndegwa. 1995. "The African Development Crisis." In *Africa*, ed. Phyllis M. Martin and Patrick O'Meara. 3rd ed., 375–394. Bloomington and Indianapolis: Indiana University Press.

Svedberg, P. 1990. "Under-Nutrition in Sub-Saharan Africa: Is there a gender bias?" *Journal of Development Studies*, 26: 469–486.

Sylla, Mohammed. Coordinateur, Volet Mali, *Projet d'appui à la lutte contre le SIDA en Afrique de l'ouest*, Bamako, Mali. 2000. Interview, June, Bamako, Mali. Cassette and unpublished notes.

Tender Proposal for the Development and Management of a "Beyond Awareness" Campaign and Media Strategy. n.d. South Africa: A Multimedia Consortium comprising CASE, DramAide, Society for Family Health, Soul City, Ulwazi Radio and Siyakha Communications.

Thompson, Robert Farris. 1973. "An Aesthetic of Cool." *African Arts* 7 (1): 40–43, 64–67, 89.

Thompson, William Irwin. 1989. *Imaginary Landscape: Making Worlds of Myth and Science.* New York: St. Martin's Press.

Togni, Lorenzo. 1997. *AIDS in South Africa and on the African Continent.* Pretoria, South Africa: Kagisco Publishers.

Tomaselli, Keyan G. 1997a. "Action Research, participatory Communication: Why Governments Don't Listen." *Africa Media Review* 11 (1): 1–9.

Tomaselli, Keyan. 1997b. Comprehensive and Integrated HIV/AIDS Prevention Campaigns Potentials for South and Southern Africa. Advisory Committee on AIDS/STDs South African Department of Health, Pretoria & Centre for Cultural and Media Studies, University of Natal, Durban. Unpublished Report.

Traoré, Salia. Economist, *Faculté des Sciences Juriduques et Economiques*, Université du Mali. 2000. Interview, June, Bamako, Mali.

Turner, Victor. 1990. "Are There Universals of performance in myth, ritual, and drama?" In *By Means of Performance*, ed. Richard Schechner and Willa Appel, 8–18. Cambridge, U.K.: Cambridge University Press.

Turner, Victor. 1982. *From Ritual to Theater.* New York: Performing Arts Journal Publications.

UNAIDS. 2000. Report on the Global HIV/AIDS Epidemic: Report and Data Tables. New York: UNAIDS. Retrieved June 2001, from www. unaids.org/epidemic update/report/index.html#table.

UNAIDS. Fact Sheet 2002, 2 July."The Impact of AIDS." Retrieved July 14, 2002, from www.unaids.org/epidemic/press.

UNAIDS. Fact Sheet. 2002, 2 July. "Accelerating Access to Treatment and Care." Retrieved July 14, 2002, from www.unaids.org/epidemic/press.

UNAIDS. 2002, July. Report on the Global HIV/AIDS Epidemic 2002: Report and Data Tables. New York: UNAIDS. Retrieved July 14, 2002, from www.unaids.org/epidemic_update/report/index.html#table.

UNICEF. 1987. *Adjustment with a Human Face*, 2 vols. New York and London: Oxford University Press.

UNICEF. 2002. *Children on the Brink: A Joint Report on Orphan Estimates and Program Strategies: Report and Data Tables.* New York: UNICEF. PDF file. Retrieved July14, 2002, from http://www/unicef.org/newline.

United Nations. 1995. *The World's Women: Trends and Statistics.* New York: United Nations.

United Nations Development Programme (UNDP). 1999. *Human Development Report: Globalization with a Human Face.* New York: United Nations Development Programme.

United Nations Development Programme (UNDP). 2000. *Human Development Report: Globalization with a Human Face.* New York: United Nations Development Programme.

United States Agency for International Development (USAID). 1999. FGC Symposium. USAID final Report. Intra-Agency Working Group on FGC. Washington, D.C.: USAID.

United States Agency for International Development (USAID). n.d. Retrieved June 2001, from http://www.usaid.gov.press/releases/.

United States Agency for International Development (USAID). 2002, 3 June. "Millennium Challenge Account Update." Retrieved August 4, 2002, from http://www/usaid.gov/press/releases/2002/fs_mea.html.

United States Department of State, Bureau of African Affairs. 2001a, May. Background Note: South Africa. Retrieved June 24, 2001, from http://www.state.gov/r/pa/bgn/index.cfm?docid=2829.

United States Department of State, Bureau of African Affairs, 2001b, December. Background Note: Mali. Retrieved August 6, 2002, from http:www.state.gov/r/pa/ie/bgn/2828/htm.

Van Gannep, Arnold. 1960. *The Rites of Passage.* Chicago: University of Chicago Press (Originally Published in 1907).

Vaughan, Peter, Everett M. Rogers, Arvind Singhal, & Ramadhan Swalehe. 2000. "Entertainment-Education and HIV/AIDS Prevention: A Field Experiment in Tanzania." *Journal of Health Communication,* 5 (Supplement): 81-100.

Wacieni, Kariamu. 1997. "False Hope: Structural Adjustment and Growth in Africa." In *Africa,* ed. F. Jefress Ramsay, 192-194. 5th ed. Guilford, Conn.: Dushkin/McGraw-Hill.

Warraq, Ibn. 1999. "Islam's Shame: Lifting the Veil of Tears." In *Women's Studies,* ed. Patricia Ojea and Barbara Quigley, 96-102. 1st ed. Guilford, Conn.: Dushin/McGraw-Hill.

Washington Post. 2000, July. "Waking Up to Devastation. AIDS Graphics." Retrieved May 30, 2002, from http://www.washingtonpost.com/wp-srv/world/daily/july00/aidsgrahpic3.htm.

Waterman, Christopher. 1990. A. *Jújù: A Social History and Ethnography of an African Popular Music.* Chicago and London. University of Chicago Press.

Weber, Max. 1958. *The Protestant Ethic and the Spirit of Capitalism.* Trans. Talcott Parsons. New York: Charles Scribner's Sons.

Whiteside, Alan. 2000. "Aids Demography." *Aids Analysis Africa,* 11, 2 (Aug./Sept.): 1, 3.

Whiteside, Alan. 2001. "The State of the Epidemic at the Beginning of 2001." *Aids Analysis Africa* 11, 5 (Feb./Mar.): 1–3.

Wilson, Des. 1987. "Traditional Systems of Communication in Modern African Development: An Analytical Viewpoint." *Africa Media Review* 1 (2): 87–104.

World Bank. 1992. Malawi Population Sector Study. Vol. 1. Main Report. Population and Human Resources Division, Southern Africa Department. Washington, D.C.: World Bank.

World Health Organization. 2001, June. Female Genital Mutilation. Retrieved June 9, 2001, from http://www.who.int/inf-fs/en/fact241.html.

World Health Organization (WHO/UNAIDS). 2002, July. HIV/AIDS in Sub-Saharan Africa. Power Point Presentation. Retrieved July 14, 2002, from www.unaids.org/edpidemic_update/ppt.

Worth, Sol. 1972. "Toward an Anthropological Politics of Symbolic Forms." In *Reinventing Anthropology,* ed. Dell Hymes, 335–64. New York: Random House.

Yahaya, Ibrahim Y. 1981. "The Hausa Poet." In *Oral Poetry in Nigeria,* ed. U. Abalogu, G. Ashiwaju, and R. Amadi-Tshiwala, 139–156. Lagos: *Nigeria Magazine.*

Xaba, Nonhlanhla. 1999. DramAide Facilitator and Research Assistant, Durban, South Africa. September, Personal Communication.

Zuma, Joel and Sibongiseni Mbambo. 1999. "*Masibambisane*" ("Let Us Unite") Original song. Private videotape recording. September 1999. Durban, South Africa.
Zuma, Joel. 1999. "Come On." Original Song. Private videotape recording. September 1999. Durban, South Africa.
Zuma, Joel. 1999. "If You Don't Know AIDS by Now." Original Song. August 1999. Private videotape recording.

Index

drumming, 87, 175, 178, 181, 187, 208